AF687104

Point of Care Ultrasound

Point of Care Ultrasound

Editor: Horton Green

AMERICAN
MEDICAL PUBLISHERS
www.americanmedicalpublishers.com

AMERICAN
MEDICAL PUBLISHERS
www.americanmedicalpublishers.com

Cataloging-in-Publication Data

Point of care ultrasound / edited by Horton Green.
p. cm.
Includes bibliographical references and index.
ISBN 979-8-88740-381-6
1. Diagnostic ultrasonic imaging. 2. Ultrasonic imaging. 3. Point-of-care testing.
4. Diagnostic imaging. 5. Ultrasonics in medicine. I. Green, Horton.
RC78.7.U4 P65 2023
616.075 43--dc23

© American Medical Publishers, 2023

American Medical Publishers,
41 Flatbush Avenue,
1st Floor, New York,
NY 11217, USA

ISBN 979-8-88740-381-6 (Hardback)

This book contains information obtained from authentic and highly regarded sources. Copyright for all individual chapters remain with the respective authors as indicated. All chapters are published with permission under the Creative Commons Attribution License or equivalent. A wide variety of references are listed. Permission and sources are indicated; for detailed attributions, please refer to the permissions page and list of contributors. Reasonable efforts have been made to publish reliable data and information, but the authors, editors and publisher cannot assume any responsibility for the validity of all materials or the consequences of their use.

Trademark Notice: Registered trademark of products or corporate names are used only for explanation and identification without intent to infringe.

Contents

Preface

An ultrasound is an imaging test that uses sound waves to generate the images of various structures inside the body. Point of care ultrasound is the use of ultrasound for making immediate decisions regarding the patient's care in emergency situations. This application of ultrasound is used for evaluating the medical condition in settings like combat zone, emergency medicine, ambulance or critical care unit. Point of care ultrasound is used for diagnosing certain pathologic conditions or injuries quickly, where other diagnostic methods will consume more time and expose the patient to greater risk. It is used for monitoring and guiding resuscitation of terminally ill patients, simultaneously confirming the clinical diagnosis to guide procedural guidance and safety. Furthermore, it is also being utilized in code blue situations, where a person has lost all signs of life. This book explores all the important aspects of point of care ultrasound in the present day scenario. It consists of contributions made by international experts. This book will prove to be immensely beneficial to students and researchers interested in this area of medical ultrasound.

The researches compiled throughout the book are authentic and of high quality, combining several disciplines and from very diverse regions from around the world. Drawing on the contributions of many researchers from diverse countries, the book's objective is to provide the readers with the latest achievements in the area of research. This book will surely be a source of knowledge to all interested and researching the field.

In the end, I would like to express my deep sense of gratitude to all the authors for meeting the set deadlines in completing and submitting their research chapters. I would also like to thank the publisher for the support offered to us throughout the course of the book. Finally, I extend my sincere thanks to my family for being a constant source of inspiration and encouragement.

Editor

1

POCUS in perioperative medicine: a North American perspective

Lorenzo De Marchi[1] and Massimiliano Meineri[2*]

Abstract

Ultrasound (US) performed at the point of care has found fertile ground in perioperative medicine. In the hands of anesthesiologists, transesophageal echocardiography (TEE) has become established as a powerful diagnostic and monitoring tool in the perioperative care of cardiac and non-cardiac patients. A number of point-of-care US (POCUS) applications are relevant to perioperative care, including airway, cardiac, lung and gastric US. Although guidelines exist to define the scope of practice for basic and advanced TEE, there remains a lack of such guidelines for perioperative point-of-care ultrasound (POCUS), despite a number of recent calls for action in the academic anesthesia community. POCUS training has been integrated into anesthesia residency curricula in Canada and the United States of America (USA). However, a nation-wide curriculum is still lacking. Many limitations to the development of perioperative POCUS curricula exist, including the need to define the scope of practice and design integrated longitudinal learning approaches. The main anesthesiologist societies in both the USA and Canada are promoting the development of guidelines and have introduced POCUS courses into their national conferences. Although bedside US imaging has been integrated into the curricula of many medical schools in North America, the need for specific national guidelines for the training and practice of POCUS in the perioperative setting by anesthesiologists is crucial to the further development of POCUS in perioperative medicine.

Keywords: Point-of-care ultrasound, Perioperative medicine, Guidelines, Hand-held ultrasound devices

Introduction

Point-of-care ultrasound (POCUS) refers to the use of ultrasound (US) examinations at a patient's bedside by a primary healthcare provider to answer a limited number of specific diagnostic questions, guide treatment and invasive procedures. In the past decade, the role of this technology during the perioperative period has become increasingly recognized.

The use of US has become an established standard of care in most operating rooms for several applications, such as regional anesthesia and central line insertion [1]. Concurrently, transesophageal echocardiography (TEE) performed by anesthesiologists has become an established practice in the cardiac operating room, supported by specific guidelines in both the United States of America (USA) and Canada [2, 3]. This has helped increase the availability of US systems in the operating room and develop specific postgraduate curricula to teach US-guided line insertion and confirmation of placement and regional blocks [4–6]. Additionally, hand-held systems have become increasingly available for many physicians and acute care teams [7, 8].

A number of specific applications of POCUS assist providers in responding to the challenges of perioperative anesthetic care. Focused cardiac US [9] has been used in the perioperative assessment of elective [10] and urgent [11] surgical cases and has significantly impacted patient management [12–14]. POCUS may also play key roles in the management of hemodynamic instability and cardiac arrest [15]. Lung US not only exhibits high accuracy in the differential diagnosis of hypoxia [16] but also has been successfully used intraoperatively to detect tracheal intubation [17], exclude main stem bronchial intubation and confirm lung isolation in thoracic surgery [18, 19]. Upper airway US has been demonstrated to be more

*Correspondence: Massimiliano.Meineri@uhn.ca
[2] Department of Anesthesia and Pain Management, Toronto General Hospital, University Health Network, University of Toronto, 200 Elizabeth Street EN 3-400, Toronto, ON M5G 2C4, Canada
Full list of author information is available at the end of the article

reliable than manual palpation in identifying the cricothyroid membrane [20] potentially reducing the risk of complications or failure in case of an emergency surgical airway.

Finally, while controversial, gastric US has become a unique tool in the hands of anesthesiologists for quantifying gastric contents and more objectively assessing aspiration risk [21]. However, this method is user dependent and subjective and is not standard of care in deciding if the patient is properly NPO.

More recently, specific perioperative scanning protocols have been proposed [22], and extensive reviews have advocated the need for anesthesiologists to perform perioperative POCUS [23]. Editorials in major anesthesia journals in the USA [24–26] and Canada [27] have clearly indicated that POCUS is the tool of the future in perioperative medicine. In 2011, an editorial by Johnson advocated for the development of POCUS into a standard of care for anesthesiologists [28]. Despite this editorial and other call for action, little progress has been made, and there exists no clear track toward a unified POCUS certification for anesthesiologists in North America.

In a recent survey of members of the Society of Cardiovascular Anesthesiologists, among 349 cardiac anesthesiologists who responded, most of whom were practicing in the USA, fewer than half had integrated focused cardiac US into their daily practice, and only 40% felt comfortable teaching this technique [29].

Although comprehensive [30] guidelines for the practice of POCUS are well established for emergency medicine and critical care in both the USA [30] and Canada [31], they are not immediately transferable to perioperative care, given the different scopes of practice. Another potential limitation restricting increases in the frequency with which POCUS is utilized is the relatively small number of anesthesiologists practicing in critical care in North America.

Where are we?

The American Society of Echocardiography and the Society of Cardiovascular Anesthesiologists have established guidelines regarding basic perioperative TEE that define the use of TEE as a monitoring tool outside of the cardiac operating room. National Board of Echocardiography certification in basic perioperative TEE is available after the completion of a written exam (for Testamur status) and the submission of a complete case log (for Diplomate status). Basic TEE certification is not supported by updated Canadian guidelines and is limited to the intraoperative setting. Training in basic perioperative TEE nonetheless requires a significant time commitment and supervision.

Basic TEE is an ideal tool for perioperative hemodynamic monitoring, assessments of volume status, guidance for fluid administration, and rescue in cases involving hemodynamic instability [32]. The integration of basic TEE training into the residency curriculum [33] should be considered to offer the full potential of this tool to the next generation of providers [23, 34].

Similarity to focused TTE [9], a more simplified "focused" TEE limited to five views with the objective of answering dichotomous questions has been successfully used in emergency medicine [35] and critical care [36]. However, the intraoperative use of this technique has not been described to date.

The feasibility and effectiveness of basic focused TTE in Canadian anesthesia residency programs were described more than 5 years ago [4]. Research has demonstrated that in the USA, a comprehensive perioperative US curriculum significantly impacted anesthesia residents' clinical assessment skills [34]. However, focused cardiac US teaching was found to be uncommon in anesthesia residency programs in the USA [37, 38], and a recent survey indicated that only 8 of 17 anesthesia residency programs in Canada offered any form of POCUS training [38]. In contrast, over 90% of cardiovascular anesthesiologists surveyed in the USA responded that focused cardiac US should be integrated into every anesthesia residency curriculum [37].

What is next?

A structured pathway for developing postgraduate curricula has been proposed for critical care anesthesiologists [39] and for specific perioperative POCUS applications [40, 41].

POCUS curriculum development for anesthesia residency programs must be considered in the context of the new framework of competency by design [42]. The current Canadian model implies that all anesthesia training is built to be tested against all applicable CanMEDS roles. POCUS appears to be relevant to all seven of these roles (medical expert, professional, communicator, collaborator, leader, scholar and professional). From this perspective, POCUS would not be regarded as a separate technical skill but would instead be integrated into daily clinical practice. This development would require a number of steps, including defining the scope of practice for perioperative POCUS and designing a longitudinal curriculum that accounts for current evidence regarding training duration and structure [4, 43], simulator use, number of scans necessary to achieve proficiency, [9, 44–46] assessments of competence [47] and skill retention [48, 49]. National or international expert consensus may be required in areas for which no supporting evidence is available.

A separate challenge is to train the trainers; this challenge will lead to the creation of a certification pathway. Definitions of learning requirements will have to consider prior US experience hands-on learning and portfolio building will be limited by access to supervision and a lack of dedicated scanning time [50].

The introduction of integrated US teaching into medical school curricula is becoming standard across North America, and current graduates are therefore being trained to integrate US into clinical decision making. Residency curricula have a mandate to build on this foundation, and practicing anesthesiologists will need to prepare themselves for new teaching challenges.

Anesthesiologists are the main players in the perioperative care of surgical patients, from preoperative assessment to post-operative pain management. Therefore, they are the natural leaders in the context of the newly proposed perioperative surgical home model. With this prospect of more comprehensive longitudinal patient management, POCUS will find a fertile field of applications, given its proven roles in facilitating problem solving [51] and ensuring patient safety [34] during the pre-, intra- and post-operative periods.

POCUS requires adequate privileges, credentialing and oversight for quality assurance. At present, privileges to perform POCUS are currently granted by individual departments. There is no exemption for POCUS; this status may be problematic for medico-legal and remuneration purposes. In Canada and the USA, local regulations require electronic image storage and written reports for billing purposes. The availability of pictures archiving and communication systems (PACS) or web-based storage systems represents a significant concern, especially for community hospitals. Given the low remuneration for POCUS exams in both Canada and the USA, it is difficult to build a business model to support the practice of these examinations and justify the setup and maintenance costs of an image storage infrastructure. However, this challenge is a major limitation with respect to quality assurance and control.

The future

An increasing number of anesthesia residency programs are integrating a mandatory POCUS curriculum. This development is echoed by increased interest in POCUS training targeted to practicing anesthesiologists. Nonetheless, guidelines are lacking.

As a start, in 2016, the Canadian Anesthesiologist's Society formed a task force to develop a perioperative POCUS consensus statement that reflected the views of POCUS experts in all academic centers across the country. The first nation-wide, full-day perioperative POCUS course was held in Vancouver in June 2016. This course addressed all perioperative POCUS applications identified by the Perioperative POCUS Consensus Group.

The Canadian Emergency Ultrasound Society (CEUS) also developed the Emergency Department Echo Course in 2001, which became the standard POCUS certification course for emergency physicians in Canada. CEUS rebranded itself as the Canadian Point of Care Ultrasound Society (CPoCUS) (https://www.cpocus.ca) in 2016, and based on the strength of its certifying platform, offers certifications to anesthesiologists by combining different modules to fit applications of interest during the perioperative period.

In contrast, no major anesthesia society in the USA has embarked on the task of defining the scope of practice for POCUS or a path towards POCUS certification.

A special POCUS interest group was established last year within the American Society of Regional Anesthesia (ASRA).

However, the 2-day workshop on POCUS in anesthesia organized for 2017 [52] specially focused on focus assessed transthoracic echocardiography (FATE) certification and did not include all of the aforementioned components.

Thus far, the only other attempt to create a comprehensive POCUS certification has been offered by the Alliance for Physician Certification & Advancement (APCA) [53], a physician-centric council spun out of the American Registry for Diagnostic Medical Sonography (ARDMS).

The APCA is currently working to provide, a POCUS Fundamental Certificate covering basic knowledge regarding US. This certificate will be followed by a series of POCUS Clinical Certificates (cardiac, GI, lung, abdominal trauma, and GU certificates, among others) [53].

The acquisition of a predetermined number of POCUS Clinical Certificates will earn the provider a certificate in POCUS specific to a determined specialty.

The first available certification will be in emergency medicine. Additional specialty-dedicated certifications, including a certification in anesthesia, are planned for development in the future.

Even if the APCA certification system does not address the extension of training necessary to reach competency in POCUS, it may nonetheless represent a useful practical tool to evaluate the results of an appropriately formulated learning curriculum. Although a minimum number of scans will likely continue to be required, the creation of a curriculum based on a competency-based education model that will be more focused on the achievement of certain milestones than a predetermined number of exams will help to finally achieve this goal.

It is hoped that the increased interest in POCUS that has recently been expressed in numerous anesthesia publications will promote a movement that will lead to the formulation of a clear curriculum and guidelines by our professional societies.

To answer to the "call to action" from Mahmood et al. in last year's June issue of *Anesthesia & Analgesia* [16], the present generation of anesthesiologists must have a well-defined and structured learning path to be able to teach subsequent generations.

Abbreviations

POCUS: point-of-care ultrasound; US: ultrasound; TEE: transesophageal echocardiography.

Authors' contributions

LDM helped create the manuscript outline, wrote part of the first draft and edited the subsequent version of the manuscript. MM conceived the original idea, helped create the manuscript outline, wrote part of the first draft and edited the subsequent version of the manuscript. All authors read and approved the final manuscript.

Author details

[1] Department of Anesthesia, Georgetown University, MedStar Georgetown University Hospital, 3800 Reservoir Road NW, CCC Building, Lower Level, Washington, DC, USA. [2] Department of Anesthesia and Pain Management, Toronto General Hospital, University Health Network, University of Toronto, 200 Elizabeth Street EN 3-400, Toronto, ON M5G 2C4, Canada.

Acknowledgements

None.

References

1. Troianos CA, Hartman GS, Glas KE et al (2012) Special articles: guidelines for performing ultrasound guided vascular cannulation: recommendations of the American Society of Echocardiography and the Society of Cardiovascular Anesthesiologists. Anesth Analg 114(1):46–72
2. Beique F, Ali M, Hynes M et al (2006) Canadian guidelines for training in adult perioperative transesophageal echocardiography. Recommendations of the Cardiovascular Section of the Canadian Anesthesiologists' Society and the Canadian Society of Echocardiography. Can J Anaesth 53(10):1044–1060
3. Hahn RT, Abraham T, Adams MS et al (2013) Guidelines for performing a comprehensive transesophageal echocardiographic examination: recommendations from the American Society of Echocardiography and the Society of Cardiovascular Anesthesiologists. J Am Soc Echocardiogr 26(9):921–964
4. Tanzola RC, Walsh S, Hopman WM et al (2013) Brief report: focused transthoracic echocardiography training in a cohort of Canadian anesthesiology residents: a pilot study. Can J Anaesth 60(1):32–37
5. Arellano R, Nurmohamed A, Rumman A et al (2014) The utility of transthoracic echocardiography to confirm central line placement: an observational study. Can J Anaesth 61(4):340–346
6. Adler AC, Jablonka DH (2016) Bedside ultrasound: a tool for assessment of IV functionality. Anesthesiology 124(4):959
7. Seward JB, Douglas PS, Erbel R et al (2002) Hand-carried cardiac ultrasound (HCU) device: recommendations regarding new technology. A report from the Echocardiography Task Force on New Technology of the Nomenclature and Standards Committee of the American Society of Echocardiography. J Am Soc Echocardiogr 15(4):369–373
8. Beaulieu Y, Marik PE (2005) Bedside ultrasonography in the ICU: part 1. Chest 128(2):881–895
9. Spencer KT, Kimura BJ, Korcarz CE et al (2013) Focused cardiac ultrasound: recommendations from the American Society of Echocardiography. J Am Soc Echocardiogr 26(6):567–581
10. Canty DJ, Royse CF, Kilpatrick D et al (2012) The impact on cardiac diagnosis and mortality of focused transthoracic echocardiography in hip fracture surgery patients with increased risk of cardiac disease: a retrospective cohort study. Anaesthesia 67(11):1202–1209
11. Botker MT, Vang ML, Grofte T et al (2014) Routine pre-operative focused ultrasonography by anesthesiologists in patients undergoing urgent surgical procedures. Acta Anaesthesiol Scand 58(7):807–814
12. Cowie B (2011) Three years' experience of focused cardiovascular ultrasound in the peri-operative period. Anaesthesia 66(4):268–273
13. Markin NW, Gmelch BS, Griffee MJ et al (2015) A review of 364 perioperative rescue echocardiograms: findings of an anesthesiologist-staffed perioperative echocardiography service. J Cardiothorac Vasc Anesth 29(1):82–88
14. Adler AC (2017) Air embolism during cardiac catheterization and the role for anesthesia use of bedside ultrasound. Anesthesiology. PMID:28562374
15. Tsou PY, Kurbedin J, Chen YS et al (2017) Accuracy of point-of-care focused echocardiography in predicting outcome of resuscitation in cardiac arrest patients: a systematic review and meta-analysis. Resuscitation 114:92–99
16. Volpicelli G, Elbarbary M, Blaivas M et al (2012) International evidence-based recommendations for point-of-care lung ultrasound. Intensive Care Med 38(4):577–591
17. Das SK, Choupoo NS, Haldar R et al (2015) Transtracheal ultrasound for verification of endotracheal tube placement: a systematic review and meta-analysis. Can J Anaesth 62(4):413–423
18. Adler AC (2017) Perioperative point of care ultrasound in pediatric anesthesiology; a case series highlighting intra-operative diagnosis of hemodynamic instability and alteration of management. J Cardiothorac Vasc Anesth. PMID:28911897
19. Díaz-Gómez J, Ripoll JG, Ratzlaff RA, Tavazzi G, Via G, Mookadam F, Ramakrishna H, FASE F (2017) Perioperative lung ultrasound for the cardiothoracic anesthesiologist: emerging importance and clinical applications. J Cardiothorac Vasc Anesth. 9:10
20. You-Ten KE, Desai D, Postonogova T et al (2015) Accuracy of conventional digital palpation and ultrasound of the cricothyroid membrane in obese women in labour. Anaesthesia 70(11):1230–1234
21. Perlas A, Mitsakakis N, Liu L et al (2013) Validation of a mathematical model for ultrasound assessment of gastric volume by gastroscopic examination. Anesth Analg 116(2):357–363
22. Adler AC, Greeley WJ, Conlin F et al (2016) Perioperative Anesthesiology UltraSonographic Evaluation (PAUSE): a guided approach to perioperative bedside ultrasound. J Cardiothorac Vasc Anesth 30(2):521–529
23. Mahmood F, Matyal R, Skubas N et al (2016) Perioperative ultrasound training in anesthesiology: a call to action. Anesth Analg 122(6):1794–1804
24. Janelle GM, London MJ (2016) Perioperative ultrasound: the future is now. Anesth Analg 122(6):1734–1736
25. Skubas NJ (2015) Teaching whole body point-of-care ultrasound: advancing the skills of tomorrow's anesthesiologists. Anesthesiology 123(3):499–500
26. Ramsingh D, Gudzenko V, Martin RD (2017) Point-of-Care Ultrasound: novel Technology to Routine Perioperative Assessment Tool. Anesth Analg 124(3):709–711
27. Denault A, Fayad A, Chen R (2013) Focused ultrasound is the next step in perioperative care. Can J Anaesth 60(8):741–747
28. Johnson DW, Oren-Grinberg A (2011) Perioperative point-of-care ultrasonography: the past and the future are in anesthesiologists' hands. Anesthesiology 115(3):460–462
29. Conlin F, Connelly NR, Eaton MP, et al. (2017) Perioperative use of focused transthoracic cardiac ultrasound: a survey of current practice and opinion. Anesth Analg. PMID:28537977
30. Marik PE, Mayo P (2008) Certification and training in critical care ultrasound. Intensive Care Med 34(2):215–217
31. Arntfield R, Millington S, Ainsworth C et al (2014) Canadian recommendations for critical care ultrasound training and competency. Can Respir J 21(6):341–345
32. American Society of Anesthesiologists CoE-PSSoTECPDA, 2015 FOR BOD/HOD information. Statement on transesophageal echocardiography (Approved by the ASA House of Delegates on October 17, 2001, and last amended on October 28, 2015) 2015

33. Smith WB, Robinson AR 3rd, Janelle GM (2015) Expanding role of perioperative transesophageal echocardiography in the general anesthesia practice and residency training in the USA. Curr Opin Anaesthesiol 28(1):95–100
34. Ramsingh D, Rinehart J, Kain Z et al (2015) Impact assessment of perioperative point-of-care ultrasound training on anesthesiology residents. Anesthesiology 123(3):670–682
35. Arntfield R, Pace J, Hewak M, et al. (2015) Focused Transesophageal Echocardiography by Emergency Physicians is Feasible and Clinically Influential: Observational Results from a Novel Ultrasound Program. J Emerg Med 50(2):286–94. PMID:26508495
36. Vieillard-Baron A, Slama M, Mayo P et al (2013) A pilot study on safety and clinical utility of a single-use 72-h indwelling transesophageal echocardiography probe. Intensive Care Med 39(4):629–635
37. Conlin F, Roy Connelly N, Raghunathan K et al (2016) Focused transthoracic cardiac ultrasound: a survey of training practices. J Cardiothorac Vasc Anesth 30(1):102–106
38. Mizubuti G, Allard R, Ho AM et al (2017) A survey of focused cardiac ultrasonography training in Canadian anesthesiology residency programs. Can J Anaesth 64(4):441–442
39. Fagley RE, Haney MF, Beraud AS et al (2015) Critical care basic ultrasound learning goals for American Anesthesiology Critical Care Trainees: recommendations from an Expert Group. Anesth Analg 120(5):1041–1053
40. Perlas A, Van de Putte P, Van Houwe P et al (2016) I-AIM framework for point-of-care gastric ultrasound. Br J Anaesth 116(1):7–11
41. Via G, Hussain A, Wells M et al (2014) International evidence-based recommendations for focused cardiac ultrasound. J Am Soc Echocardiogr 27(7):683 e1–683 e33
42. Fraser AB, Stodel EJ, Jee R et al (2016) Preparing anesthesiology faculty for competency-based medical education. Can J Anaesth 63(12):1364–1373
43. Poelaert J, Mayo P (2007) Education and evaluation of knowledge and skills in echocardiography: how should we organize? Intensive Care Med 33(10):1684–1686
44. Millington SJ, Hewak M, Arntfield RT et al (2017) Outcomes from extensive training in critical care echocardiography: identifying the optimal number of practice studies required to achieve competency. J Crit Care 40:99–102
45. Arzola C, Carvalho JC, Cubillos J et al (2013) Anesthesiologists' learning curves for bedside qualitative ultrasound assessment of gastric content: a cohort study. Can J Anaesth 60(8):771–779
46. Gaspar HA, Morhy SS, Lianza AC et al (2014) Focused cardiac ultrasound: a training course for pediatric intensivists and emergency physicians. BMC Med Educ 14:25
47. Millington SJ, Arntfield RT, Hewak M et al (2016) The Rapid Assessment of Competency in Echocardiography Scale: validation of a Tool for Point-of-Care Ultrasound. J Ultrasound Med Off J Am Inst Ultrasound Med 35(7):1457–1463
48. Kimura BJ, Sliman SM, Waalen J et al (2016) Retention of Ultrasound Skills and Training in "Point-of-Care" Cardiac Ultrasound. J Am Soc Echocardiogr 29(10):992–997
49. Gaspar HA, Brunow de Carvalho W, Delgado AF (2016) How to train and maintain pediatric intensivists updated in focused cardiac ultrasound? Pediatr Crit Care Med 17(10):1015
50. Patrawalla P, Eisen LA, Shiloh A et al (2015) Development and validation of an assessment tool for competency in critical care ultrasound. J Grad Med Educ 7(4):567–573
51. Vignon P (2012) PRO: physician-performed ultrasound: the time has come for routine use in acute care medicine. Anesth Analg 115(5):999–1003
52. Perioperative Point-of-Care Ultrasound SIG ASoRA. Introduction to Perioperative Point-of-Care Ultrasound. February 25–26, 2017. https://www.asra.com/page/189/perioperative-point-of-care-ultrasound-sig
53. APCA AfPCaA-. Point-of-Care Ultrasound (POCUS) Academy. https://www.apca.org/pocus#!prerequisites-specialtycertifications

2

Diagnostic performance of abdominal point of care ultrasound performed by an emergency physician in acute right iliac fossa pain

Jean-Eudes Bourcier[1*], Emeric Gallard[1], Jean-Philippe Redonnet[1], Magali Majourau[1], Dominique Deshaie[1], Jean-Marie Bourgeois[2], Didier Garnier[1] and Thomas Geeraerts[3]

Abstract

Background: Right iliac fossa abdominal pain is a common reason for emergency ward admissions, its etiology is difficult to diagnose. It can be facilitated by an imaging examination, such as a Computerized Tomography scan which exposes the patient to ionizing radiation and implies delays. A bedside ultrasound performed by emergency physicians could avoid these issues. The aim of our study was to assess the performance of ultrasound carried out at the patient's bedside by an emergency physician compared with a clinical-laboratory examination for the diagnosis of a surgical pathology in right iliac fossa pain.

Methods: This is a single-center prospective cohort study conducted in an Emergency Department receiving 19,000 patients per year. All patients presenting pain in the right iliac fossa were included by four (out of ten) emergency physicians certified in an ultrasound examination. A full grid pattern scan ultrasound of the abdominal cavity with analysis of the right iliac fossa was performed. The primary outcome was to compare the diagnosis performance of bedside ultrasound and clinical-laboratory examination to detect a surgical pathology. Two emergency physicians who did not participate in the study made the final diagnosis (i.e., surgical or non-surgical pathology) by reviewing the entire medical chart of each patient.

Results: From January 2011 to July 2013, 158 patients with a median age of 17 [13–32] years were analyzed. The diagnosed cases were: appendicitis (53), non-specific abdominal pain (48), lymphadenitis (22), ileitis (11), complicated ovarian cysts (7), neoplasias (5), inflammatory or infectious colitis (5), inguinal herniations (3), bowel obstructions (2), and salpingitis (2). The accuracy of ultrasound diagnoses was 0.89 (95% CI 0.84–0.94) versus 0.70 (95% CI 0.57–0.82) for diagnoses based on clinical-laboratory examination only ($p < 0.001$).

Conclusion: Bedsides, ultrasound allows an accurate diagnosis of a surgical pathology in 89% of cases, which is more efficient than the clinical-laboratory examination.

Keywords: Bedside ultrasound, Abdominal pain, Appendicitis, Diagnostic methods

*Correspondence: je.bourcier@gmail.com
[1] Emergency, Anesthesiology and Critical Care Department, Lourdes Hospital, 2 Avenue Alexandre Marqui, 65100 Lourdes, France
Full list of author information is available at the end of the article

Introduction

Abdominal pain is the third most common reason for attending a hospital emergency ward [1]. Even though in 40% of cases the clinical picture is benign and without a precise etiology; in cases requiring emergency surgery, any delay in treatment can result in an increase in morbidity or mortality. The pain in the right iliac fossa represents a specific problem in regard to appendicitis, as the diagnosis is sometimes hard to make, with a clinical exam and a laboratory test alone [2, 3]. On their own, clinical examinations perform relatively poorly, with sensitivity and specificity ranging from 50 to 86% [4], thus warranting introduction of decisions scores. For instance, the Alvarado or Appendicitis Inflammatory Response (AIR) score, that couple clinical and laboratory assessments have sensitivity and specificity close to 90% according to some papers [5–9]. All the international guidelines are in support of the use of complementary examinations, and particularly of imaging, for undertaking a diagnosis of pain in the right iliac fossa [10–12]. The abdominal computerized tomography (CT) scan with injection of a contrasting agent is the standard imaging method, although it has drawbacks with regard to availability and the associated radiation [13, 14]. Recently, imaging by magnetic resonance has become more common, particularly with children and pregnant women, although its availability is even more limited than for the CT scan [15–17]. Abdominal ultrasound has the advantage of being inexpensive and it does not involve ionizing radiation, although its performance remains operator dependent [18]. In practice, however, a radiologist cannot always be available on short notice, which can lead to diagnostic delays that may have detrimental consequences for the patient [19]. That is why an abdominal ultrasound performed by the emergency physician at the patient's bedside in addition to clinical and biological data could be helpful in detection of a surgical pathology more efficiently. Of course, it remains dependent on the extent of training and the reliability of the interpretation of the imaging results by a non-specialist in radiology. Some studies have showed the reliable accuracy in the diagnosis of acute appendicitis, with a bedside ultrasound performed in emergency ward [20, 21].

The aim of our study was to assess the performance of abdominal ultrasound carried out at the patient's bedside by an emergency physician compared with a clinical-laboratory examination, for the diagnosis of a surgical pathology in right iliac fossa. Our hypothesis was that ultrasound would improve diagnostic performance.

Materials and methods

Study design

This prospective cohort study was carried out in the emergency ward of a general hospital center that has 19,000 admissions per year.

Ethics approval

The protocol for the study was approved by the Ethics Committee of Lourdes hospital (PV N°14244) and follows the World Medical Association's Declaration of Helsinki. It did not require written consent since the standard treatment procedures were not altered in order to perform the study.

Patients

From January 2011 to July 2013, all patients (children and adults) presented to the emergency department with as main symptom an acute pain of the right iliac fossa were included if a physician trained in use of ultrasound was present.

Clinical and laboratory examination

The history of the patient and the clinical examination strived to characterize the surgical origin of the pain by relying on standard functional and physical symptoms (e.g., signs of occlusion or localized peritonitis, nausea, vomiting, a palpable mass, abdominal pain, rebound tenderness, etc.). Urological and/or gynecological symptoms were also probed for, depending on the symptoms. A point of care urinalysis was also performed at the admission.

Systematic common laboratory testing upon admission was composed of a blood count, a test for C-reactive protein levels, as well as a blood electrolytes test, and a test of kidney function. Depending on the patient history and clinical findings, a Human Chorionic Gonadotropin (β-HCG) test, a liver and pancreatic assessment, a hemostasis assessment, a blood group typing, or any other laboratory test deemed to be of use by the emergency physician were added.

Upon assessment of all these items, the physician had to make a suspected clinical-laboratory diagnosis: surgical pathology (i.e., requiring a surgical treatment) or medical pathology (i.e., requiring a medical treatment).

Ultrasound data

After having undergone basic training in the use of abdominal ultrasound imaging, the emergency physicians who included patients for this study had to have at least 2 years of experience with emergency ultrasound use. This was first broken down into training sessions in a certified center over 7 days and then by e-learning for 1 year. This training was based on the specifications of the American College of Emergency Physicians [22]. This course was completed by supervised training over a 6-month period that involved receiving ultrasound images with validation of the observed anomalies made by a radiologist.

Following the clinical examination and the laboratory testing, the emergency physician performed an ultrasound at the patients' bedside (using an M Turbo miniaturized ultrasound device from FUJIFILM SONOSITE©, Bothell, WA, USA).

The examination consisted of an initial grid pattern of the abdominal cavity using a convex abdominal probe (3.5 MHz), which permitted to search peritoneal effusion, masses. A scan of the two kidneys, liver, biliary tracts and aorta was equally performed. Because of the lack of a vaginal probe, pelvic analysis was performed by an abdominal probe. The emergency physician used the surface probe (7.5 MHz) to complete the scan, guided by the site of the pain, the analysis then focused on the right iliac fossa. Gradual compression was applied as described by Ooms [23, 24]: the normal digestive structures, which contain air, disappear from the screen upon compression. Furthermore, their wall is thin, with a thickness of less than 3 mm. By contrast, an inflamed digestive tract is not compressible, and it is painful upon application of pressure, while also exhibiting a thickened wall.

Other pathological images can also be seen, such as an intra-peritoneal effusion, an obstruction syndrome, inflammatory adenopathies, and complicated ovarian cyst [25–27] (Fig. 1).

In all cases, the emergency physician attempted to adequately discern the appendix. A diagnosis of appendicitis was made in conjunction with more than two of the following images: a double cockade cross-sectional appearance of the appendix of more than 6 mm in diameter, ending as a sleeve in a longitudinal section, a non-compressible nature, and association or not of a peri-appendicular effusion. In case of normal appendix viewed (none of previous images), this diagnosis was excluded (Fig. 2).

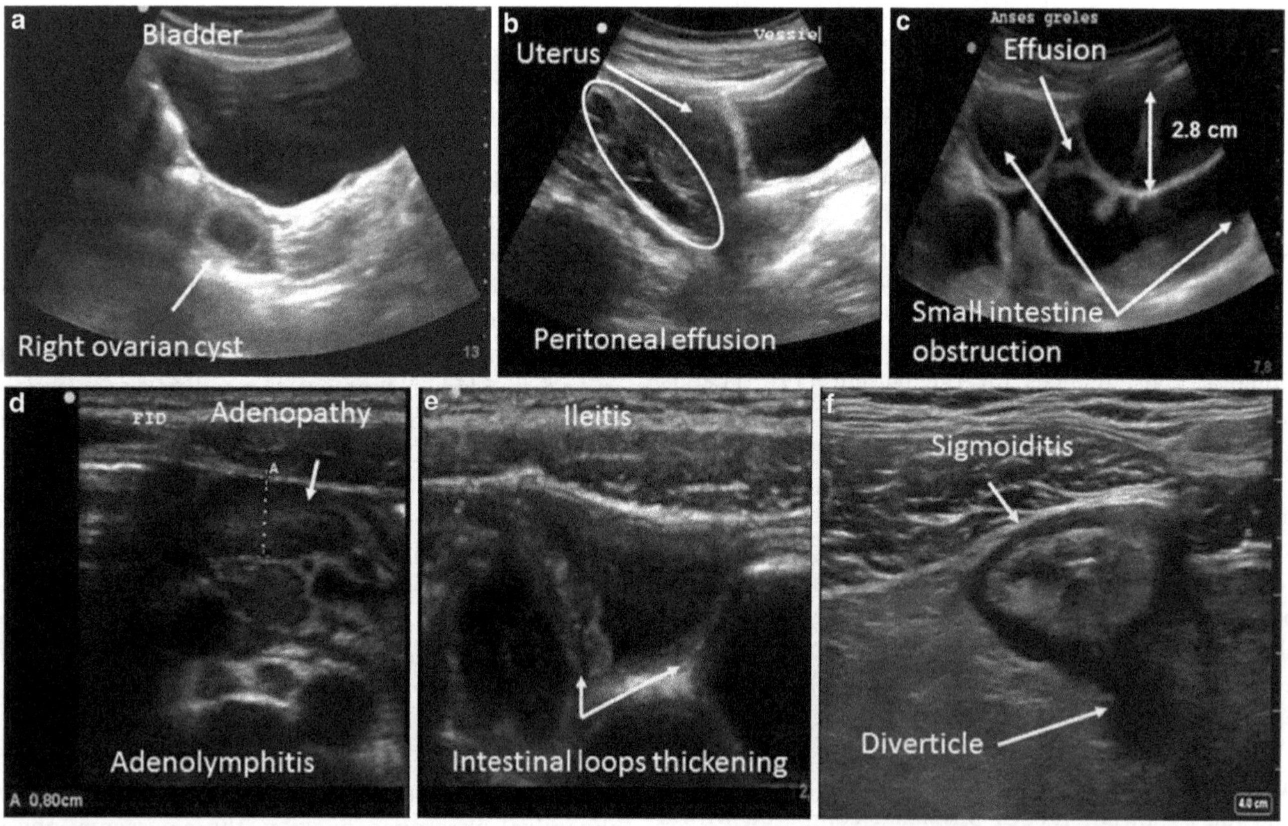

Fig. 1 Examples of abnormal ultrasound images: **a** a latero-uterine mass with a sonolucent liquid content suggestive of a complicated ovarian cyst, **b** isolated peritoneal effusion (often at the bottom of the Douglas pouch), **c** appearance of a small intestinal occlusion (widening of the intestinal loops by more than 2.5 cm, with a liquid content and possible inter-loop effusion), **d** adenopathies (hypoechoic oval images greater than 5 mm in terms of the antero-posterior diameter, sensitive to passage of the probe, and enhanced by color Doppler), **e** thickening of the last small intestinal loops suggestive of ileitis (thickening by more than 3 mm of the wall of the digestive tract), **f** circumferential widening of the colon wall (a pseudo-kidney appearance) suggestive of an inflammation or an infection

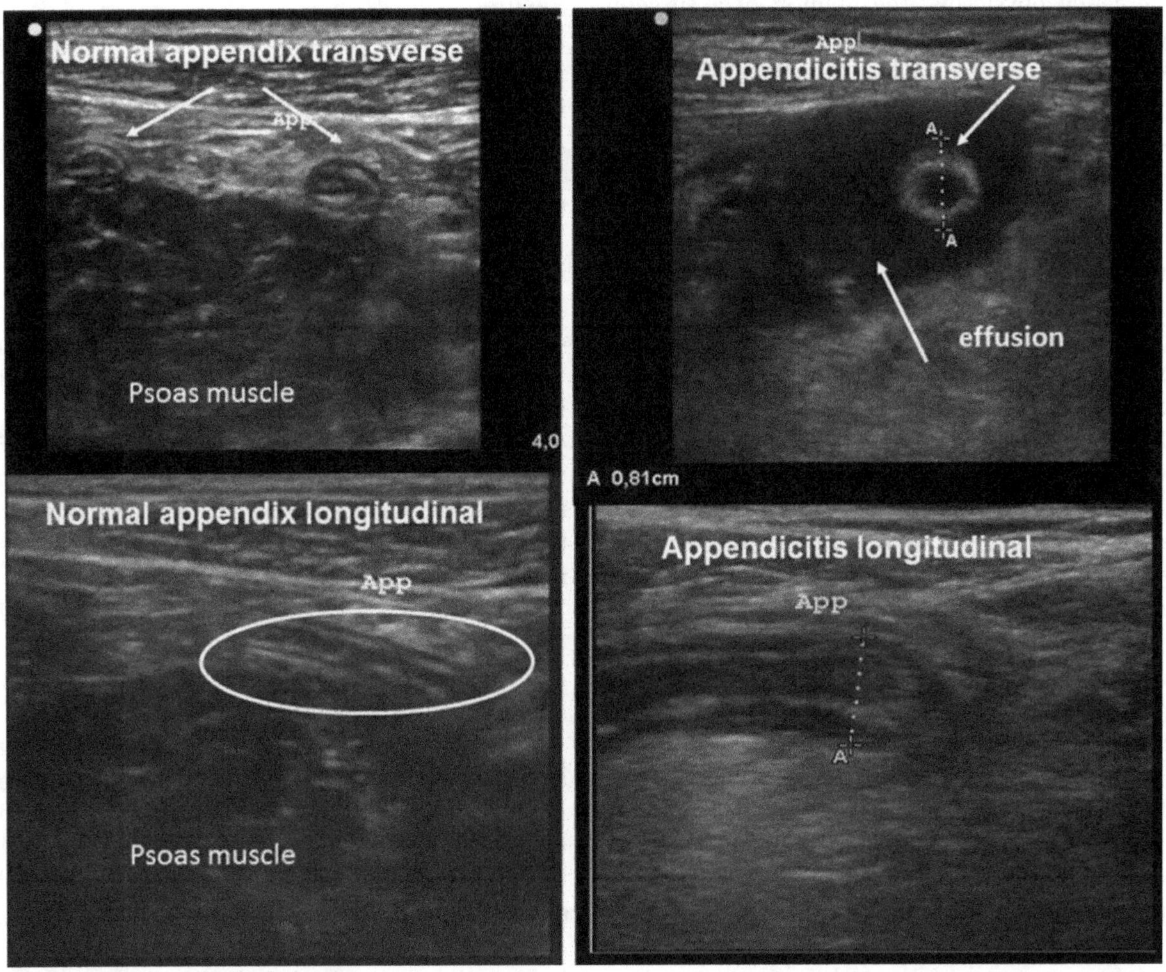

Fig. 2 Ultrasound appearance of a normal appendix and a pathological one

Upon completion of the examination, the practitioner provided a full written report regarding the ultrasound that fully detailed all of their findings. In case of a visually diseased appendix, intestinal occlusion, or peritoneal effusion, the ultrasound indicated a surgical pathology. In case of a normal appearing appendix, or other images indicative of pathologies, the ultrasound indicated a medical pathology.

After making the clinical-laboratory diagnosis, and the ultrasound diagnosis, the emergency physician in charge of the patient could ask for an abdominal CT scan and/or the opinion of a surgeon if he deemed it necessary, in particular to decide on the continuation of the patient's care.

Final diagnosis

The final diagnosis was the etiologic diagnosis of right iliac fossa pain (i.e., surgical or medical pathology). A surgical pathology was defined by a pathology requiring surgical treatment like laparoscopy or laparotomy which was decided and performed by the surgeon. Medical pathology was defined by a pathology requiring medical treatment (non-surgical).

Two emergency physicians who did not participate in the study made the final diagnosis by reviewing the entire medical chart of each patient, taking into account their evolution. They had to classify patients into two groups: surgical or medical pathology. In each group, the etiologic diagnosis was investigated.

For the patients who underwent surgery, the final diagnosis relied on an analysis of the surgical report and of the histological examination in case of surgical exeresis. For the patients who were hospitalized without undergoing surgery, the final diagnosis was based on the final hospitalization report. When patients were not hospitalized, they were contacted 2 months after discharge, and the diagnosis made when they left the emergency ward was then confirmed or not by their medical progress. Indeed, a surgical pathology was excluded if there was no re-hospitalization in our institution or another. In case of discrepancy between the two emergency physicians, the opinion of a surgeon from our institution could be taken into consideration.

Consequently, the performance of abdominal ultrasound was compared to the performance of clinical-laboratory examination for the diagnosis of a surgical pathology.

Statistical analyses

The quantitative variables were expressed as mean ± SD for normally distributed variables and otherwise as a median with interquartile range. Qualitative variables were expressed as numerical values and as percentages.

The diagnostic performances of the ultrasound and the clinical and laboratory examination were expressed as sensitivity (Se), specificity (Sp), positive predictive value (PPV), negative predictive value (NPV) with their [confidence intervals at 95%]. A Youden's index and an accuracy were calculated. The Youden's index is defined by (sensitivity + specificity − 1), and the performance of the examination was deemed to be better when the Youden's index is close to 1. Accuracy was defined as the percentage of properly classified cases upon completion of examinations for which the performance was tested.

The relative accuracies of the ultrasound and of the clinical-laboratory diagnosis were compared using a McNemar's test, with a threshold for significance set at $p = 0.05$.

No power analysis was performed because of the absence of previous studies comparing abdominal ultrasound by emergency physician and standard examination (clinic + laboratory) in the management of right iliac fossa pain.

Results

Four emergency physicians (of ten in the department) met the training requirements and thus participated in the study.

Ultimately, 158 patients were analyzed (sex ratio = 1) who were 17 [13–32] years old. Of these, 69 patients (44%) were hospitalized and 89 (56%) were sent home. The time spent in the emergency ward was 167 ± 51 min. The mean Body Mass Index was 21 ± 4 kg m^{-2}.

The final diagnoses made included 53 cases of appendicitis (33%), 48 (31%) cases of non-specific abdominal pain (NSAP), 22 cases of adenolymphitis (14%), 11 cases of ileitis(7%), 7 complicated ovarian cysts (5%), 5 (3%) newly discovered neoplasias (4 colon, 1 pancreatic), 5 (3%) cases of inflammatory or infectious colitis (3 sigmoidal, 2 inflammatory colitis), 3 (2%) inguinal herniation's, 2 (1%) bowel obstructions (one by a bridle and one by a neoplastic growth) and 2 (1%) salpingitis.

The sample characteristic is presented in STARD flow diagram (Fig. 3).

Detailed images viewed on ultrasound compared to the final diagnosis are reported in Table 1.

Out of the 56 patients with an appendicitis diagnosed by ultrasound, 44 (84%) were taken directly to the operating room after surgical advice in the emergency department. There were four false-positive ultrasounds where the final diagnosis turned out to be one NSAP and three adenolymphitis.

None of these four patients underwent an operation, because they were examined by the surgeon on duty. This one decided to supervise three patients in the surgery

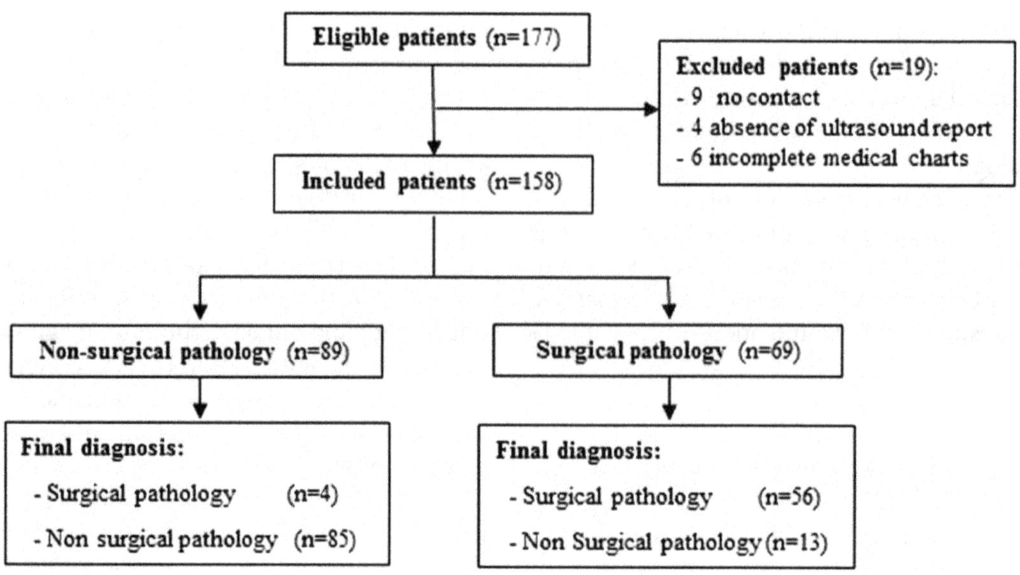

Fig. 3 STARD flow diagram

Table 1 Comparison of ultrasound diagnosis and final diagnosis

			ULTRASOUND DIAGNOSIS							
			MEDICAL PATHOLOGIES n= 89					SURGICAL PATHOLOGIES n= 69		
			Normal n = 46	Adenopathy n = 25	Ileitis n= 9	Colic wall thickening n = 5	latero-uterine mass n = 4	Appendicitis n = 56	Obstruction n = 3	Effusion n = 10
FINAL DIAGNOSIS	MEDICAL PATHOLOGIES n= 98	NSAP n = 48	36	9				1		2
		Adenolymphitis n = 22	3	13				3		3
		Ileitis n=11	2		9					
		Complicated ovarian cyst n=7		2			3			2
		Colitis n = 5	1	1		2			1	
		Discovery of cancer n = 5	1			3				1
	SURGICAL PATHOLOGIES n= 60	Complicated hernia n=3	3							
		Flange obstruction n=1							1	
		Salpingitis n=2					1			1
		Cancerous obstruction n=1							1	
		Appendicitis n= 53						52		1
		CT scans n = 34	9	3		5	4	5	3	5

department. Concerning the fourth he asked for a CT scan.

Among the 89 patients for whom the bedside ultrasound did not find a surgical pathology, there were four false negative. The diagnosis was corrected by surgeon on duty for two of them and by a CT scan for two others. For the other eighty-five patients (true negative), none had to later undergo an operation or be re-hospitalized.

The clinical-laboratory diagnosis compared to the final diagnosis is shown in Table 2.

The compared performances of bedside ultrasound and clinical-laboratory approach according to the diagnosis of a surgical pathology are reported in Table 3.

Discussion

In our study of patients exhibiting pain in the right iliac fossa, an ultrasound performed by the emergency physician allowed for the diagnosis of a surgical pathology with an accuracy rate of 89%. This amounts to a significant gain in performance relative to clinical-laboratory examinations, since the latter has an accuracy rate of 70%.

The performance of the clinical-laboratory approach is relatively modest, perhaps because there is still ample room for improvement in terms of the clinical examination. This is indeed suggested by studies of this approach, and Alvarado or AIR score also yields extremely variable results [28–31]. These scores are

Table 2 Comparison of the clinical-laboratory diagnosis and the final diagnosis

			CLINICAL LABORATORY DIAGNOSIS	
			MEDICAL PATHOLOGIES n= 87	SURGICAL PATHOLOGIES n= 71
FINAL DIAGNOSIS	MEDICAL PATHOLOGIES n= 98	NSAP n = 48	36	12
		Adenolymphitis n = 22	15	7
		Ileitis n=11	8	3
		Complicated ovarian cyst n=7	6	1
		Colitis n = 5	1	4
		Discovery of cancer n = 5	3	2
	SURGICAL PATHOLOGIES n= 60	Complicated hernia n = 3	3	
		Flange obstruction n=1		1
		Salpingitis n=2		2
		Cancerous obstruction n=1		1
		Appendicitis n= 53	15	38
		CT scans n = 34	21	13

used to determine likelihood of appendicitis. However, this affection is not the only one that can underlie pain located in the right iliac fossa, thus explaining the lower performance with a cohort of right iliac fossa pain comprising different pathologies. When the final diagnosis was appendicitis, only 38 out of 53 cases were suspected by the clinical-laboratory examination, which seem to confirm that these scores are not foolproof. Analysis of the results shows that the highest levels of false positives were encountered above all in cases of adenolymphitis and ileitis, or in cases of colitis (inflammatory or infectious). This can undoubtedly be explained by the early appearance of these affections with surgical pathology such as appendicitis.

As for the 13 patients for whom the ultrasound diagnosis indicated a surgical pathology, although the final

Table 3 Performance of ultrasound and clinical-laboratory examination according to the final diagnosis of surgical pathology

	Sensitivity [95% CI]	Specificity [95% CI]	PPV [95% CI]	NPV [95% CI]	Youden	Accuracy * [95% CI]
Ultrasounds	0.93 [0.87, 0.99]	0.87 [0.79, 0.93]	0.81 [0.72, 0.90]	0.95 [0.91, 0.99]	0.80	0.89 [0.84, 0.94]
Clinical-laboratory examination	0.7 [0.58, 0.81]	0.7 [0.60, 0.78]	0.59 [0.46, 0.69]	0.79 [0.7, 0.87]	0.4	0.70 [0.57, 0.82]

95% CI: confidence interval; PPV: positive predictive value; NPV: negative predictive value

* $p < 0.05$

diagnosis was in fact a non-surgical pathology, none incorrectly underwent surgery. This was thanks to reassessment by the surgeon on duty, who either monitored them in the surgery department, or who ordered a CT scan that allowed the diagnosis to be corrected or to be made with a greater degree of accuracy. In case of discordant ultrasound/clinical–biological results, the reassessment of the surgeon evaluation was considered as the reference method.

The performances of the ultrasound carried out by the emergency physician are comparable to those found in the literature when a radiologist performed the ultrasound: i.e., a specificity of 70 to 90% and a sensitivity of 85 to 100%. These works compared accuracy of an ultrasound with the surgery results or a CT scan only in appendicitis diagnosis [24, 32]. By contrast, assessments regarding the performance of ultrasounds by doctors who are not radiologists encountered highly variable results (sensitivity from 60 to 90%) [33–35]. This was probably related to the fact that the duration of learning to research appendicitis was too short; however, the emergency ultrasound guidelines do not yet cover this area [22].

The fact that the emergency physician performs the ultrasound themselves will strengthen the notion of the pain in the right iliac fossa being innocuous when they do not see an abnormal image and, by contrast, tend to confirm or give rise to suspicion of a serious diagnosis when they obtain an abnormal image. This is the case for appendicitis, unlike with other pathologies, where a typical image usually is enough to confirm a diagnosis. Indeed, colonic afflictions (inflammatory, infectious, or neoplastic) translate into a non-specific thickening of the wall. Similarly, a peritoneal effusion, even when in isolation, is reason for the practitioner to be cautious since it should be considered as a sign of a surgical pathology until proven otherwise. These elements are reason to prescribe complementary assessments or to seek specialist advice.

Thus, this strategy allowed scanning to be optimized, with the irradiative examination given to 28% of the patients in our study, whereas in North American register, a CT scan was performed for 43% of patients who suffered from abdominal pain [36, 37].

Furthermore, this ultrasound-clinical process optimizes the processing of the patient by avoiding incorrect conclusions being made with regard to the cause of harmless abdominal pain, and by unnecessarily resulting in invasive procedures or hospitalization. As such, none of the 86 patients who were processed by the emergency department secondarily presented surgical pathologies.

With regard to the 60 patients in our cohort who underwent a surgical treatment, the use of an ultrasound resulted in rectifying the diagnosis for 14 (23%) patients for which the clinical-laboratory approach concluded with a non-surgical pathology.

These findings could encourage a two-step approach, with first clinical-laboratory and bedside ultrasound examination and secondarily a CT scan and/or surgical advice for management of right iliac fossa pain [38].

Limitations

As this is a monocentric study with a relatively limited number of participants, it is difficult to extrapolate the results of this work to the entire specialty.

Our results are probably not transferable to less well-trained operators. Nonetheless, the results of this work are reason to encourage further training efforts.

In the present sample of patients, no pyelonephritis or ureteral colic was observed. This could be related to strict inclusion criteria (main symptom of acute pain of the right iliac fossa). The number of patients included in the study did not reflect the prevalence of right iliac fossa pain in the emergency department over 30 months because only 4 of 10 EP could participate in the study.

Despite a good performance by the ultrasound-clinical strategy, there were still 17 diagnostic errors (thirteen false positives and four false negatives).

Three of the four surgical pathologies not detected by the ultrasound were strangulated inguinal hernia, probably explained by the fact that the ultrasound scan was not carried out in this area. It should be noted that clinical examinations for this affliction were equally inadequate. This highlights the importance of systematically exploring this area, with a careful physical examination and a focus with an ultrasound probe.

The 13 false positives were largely dominated by the presence of a non-specific peritoneal effusion in eight (61%) cases. Indeed, the cohort included only two cases out of 10 where those in fact revealed a surgical pathology. This is why it seems reasonable to retain this warning sign, since it motivates further exploration. Regarding the four false positives for appendicitis, it was the reassessment by the surgeon that allowed a cutoff decision to be made. The latter hence has a central role in the assessment of acute abdominal pains [39, 40].

Our analysis of the performance of the ultrasound was based on whether an anomaly was seen rather than whether an accurate diagnosis was made. This is particularly true in case of peritoneal effusion which can be indirect sign of a surgical pathology. This choice potentially leads to an overestimation of the merit of the ultrasound performed by the emergency physician.

As this study was not comparative, it does not allow for the contribution of the ultrasound to the diagnostic performance of the emergency physician to be appraised.

For that it would have been necessary to compare the treatment with a typical process whereby the examinations were performed by a radiologist.

Similarly, it was not possible to assess the gain in terms of the effect on the duration of the stay in the emergency department.

The emergency physicians were aware of clinical-laboratory results when ultrasounds were performed. This could have influenced the results. Indeed, confirmation of the final diagnosis by the two independent doctors was performed retrospectively, as was the case for the complementary examinations, of which the bedside ultrasound could influence the diagnosis. Yet this is so for all the complementary examinations (laboratory tests and CT scans) which form an integral part of the diagnostic process. Furthermore, this limitation does not apply to the patients who underwent surgery. Aside from surgical, anatomical–pathological, or scan-based findings, confirmation of the final diagnosis was not supported by items that could not be questioned. Indeed, it is ethically questionable to perform a CT for all patients or to make surgical exploration like laparoscopy in order to exclude a surgical pathology in case of adenolymphitis, ileitis or NSAP for example. Yet this limitation can be found in most of the studies treating abdominal pains, and particularly in the case of a non-surgical diagnosis [41, 42].

Conclusion

The diagnosis accuracy of an abdominal ultrasound performed by an emergency physician is 89% compared to an accuracy of 70% by a clinical-laboratory examination alone, for the diagnosis of a surgical pathology in case of right iliac fossa pain.

Abbreviations

CT: Computerized Tomography; PPV: positive predictive value; NPV: negative predictive value.

Authors' contributions

JEB, EG, JPR and MM collected the data. DD, JMB, DG and TG analyzed the data. All authors read and approved the final manuscript.

Author details

[1] Emergency, Anesthesiology and Critical Care Department, Lourdes Hospital, 2 Avenue Alexandre Marqui, 65100 Lourdes, France. [2] CFFE (Centre Francophone de Formation en Echographie), Nîmes, France. [3] Anesthesiology and Critical Care Department, Toulouse University Hospital, University Toulouse III Paul Sabatier, Toulouse, France.

Acknowledgements

Not applicable.

References

1. Stone R (1998) Acute abdominal pain. Lippincotts Prim Care Pract 2(4):341–357
2. Petroianu A (2012) Diagnosis of acute appendicitis. Int J Surg 10(3):115–119
3. Powers RD, Guertler AT (1995) Abdominal pain in the ED: stability and change over 20 years. Am J Emerg Med 13(3):301–303
4. Irvin TT (1989) Abdominal pain: a surgical audit of 1190 emergency admissions. Br J Surg 76(11):1121–1125
5. Kim HC, Yang DM, Lee CM, Jin W, Nam DH, Song JY et al (2011) Acute appendicitis: relationships between CT-determined severities and serum white blood cell counts and C-reactive protein levels. Br J Radiol 84(1008):1115–1120
6. Shindoh J, Niwa H, Kawai K, Ohata K, Ishihara Y, Takabayashi N et al (2011) Diagnostic power of inflammatory markers in predicting severity of appendicitis. Hepatogastroenterology 58(112):2003–2006
7. Wu H-P, Chen C-Y, Kuo I-T, Wu Y-K, Fu Y-C (2012) Diagnostic values of a single serum biomarker at different time points compared with Alvarado score and imaging examinations in pediatric appendicitis. J Surg Res 174(2):272–277
8. Alvarado A (1986) A practical score for the early diagnosis of acute appendicitis. Ann Emerg Med 15(5):557–564
9. Kollár D, McCartan DP, Bourke M, Cross KS, Dowdall J (2015) Predicting acute appendicitis? A comparison of the Alvarado score, the Appendicitis Inflammatory Response Score and clinical assessment. World J Surg 39(1):104–109
10. Howell JM, Eddy OL, Lukens TW, Thiessen MEW, Weingart SD, Decker WW et al (2010) Clinical policy: critical issues in the evaluation and management of emergency department patients with suspected appendicitis. Ann Emerg Med 55(1):71–116
11. Bhangu A, Søreide K, Di Saverio S, Assarsson JH, Drake FT (2015) Acute appendicitis: modern understanding of pathogenesis, diagnosis, and management. Lancet 386(10000):1278–1287
12. Di Saverio S, Birindelli A, Kelly MD, Catena F, Weber DG, Sartelli M et al (2016) WSES Jerusalem guidelines for diagnosis and treatment of acute appendicitis. World J Emerg Surg 11:34
13. Poortman P, Lohle PNM, Schoemaker CMC, Oostvogel HJM, Teepen HJLJM, Zwinderman KAH et al (2003) Comparison of CT and sonography in the diagnosis of acute appendicitis: a blinded prospective study. AJR Am J Roentgenol 181(5):1355–1359
14. Brenner DJ, Hall EJ (2007) Computed tomography–an increasing source of radiation exposure. N Engl J Med 357(22):2277–2284
15. Kearl YL, Claudius I, Behar S, Cooper J, Dollbaum R, Hardasmalani M et al (2016) Accuracy of magnetic resonance imaging and ultrasound for appendicitis in diagnostic and nondiagnostic studies. Acad Emerg Med 23(2):179–185
16. Aspelund G, Fingeret A, Gross E, Kessler D, Keung C, Thirumoorthi A et al (2014) Ultrasonography/MRI versus CT for diagnosing appendicitis. Pediatrics 133(4):586–593
17. Fonseca AL, Schuster KM, Kaplan LJ, Maung AA, Lui FY, Davis KA (2014) The use of magnetic resonance imaging in the diagnosis of suspected appendicitis in pregnancy: shortened length of stay without increase in hospital charges. JAMA Surg 149(7):687–693
18. Pinto F, Pinto A, Russo A, Coppolino F, Bracale R, Fonio P et al (2013) Accuracy of ultrasonography in the diagnosis of acute appendicitis in adult patients: review of the literature. Crit Ultrasound J 5(Suppl 1):S2
19. Flum DR, Morris A, Koepsell T, Dellinger EP (2001) Has misdiagnosis of appendicitis decreased over time? A population-based analysis. JAMA 286(14):1748–1753
20. Mallin M, Craven P, Ockerse P, Steenblik J, Forbes B, Boehm K et al (2015) Diagnosis of appendicitis by bedside ultrasound in the ED. Am J Emerg Med 33(3):430–432
21. Gungor F, Kilic T, Akyol KC, Ayaz G, Cakir UC, Akcimen M et al (2017) Diagnostic value and effect of bedside ultrasound in acute appendicitis in the emergency department. Acad Emerg Med 24(5):578–586
22. Guidelines Ultrasound (2017) Emergency, point-of-care and clinical ultrasound guidelines in medicine. Ann Emerg Med 69(5):e27–e54
23. Ooms HW, Koumans RK, Ho You PJK, Puylaert JB (1991) Ultrasonography in the diagnosis of acute appendicitis. Br J Surg 78(3):315–318
24. van Randen A, Bipat S, Zwinderman AH, Ubbink DT, Stoker J, Boermeester MA (2008) Acute appendicitis: meta-analysis of diagnostic performance of CT and graded compression US related to prevalence of disease. Radiology 249(1):97–106
25. Valette PJ, Rioux M, Pilleul F, Saurin JC, Fouque P, Henry L (2001) Ultrasonography of chronic inflammatory bowel diseases. Eur Radiol 11(10):1859–1866

26. Puylaert JB (1986) Mesenteric adenitis and acute terminal ileitis: US evaluation using graded compression. Radiology 161(3):691–695
27. Lambert MJ, Villa M (2004) Gynecologic ultrasound in emergency medicine. Emerg Med Clin North Am 22(3):683–696
28. Stephens PL, Mazzucco JJ (1999) Comparison of ultrasound and the Alvarado score for the diagnosis of acute appendicitis. Conn Med 63(3):137–140
29. Kularatna M, Lauti M, Haran C, MacFater W, Sheikh L, Huang Y et al (2017) Clinical prediction rules for appendicitis in adults: which is best? World J Surg 41(7):1769–1781
30. Ohmann C, Yang Q, Franke C (1995) Diagnostic scores for acute appendicitis. Abdominal Pain Study Group. Eur J Surg 161(4):273–281
31. Meltzer AC, Baumann BM, Chen EH, Shofer FS, Mills AM (2013) Poor sensitivity of a modified Alvarado score in adults with suspected appendicitis. Ann Emerg Med 62(2):126–131
32. Puylaert JB, Rutgers PH, Lalisang RI, de Vries BC, van der Werf SD, Dörr JP et al (1987) A prospective study of ultrasonography in the diagnosis of appendicitis. N Engl J Med 317(11):666–669
33. Fox JC, Solley M, Anderson CL, Zlidenny A, Lahham S, Maasumi K (2008) Prospective evaluation of emergency physician performed bedside ultrasound to detect acute appendicitis. Eur J Emerg Med 15(2):80–85
34. Lam SHF, Grippo A, Kerwin C, Konicki PJ, Goodwine D, Lambert MJ (2014) Bedside ultrasonography as an adjunct to routine evaluation of acute appendicitis in the emergency department. West J Emerg Med 15(7):808–815
35. Elikashvili I, Tay ET, Tsung JW (2014) The effect of point-of-care ultrasonography on emergency department length of stay and computed tomography utilization in children with suspected appendicitis. Acad Emerg Med 21(2):163–170
36. Kocher KE, Meurer WJ, Fazel R, Scott PA, Krumholz HM, Nallamothu BK (2011) National trends in use of computed tomography in the emergency department. Ann Emerg Med 58(5):452–462.e3
37. Larson DB, Johnson LW, Schnell BM, Salisbury SR, Forman HP (2011) National trends in CT use in the emergency department: 1995–2007. Radiology 258(1):164–173
38. Poortman P, Oostvogel HJM, Bosma E, Lohle PNM, Cuesta MA, de Lange-de Klerk ESM et al (2009) Improving diagnosis of acute appendicitis: results of a diagnostic pathway with standard use of ultrasonography followed by selective use of CT. J Am Coll Surg 208(3):434–441
39. McCartan DP, Fleming FJ, Grace PA (2010) The management of right iliac fossa pain—is timing everything? Surgeon 8(4):211–217
40. Cavuşoğlu YH, Erdoğan D, Karaman A, Aslan MK, Karaman I, Tütün OC (2009) Do not rush into operating and just observe actively if you are not sure about the diagnosis of appendicitis. Pediatr Surg Int 25(3):277–282
41. Laméris W, van Randen A, van Es HW, van Heesewijk JPM, van Ramshorst B, Bouma WH et al (2009) Imaging strategies for detection of urgent conditions in patients with acute abdominal pain: diagnostic accuracy study. BMJ 338:b2431
42. Dahabreh IJ, Adam GP, Halladay CW, Steele DW, Daiello LA, Wieland LS, et al (2015) Diagnosis of right lower quadrant pain and suspected acute appendicitis [Internet]. Rockville (MD): Agency for Healthcare Research and Quality (US). (AHRQ Comparative Effectiveness Reviews). http://www.ncbi.nlm.nih.gov/books/NBK355441/. Accessed 5 June 2018

How POCUS picks up a rare mimickers of acute appendicitis in the emergency department

Shihab Al Sheikh*, Mariam Al Ali, Dhanya Sochel Kiran and Mohsen Al Tabatabai

Abstract

Background: Appendicitis is the most common surgical abdominal emergency. Punctual diagnosis and rapid operative treatment of acute appendicitis are critically important, as it reduces the risk of complications, associated with greater morbidity and cost of care. The clinical diagnosis of acute appendicitis can be difficult and confusing. Due to some typical presentation and mimic, several abdominal conditions are left undiagnosed. POCUS has comparatively acceptable sensitivity and high specificity for diagnosing acute appendicitis, and early practice POCUS has a standalone test to rule out acute appendicitis.

Case presentation: A 43-year-old man presented with a 3-day history of abdominal pain rated 5/10 in intensity which had localized to the right iliac fossa by the time he attended our emergency. He described the acute pain as sharp in nature, colicky without the presence of any radiation. The pain was associated with nausea, but there was no vomiting. On clinical examination, the patient was stable at first, had a normal temperature with tenderness and guarding the right iliac fossa under nearby normal laboratory investigation.

Conclusion: The importance of POCUS in scanning right iliac fossa for patients present with signs and symptoms that are mimicking acute appendicitis for diagnosing a rare pathology and avoiding the risk of ionizing radiation hazards and unnecessary surgical intervention.

Keywords: POCUS, Point of care ultrasound, Acute appendicitis mimicker, Computed tomography, Emergency department

Background

Appendicitis is the most common surgical abdominal emergency worldwide with more than 250,000 people diagnosed annually, and 7% of the population having the disease in their lifetimes [1]. A life table model suggests that the lifetime risk of appendicitis is 8.6% for males and 6.7% for females; the lifetime risk of appendectomy is 12.0% for males and 23.1% for females [2]. Punctual diagnosis and rapid operative treatment of acute appendicitis are critically important, as it helps in the reduction of the risk in case of certain complications, associated with greater morbidity and cost of care [3, 4]. The clinical diagnosis of acute appendicitis can be difficult and confusing due to an atypical presentation and mimic several abdominal conditions [5]. Patients with many other disorders have symptoms similar to those of appendicitis, such as acute gastrointestinal diseases like Crohn's disease, infectious enterocolitis, mesenteric adenitis, cecal diverticulitis, Meckel's diverticulitis, epiploic appendagitis, and omental infarcts can present with right lower quadrant. In addition, acute genitourinary diseases, like pyelonephritis and ureterolithiasis, also have similar symptoms. In a young woman, acute gynecological disease processes, such as ovarian torsion, hemorrhagic ovarian cyst, pelvic inflammatory disease, and ectopic

*Correspondence: shihab963@gmail.com
Emergency Department, Rashid Hospital Trauma Center, Dubai, United Arab Emirates

pregnancy, should also be considered within the differential diagnosis [6].

In 1981, Preusser published a first case report in an 87-year-old man, with typical symptoms and clinical signs of acute appendicitis where he was able to demonstrate the swollen and fluid-filled appendix by sonography that was confirmed at operation [7]. Pyualert et al. 5 years later described the 'graded compression technique' for the sonographic examination of the appendix with high-frequency transducer [8]. The POCUS for the diagnosis of appendicitis has reported sensitivities of 75% to 90%, specificities of 83% to 95%, positive LR of 4.5 to 5.8, negative LRs of 0.19 to 0.27, and positive predictive value of 90% [9].

Case presentation

A 43-year-old man presented with a 3-day history of abdominal pain rated 5/10 in intensity which occurred at the right iliac fossa by the time he attended our emergency. He described the acute pain, colicky, and there was no radiation. The pain was associated with nausea, but no vomiting occurred. He had no bowel or urinary symptoms and no previous abdominal problems. He had no significant past medical and family history.

On examination: vital signs were temperature: 36.8 °C, pulse: 80 per min, blood pressure: 116/78, SPo2: 99%. Abdominal examination findings revealed a soft abdomen with tenderness and guarding in the right iliac fossa. There was no rebound tenderness. Rovsing's, psoas and obturator signs were negative.

Investigation

Laboratory investigations revealed his peripheral white blood cell count to be 9.900/μL and the neutrophil level was 7.400/μL (3.9–11.0/μL). His serum C-reactive protein level was 0.6 mg/L (<0.5 mg/L), and serum creatinine was 1.2 mg/dL (0.7–1.2 mg/dL). Urine analysis has revealed that blood by strips 5+, RBC/HPF 10–15, WBC/HPF 0–s5 and epithelial cells are few in number.

According to the physical examination and lab tests, acute appendicitis was the most likely form of diagnosis. POCUS was done using a curvilinear probe and started in the right lower quadrant at the point of maximum tenderness. This was mainly carried out to explore the inflamed appendix, where we found a kidney-shaped mass at the right iliac fossa. An appendix could not be visualized in a clear manner. Thus, we scanned both flanks and found that the right kidney was absent, while the location of the left kidney was normal. This alarmed us of the ectopic right pelvic kidney (Fig. 1). On detailed evaluation, we identified the mass as a kidney with mild hydronephrosis (Fig. 2). After the pain was managed with adequate analgesics, we proceeded to do a CT with contrast. This revealed a normal left kidney and right ectopic kidney which had 2 small stones of size 3 mm and 6 mm at its renal pelvis and pelviureteric junction. It was also observed that the left kidney was affected by secondary mild hydronephrosis, where the appendix is normal (Fig. 3).

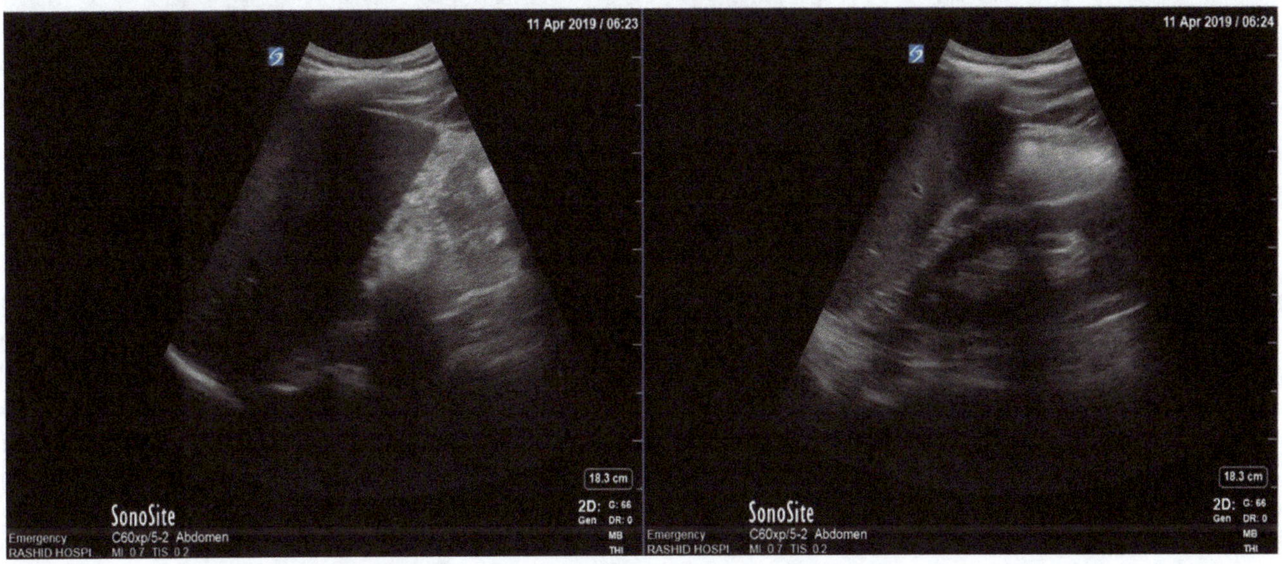

Fig. 1 Left side showing the absence of the right kidney where the left kidney in the normal position

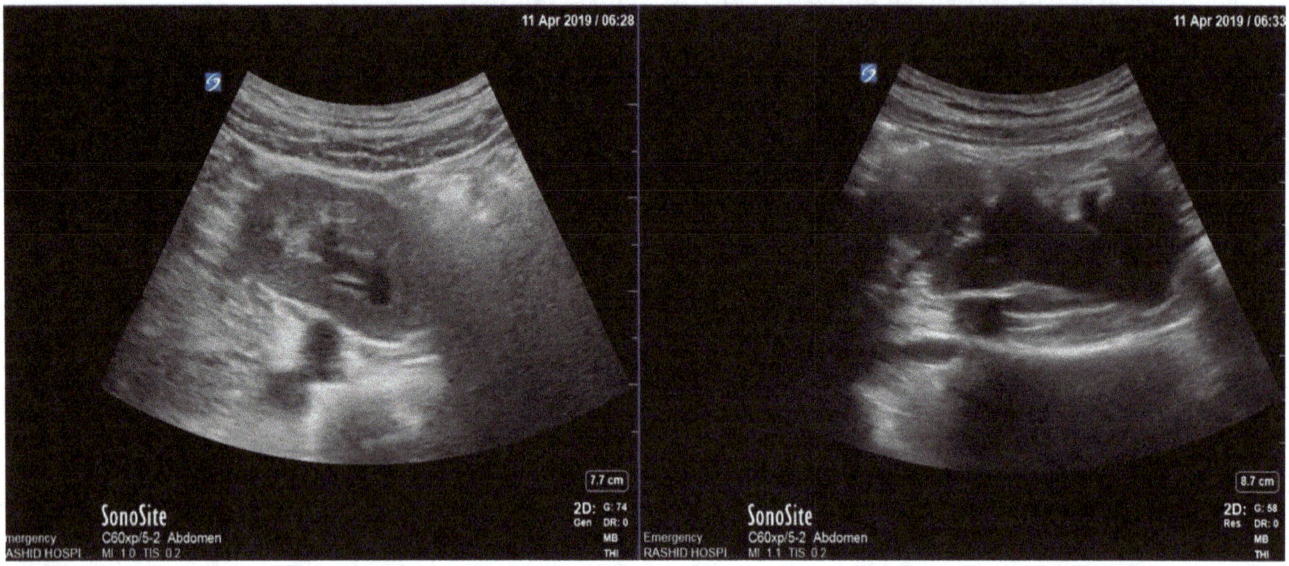

Fig. 2 Left side showing the transverse section through the right ectopic kidney and right side through the longitudinal section

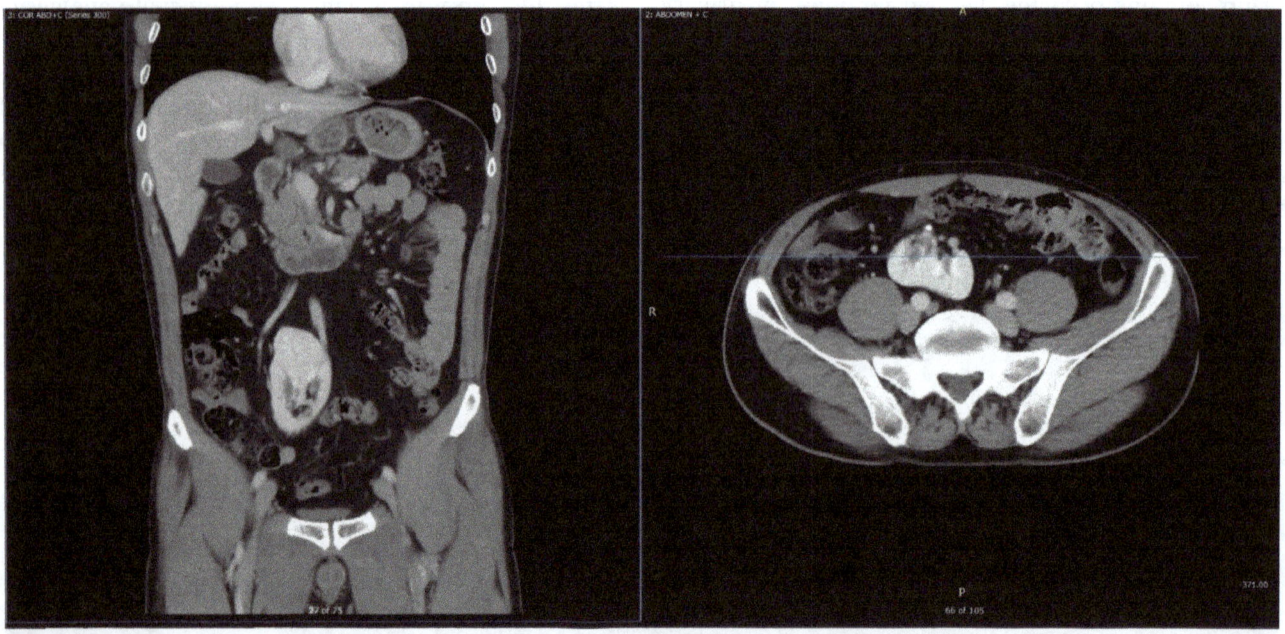

Fig. 3 CT abdomen, showing anterior malrotated ectopic right kidney with small stone at pelviureteric junction

Discussion

The first observation on the solitary ectopic pelvic kidney was made by Henot in 1830. It was made on an autopsy of 8 months of age whose sex was indefinite owing to the absence of the genitalia [10]. Necropsy records were derived from many sources which had indicated that ectopic kidney is found once in from 2150 to 3000 [11]. There are many factors that inhibit the kidney from gradual ascend to the abdomen and away from the midline. The factors can be in the form of ureteral bud maldevelopment, defective metanephric tissue, genetic abnormalities, maternal illness and teratogenic causes [12]. Clinically the renal ectopia is more readily recognized in females because they undergo uro-radiological evaluation more frequently than that of males. As a result of which, a higher rate of urinary tract infection gets associated with genital anomalies [13]. Ectopic kidneys are usually smaller than the normal size of kidneys. The renal pelvis is usually anterior to the parenchyma because it is incompletely rotated. It has been observed that the major portion of the ectopic kidneys is clinically asymptomatic. Ectopic kidneys are no more susceptible to disease than normal. Exceptions are there such as hydronephrosis development, renal stones formation, and urinary tract infections [14].

In our case, the unnecessary surgical operation was avoided by just 2 min. With the implementation of POCUS and diagnosis, it was confirmed that CT abdomen with IV contrast. Ultrasound can recognize the ectopic kidney by its overall similarity in shape, size and structure to normal kidneys. However, the pelvic kidneys might get developed with unusual shapes and degrees of rotation can form. Moreover, it may show some dilatation of the collecting system [15]. These unusual features may make an ectopic kidney difficult to recognize as a kidney, especially if an unexpected finding is observed which might present a mass during an examination. This can be highly confusing, as it can have similarities with appendicular mass, bowel tumors, and pelvic lymphadenopathy. Here the color Doppler is of great value as it demonstrates a normal vascular architecture that is compatible with renal vessels [16] (Fig. 4).

Both POCUS and abdominal helical computed tomography (CT) are essential tools in managing the patient who is affected with acute abdominal pain in the emergency department. Both are considered to have acceptable sensitivities, specificities, and positive and negative predictive values. It has been regarded that CT to be more superior in numerous studies [17]. Although with the advantage of the high sensitivity of abdominal CT, there are mainly three disadvantages of the abdominal CT. The first is exposing the patient to the risk of ionizing radiation, with an estimated 2% of future cancers being triggered just by CT scans [18]. The second disadvantage is that the CT abdomen is highly expensive and is not accessible in all medical providing institutions primarily in developing countries. Finally, prolonged emergency department stays when CT abdomen order with oral and/or rectal administration. It has also been inculcated that there is a risk of allergic reaction and nephrotoxicity from IV contrast administration. The advantages of the POCUS are lack of ionizing radiation, noninvasive, simple to handle, document the entire ultrasound finding, widely available, real-time imaging, portable and cheap. Furthermore, repetitive ultrasound examinations can be done easily simultaneously which leads to enhancing clinicians' ability to perform serial reassessments and assists in further management. POCUS is recognized to be useful in children and pregnant patients and is one of the principal modality for these patients based on the American College of Radiology guidelines [19]. The disadvantages are decrease sensitivity, lack of operator experience, patient factors like obesity. A few of the other disadvantages can be superimposed bowel gas or typically located appendix. There can also be greater pain during the application of the graded compression process. Poortman et al. [20] concluded that a diagnostic pathway includes the initial US and complimentary CT in patients with negative or inconclusive US. The results yield high diagnostic accuracy in the management of acute appendicitis without adverse events.

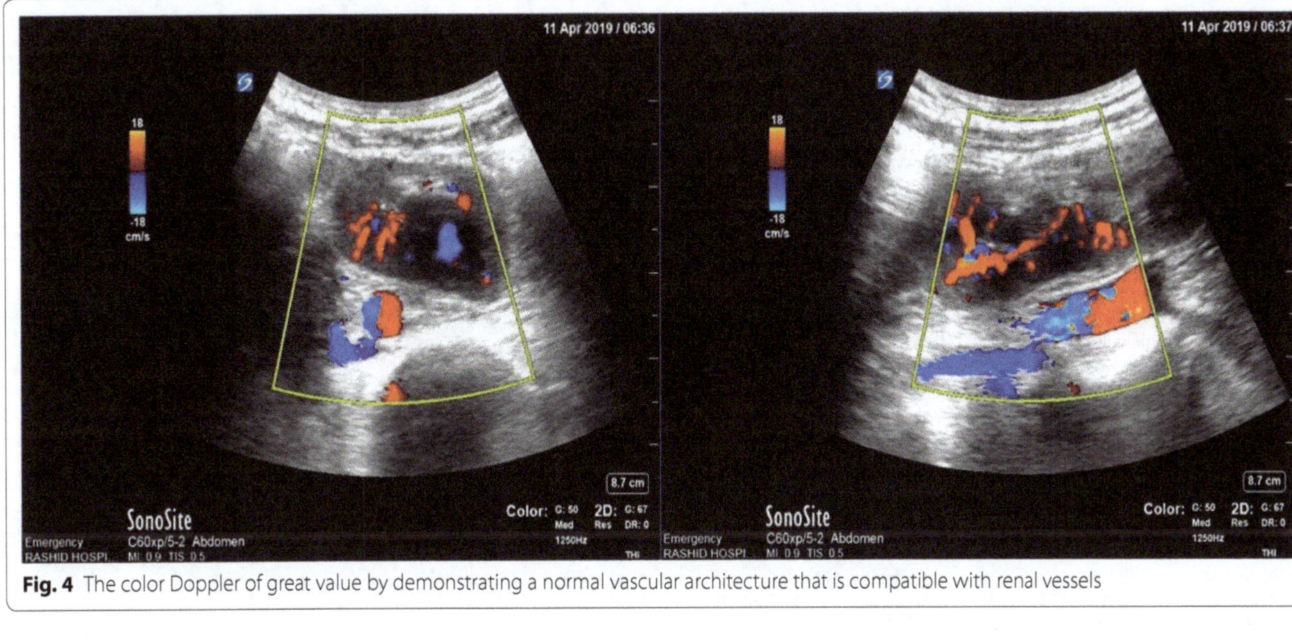

Fig. 4 The color Doppler of great value by demonstrating a normal vascular architecture that is compatible with renal vessels

Conclusion

This case report highlights the importance of POCUS for scanning the right iliac fossa for patients with suspicion of acute appendicitis before any hazardous ionizing radiation imaging or surgical intervention. Thus, it can be considered that the calculus of renal pain of an ectopic right pelvic kidney in the differential diagnosis falls under the list of right iliac fossa pain.

Abbreviations

POCUS: point-of-care ultrasound; CT: computed tomography; IV: intravenous.

Acknowledgements

This work has not been presented at any conference.

Authors' contributions

SAS and DSK observed the case, performed the ultrasound examinations, collected the data and drafted the manuscript. MAA and MAT contributed significantly to the drafting and editing of the manuscript, performed the literature review. All authors read and approved the final manuscript.

References

1. Mallin M, Craven P, Ockerse P, Steenblik J, Forbes B, Boehm K, Youngquist S (2015) Diagnosis of appendicitis by bedside ultrasound in the ED. Am J Emerg Med 33(3):430–432
2. Addiss DG, Shaffer N, Fowler B, Tauxe R (1990) The epidemiology of appendicitis and appendectomy in the United States. Am J Epidemiol 132(5):910–925
3. Flum D, Koepsell T (2002) The clinical and economic correlates of misdiagnosed appendicitis. Arch Surg 137(7):799–804
4. French A (2008) Diagnosing acute appendicitis in adults: accuracy of color Doppler sonography and MDCT compared with surgery and clinical follow-up. J Emerg Med 35(3):350–351
5. Karamanakos S, Sdralis E, Panagiotopoulos S, Kehagias I (2010) Laparoscopy in the emergency setting. Surg Laparosc Endosc Percutan Tech 20(2):119–124
6. Thompson J, Selvaraj D, Nicola R (2014) Mimickers of acute appendicitis. J Am Osteopath Coll Radiol 3(4):10–21
7. Perusser R (1981) Ultrasonic diagnosis of acute suppurative appendicitis: a case report. Wiener Klinische Wochenschrift 93(18):587–588
8. Puylaert J (1986) Acute appendicitis: US evaluation using graded compression. Radiology 158(2):355–360
9. Van Randen A, Laméris W, van Es H, Van Heesewijk H, Van Ramshorst B, ten Hove W, Bouma W, van Leeuwen M, Van Keulen E, Bossuyt P, Stoker J, Boermeester M (2011) A comparison of the accuracy of ultrasound and computed tomography in common diagnoses causing acute abdominal pain. Eur Radiol 21(7):1535–1545
10. Butler T (1951) Solitary ectopic pelvic kidney. With a report on a case associated with incomplete rotation of the gut. Br J Surg 38(152):522–525
11. Stevens A (1937) Pelvic single kidneys. J Urol 37(5):610–618
12. Rascher W, Rosch W (2005) Congenital abnormalities of the urinary tract, 1st edn. Oxford textbook of clinical nephrology. Oxford University Press, Oxford, pp 1402–1412
13. Campbell M, Wein A, Kavoussi L (2007) Campbell-Walsh urology. Saunders Elsevier, Philadelphia
14. Gleason P, Kelalis P, Husmann D, Kramer S (1994) Hydronephrosis in renal ectopia: incidence, etiology, and significance. J Urol 151(6):1660–1661
15. Sanders R (1984) Normal ultrasonic anatomy of the genitourinary system, ultrasound in urology, 2nd edn. Williams & Wilkins, Baltimore, p 76
16. Mascatello V, Lebowitz R (1976) Malposition of the colon in left renal agenesis and ectopia. Radiology 120(2):371–376
17. Reich B, Zalut T, Weiner S (2011) An international evaluation of ultrasound vs. computed tomography in the diagnosis of appendicitis. Int J Emerg Med 4(1):68
18. Brenner D, Hall E (2007) Computed tomography—an increasing source of radiation exposure. N Engl J Med 357(22):2277–2284
19. Albakri I, Al-Qahtani R, Alsharif M (2017) Ultrasound and computed tomography in abdominal and pelvic diagnoses. Egypt J Hosp Med 69(7):2777–2782
20. Poortman P, Oostvogel H, Bosma E, Lohle P, Cuesta M, de Lange-de Klerk E, Hamming J (2009) Improving diagnosis of acute appendicitis: results of a diagnostic pathway with standard use of ultrasonography followed by selective use of CT. J Am Coll Surg 208(3):434–441

4

Clinical measurements obtained from point-of-care ultrasound images to assess acquisition skills

Brian P. Lucas[1,2*], Antonietta D'Addio[2], Clay Block[1,2], Harold L. Manning[2,3], Brian Remillard[2,3] and James C. Leiter[2,3]

Abstract

Background: Current methods of assessing competence in acquiring point-of-care ultrasound images are inadequate. They rely upon cumbersome rating systems that do not depend on the actual outcome measured and lack evidence of validity. We describe a new method that uses a rigorous statistical model to assess performance of individual trainees based on the actual task, image acquisition. Measurements obtained from the images acquired (the actual desired outcome) are themselves used to validate effective training and competence acquiring ultrasound images. We enrolled a convenience sample of 21 spontaneously breathing adults from a general medicine ward. In random order, two trainees (A and B) and an instructor contemporaneously acquired point-of-care ultrasound images of the inferior vena cava and the right internal jugular vein from the same patients. Blinded diameter measurements from each ultrasound were analyzed quantitatively using a multilevel model. Consistent mean differences between each trainee's and the instructor's images were ascribed to systematic acquisition errors, indicative of poor measurement technique and a need for further training. Wider variances were attributed to sporadic errors, indicative of inconsistent application of measurement technique across patients. In addition, the instructor recorded qualitative observations of each trainee's performance during image acquisition.

Results: For all four diameters, the means and variances of measurements from trainee A's images differed significantly from the instructor's, whereas those from trainee B's images were comparable. Techniques directly observed by the instructor supported these model-derived findings. For example, mean anteroposterior diameters of the internal jugular vein obtained from trainee A's images were 3.8 mm (90% CI 2.3–5.4) smaller than from the instructor's; this model-derived finding matched the instructor's observation that trainee A compressed the vein during acquisition. Instructor summative assessments agreed with model-derived findings, providing internal validation of the descriptive and quantitative assessments of competence acquiring ultrasound images.

Conclusions: Clinical measurements obtained from point-of-care ultrasound images acquired contemporaneously by trainees and an instructor can be used to quantitatively assess the image acquisition competence of specific trainees. This method may obviate resource-intensive qualitative rating systems that are based on ultrasound image quality and direct observation, while also helping instructors guide remediation.

Keywords: Clinical competence, Point-of-care systems, Anthropometry, Ultrasonography, Multilevel analysis

*Correspondence: brian.p.lucas@dartmouth.edu
[2] Geisel School of Medicine at Dartmouth College, Hanover, NH, USA
Full list of author information is available at the end of the article

Background

Point-of-care ultrasound images should reflect patient anatomy and physiology at a given moment in time. Clinical measurements obtained from ultrasound images, however, are known to be highly operator-dependent [1]. The trueness of clinical measurements obtained from ultrasound images should, therefore, be a part of assessments of competence in acquiring them [2]. Reference standards of 'truth' are hard to come by, however [3]. Advanced imaging, such as computed tomography or magnetic resonance, is not practical for everyday assessments [4], especially since many point-of-care ultrasound targets are dynamic and require contemporaneous reference standards. Thus, after training programs in point-of-care ultrasound, assessments of trainee competence have not been based on clinical measurements but instead on perceived manual skills or image quality. One potential solution is to have instructors acquire ultrasound images on the same patients at the same time as the trainees under assessment. Clinical measurements obtained from these contemporaneously acquired ultrasound images of an instructor can then serve as reference standards.

Methods

We describe a method of assessing image acquisition competence for two central veins that are commonly used in bedside assessments of central venous pressure: the inferior vena cava and the right internal jugular vein. Central veins are ideal for studying image acquisition techniques because measurements obtained from ultrasound images of central veins are highly operator-dependent [5]. Our method of performance assessment is derived from statistical modeling of measurements obtained from ultrasound images that were contemporaneously acquired by an instructor and two trainees. We first use this quantitative statistical model to partition measurement errors of ultrasound acquisition for each specific trainee. We then validate these model-derived errors against the instructor's direct observations of each trainee's technique acquiring ultrasound images.

Setting and participants

We conducted this cross-sectional study at a 76-bed, rural, Veterans Affairs hospital during 2 months in 2015. A board-certified internal medicine physician with over 10 years of experience in point-of-care ultrasound [6] served as the instructor. The two trainees were clinical research coordinators who underwent a training program in point-of-care ultrasound. (Details about the training program can be found in Additional file 1: Table S1). The instructor identified a convenience sample of spontaneously breathing adult general medicine inpatients who could comfortably lie supine and had no abdominal or neck tenderness. Given that no identifying information was collected, our internal review board approved participation if patients gave verbal informed consent.

Ultrasound images

In randomized order and within minutes of each other, each trainee and the instructor acquired ultrasound images on each participant. A full description of the acquisition protocol is presented elsewhere [7]. Briefly, the M-Turbo™ ultrasound (Fujifilm Sonosite, Inc., Bothwell, Washington) was used to acquire 10-s 2-dimensional gray-scale (B-mode) video sequences. A 1–5 MHz phased-array transducer was used to acquire the longitudinal axis of the inferior vena cava from the subcostal window, and a 6–13 MHz linear transducer was used to acquire the transverse axis of the right internal jugular vein from the anterior cervical triangle. Each operator was free to adjust the ultrasound device to optimize the ultrasound image. The image acquisition by all three operators took no more than 10–15 min in any given participant.

All acquired ultrasound images were transferred to a desktop computer without identifying information to ensure that interpretations were not biased by whoever acquired the ultrasound images. The entire 10 s clip of each image was reviewed, and uninterpretable ultrasound images (Additional file 1: Figure S1) were discarded through consensus opinion in group review. All remaining images were randomly arranged and independently interpreted by each trainee and the instructor three times to both limit the influence of outlying measurements and increase the stability of our statistical models. Each vein type was, therefore, measured nine times. The inferior vena cava diameter was measured 3–4 cm from the junction of the right atrium at maximum and minimum excursions, corresponding to end-expiration and end-inspiration, respectively [8]. The mediolateral diameter of the right internal jugular vein was measured when its area was largest, corresponding to end-expiration; from the same still frame, the anteroposterior diameter was measured perpendicular to the midway point of the mediolateral diameter. All diameters were measured from inner edge to inner edge of each vessel.

Model-derived acquisition-level measurement errors

We constructed a theoretical measurement model from principles of error analysis [9] and generalizability theory [10] with several standard assumptions (Fig. 1). First, we assumed that measurements reflected not only each patient's true vein diameters, but also how the ultrasound images were acquired [11]. Second, we ascribed differences between ultrasound images that were acquired on the same patients to acquisition technique rather

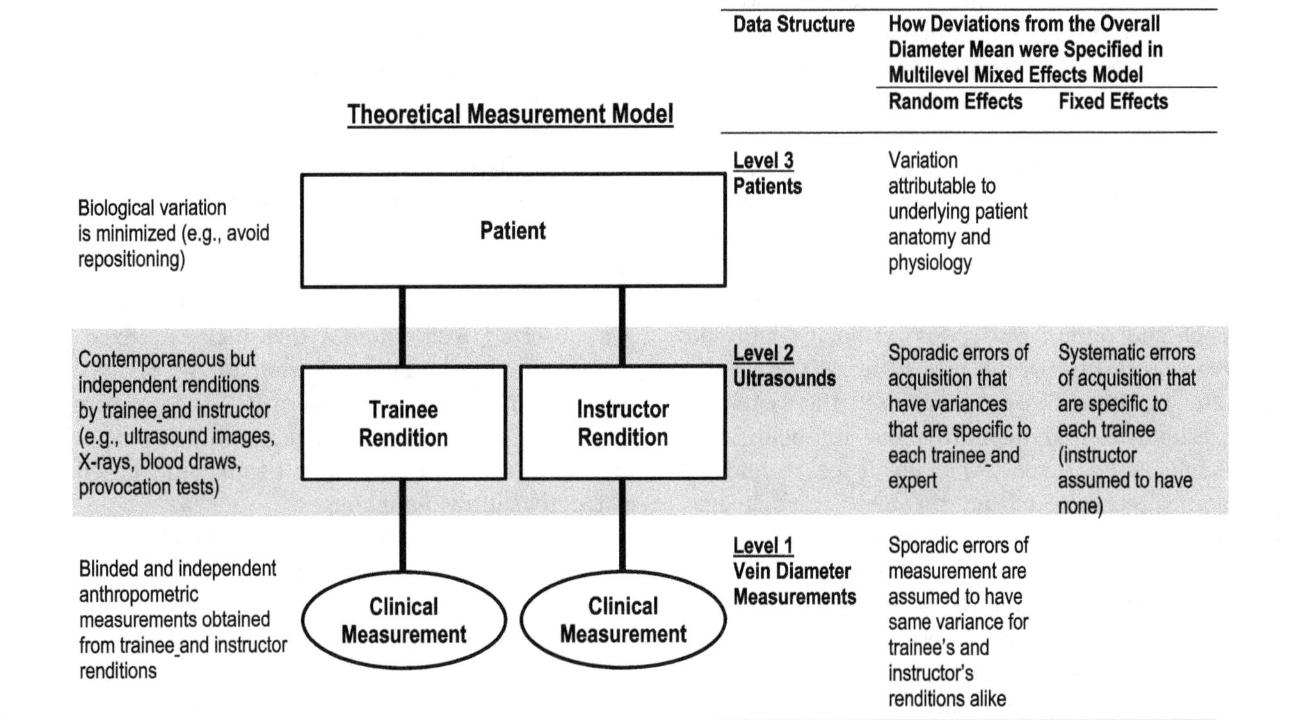

Fig. 1 Theoretical measurement model and corresponding specification of multilevel statistical models. *Rectangles* represent groupings (or 'clusters'), the *ovals* represent vein diameter measurements (the most granular unit of analysis), and *connecting lines* represent nested relationships. In the mixed-effect models, groupings were defined by both random effects and, at level 2 only, fixed effects. There were two fixed effects at level 2, one for each trainee that represented the adjusted differences between diameter means obtained from instructor-acquired ultrasound images. Because instructor-acquired ultrasound images served as the reference standard, the models assume that the instructor made no systematic errors of acquisition. (See text for additional assumptions made for this model.)

than substantive biological changes; biological variability within each patient was an improbable source of variation because ultrasound images were acquired contemporaneously and in random order without patient repositioning and while each patient's volume status was stable [12]. Third, we regarded the instructor's ultrasound images as the truest representation of each patient's vein diameters for that moment in time [13]. Fourth, we assumed that the type of difference between trainee- and instructor-acquired ultrasound images (fixed or random) reflected the type of errors being committed by trainees during acquisition: fixed differences reflected systematic errors and random differences reflected sporadic errors [14]. Fifth, we assumed that the techniques used to obtain measurements from images were unaffected by whoever acquired the images, because the person making those measurements was blind to information about who acquired them. Last, we considered diameter measurements on the same ultrasound to be independent of each other because the instructor and trainees worked alone, each obtaining repeated measurements on different days to limit recall of earlier measurements [15]. From this model we devised corresponding statistical models for each of the four vein diameter types. Parameters from the statistical models reflected errors attributable to trainee A's and trainee B's images. The primary advantage of this approach is in both quantifying and classifying specific errors of ultrasound acquisition that can then be used to guide the type of remediation best suited to each trainee.

Under an assumption that acquisition technique contributed to measurement error [12], we focused on two comparisons that represented two types of trainee acquisition errors: differences in diameter means reflected one or more systematic errors and differences in the variances of those means reflected one or more sporadic errors. To gauge the magnitude of each trainee's model-derived acquisition errors, we used thresholds based on the theory of measurement error that have been used for many other types of clinical measurements [9, 16]. We defined each trainee's *systematic* errors to be acceptable if the magnitude of these errors was less than half a standard deviation of the mean diameter measurements obtained from the instructor's ultrasound images. Since diameter measurements follow a normal distribution [17], systematic errors of this relative magnitude will misclassify 1 out of 15 vein diameters whenever a reference range is defined as 2 standard deviations above and below a mean [16]. We defined each trainee's *sporadic* errors to be acceptable when the variance of these errors was less than a quarter of the variance of diameter measurements obtained from the instructor's ultrasound images across all patients. (This heuristic is based on the simplification that roughly half of the overall variance in measurements is due to variance of measurements within patients.) Sporadic errors with this relative dispersion will add no more than 40% to the overall variability of diameter measurements [16].

We used these thresholds to construct zones of equivalence and noninferiority for systematic and sporadic errors, respectively. Because systematic errors are meaningful in either direction, we used the systematic error thresholds as margins both above and below zero, thereby delineating a zone of equivalence around the adjusted mean obtained from the instructor's images. For sporadic errors, because variance is inherently 'one-sided' (as it is a squared quantity), we used sporadic error thresholds as single margins above zero, delineating the upper bound of zones of noninferiority. We considered model-derived errors to be significant if 90% confidence intervals (CIs) around the point estimates, using two-sided CIs for systematic errors and one-sided CIs for sporadic errors, fell outside zones of equivalence and noninferiority, respectively.

Instructor-observed acquisition deficiencies

Before the model-derived sources of acquisition errors became available, the instructor observed each trainee's acquisition technique (Additional file 1: Table S1). The instructor categorized potential deficiencies of each trainee into three domains: placing the ultrasound transducer, confirming visualization, and optimizing ultrasound quality. To avoid influencing each other, the trainees neither observed each other nor the instructor during acquisition of the ultrasound images; nor did they discuss acquisition techniques while awaiting their respective turns to acquire images outside each patient's room.

Statistical analysis

Our participant sample size was based on the statistical consideration that at least 12 patients would be needed for unbiased variance estimations [18]; we enrolled more than 12 patients to ensure that we acquired enough evaluable images over a 12-h timeframe. For each diameter measurement, we constructed a separate mixed-effects multilevel model.

The experimental design led to a hierarchical data structure in which the vein diameter measurements themselves where one level nested within the ultrasound image which were in turn nested within the patients (Fig. 1). Patient- and measurement-level random effects were weighted averages (so-called random intercepts), but ultrasound-level random effects were specific to the instructor and the trainee (random coefficients), allowing the magnitude of sporadic errors of acquisition (the variances of ultrasound image random effects) to be compared between the instructor and each trainee. We represented each trainee's systematic errors of acquisition using fixed effects to allow us to focus specifically on the acquisition performance of the each of the trainees [19]. Intraclass correlation coefficients (ICCs) were derived from models that included fixed effects representing each trainee's systematic errors of acquisition; this inclusion makes these ICCs so-called 'consistency ICCs' [20] because they represent the proportion of total variance that is attributable to patients based on the instructor's ultrasound images.

For model estimation in our multilevel mixed-effects model, we used a Bayesian estimator because maximum likelihood estimators often fail to converge in three-level models of moderate size. We used the runmlwin [21] command within Stata, version 15.1 (StataCorp, College Station, TX) to run Markov chain Monte Carlo procedures in MLwiN software, version 3.01 (Centre for Multilevel Modeling, Bristol, UK). We used noninformative (or diffuse) priors. Such priors allow the data to drive the results, which will be numerically equivalent to those based on maximum likelihood [22]. Thus, we refer to central ranges of our posterior distributions as 'confidence intervals,' even though they are technically Bayesian 'credibility intervals.' We report posterior medians rather than means or modes, because medians are less biased for variance components [18].

Results

Among 21 participants, the instructor and trainees acquired a total of 39 interpretable inferior vena cava ultrasound images from 16 participants (mean 2.4 examinations per participant, interquartile range [IQR] 2–3) and 48 interpretable internal jugular vein ultrasound images from 18 participants (mean 2.7 examinations per participant, IQR 2–3; Additional file 1: Figure S1). Because the instructor and each trainee obtained diameter measurements from each ultrasound three times, the dataset consisted of 351 inferior vena cava and 432 internal jugular vein ultrasound diameter measurements. The mean inferior vena cava right internal jugular vein diameters (footnote to Fig. 2) suggest that patients had intermediate central venous pressures on average [23, 24]. Nevertheless, the ICCs indicate that 63–88% of variation among vein diameters was attributable to differences between patients (footnote to Fig. 3).

None of the four diameter means obtained from images acquired by trainee A were equivalent to the instructor's,

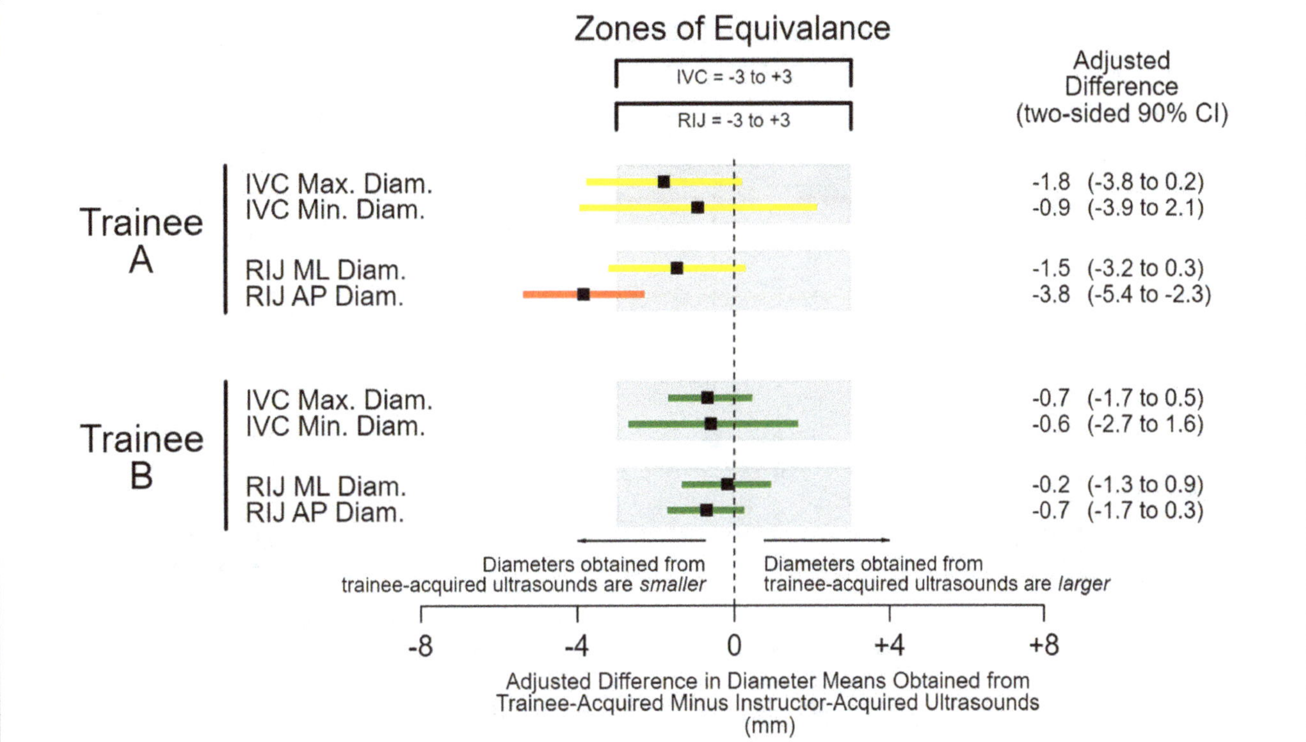

Fig. 2 Trainees' model-derived acquisition-level systematic errors. Shaded areas represent zones of equivalence, which are bounded in each direction by half a standard deviation of mean diameter measurements obtained from the instructor's ultrasound images (see text for rationale). Color-coded error bars indicate two-sided 90% confidence intervals (CI) that are red if CIs and the point estimates of the mean values are outside equivalence zones; yellow if CIs are outside but point estimates are within the zones; and green if CIs are entirely within the zones. The vertical dashed line represents the adjusted means of diameters obtained from the instructor's ultrasound images: IVC maximum 16.2 mm (95% CI 13.3–19.1 mm); IVC minimum 10.3 mm (95% CI 6.7–13.9 mm); RIJ mediolateral 14.4 mm (95% CI 11.7–17.0 mm); and RIJ anteroposterior 11.6 mm (95% CI 9.8–13.5 mm). *IVC* inferior vena cava, *RIJ* right internal jugular, *max.* maximum, *min.* minimum, *ML* mediolateral, *AP* anteroposterior, *diam.* diameter

including the mean of the right internal jugular anteroposterior diameter (−3.8 mm), which fell below the lower equivalence margin of −3 mm (Fig. 2). In contrast, all four diameter means obtained from trainee B's images were equivalent to the instructor's. A similar pattern was seen with variances. The confidence intervals for all four variances of diameter means obtained from trainee A's images fell outside the noninferiority zones, making them meaningfully larger than the instructor's; in fact, even the point estimates fell outside the noninferiority zone for inferior vena cava diameters, (Fig. 3). In contrast, all four variances of diameter means from Trainee B's images were noninferior to the instructor's.

Likely proximate effects of the deficiencies of trainees' acquisition techniques on the measured diameters are listed in Table 1. These qualitative, instructor-observed deficiencies were mapped to the quantitative, model-derived acquisition-level measurement errors. For example, under the assumption that faulty techniques impact ultrasound depictions of vein dimensions, which in turn affect the eventual measurements obtained from those ultrasound images, the deficiencies of trainee A's techniques likely caused the depiction in the ultrasound images of the anteroposterior diameters of the right internal jugular vein to be smaller than they truly were.

Discussion

We conducted a performance evaluation of ultrasound image acquisition in which the assessment of competence was (a) based on actual performance of the skill being taught, ultrasound image acquisition, and (b) based on clinically meaningful measurements that are derived from the images acquired. Such a direct performance assessment has an advantage over indirect assessment, including direct observations of technique, because the actual results obtained from the activity for which the trainee is being trained are evaluated [2].

Ultrasound measurements of central veins vary greatly between patients. It is worth noting that this variability was incorporated into our statistical model by accounting for the 'clustering' of ultrasound images within each patient. This accounting makes the assessment of the acquisition skills of the individual trainees or instructor immune to the large variability of central venous

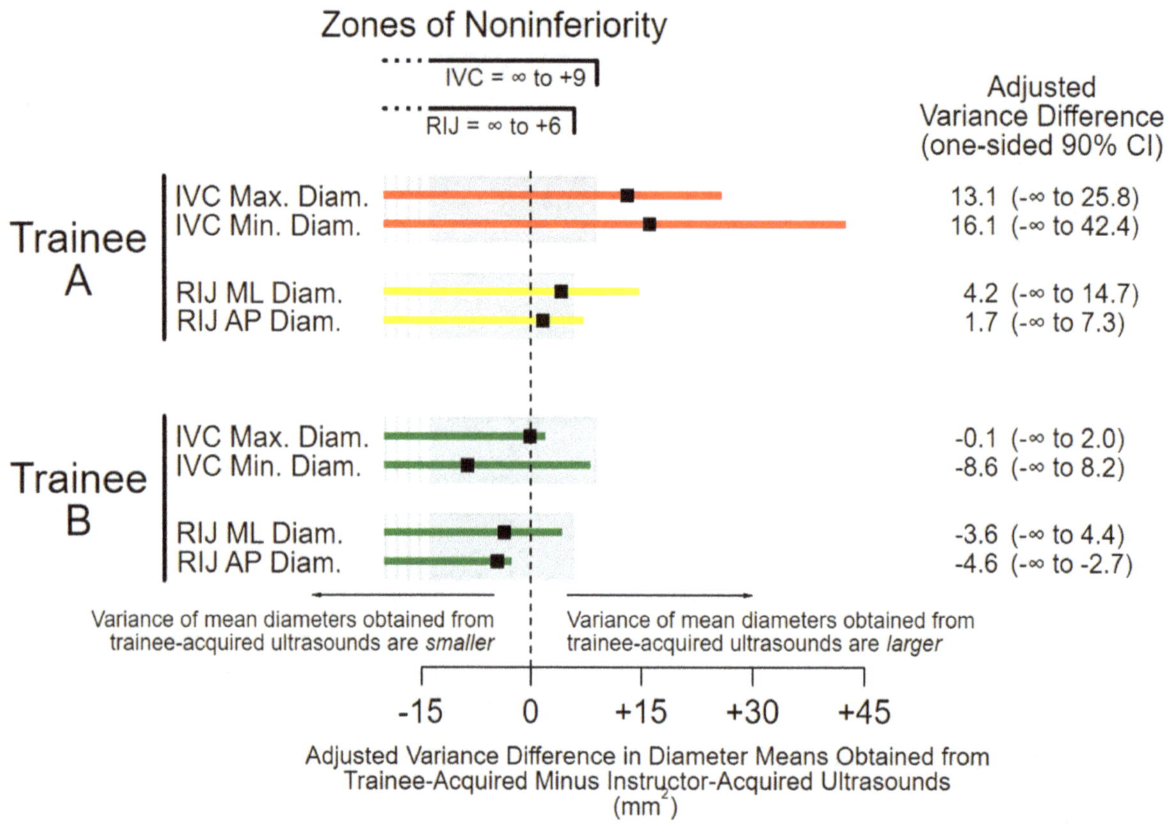

Fig. 3 Trainees' model-derived acquisition-level sporadic errors. Shaded areas represent noninferiority zones, which are bounded only in the direction of larger trainee variance by a quarter of the variance of diameter measurements obtained from the instructor's ultrasound images (see text for rationale). Color-coded error bars indicate one-sided 90% confidence intervals (CIs) that are red if CIs and the point estimates of variance values are outside noninferiority zones; yellow if CIs are outside but point estimates are within the zones; and green if CIs are entirely within the zones. The vertical dashed line represents the variance in diameter means obtained from instructor-acquired ultrasound images. With the instructor obtaining ultrasound images, intraclass correlation coefficients (the fractions of total variance attributable to patients) for IVC and RIJ veins were 0.88 (95% CI 0.65–0.95) and 0.69 (0.35–0.93) for max. and min. diameters; and 0.83 (0.59–0.99) and 0.63 (0.38–0.83) for ML and AP diameters, respectively. *IVC* inferior vena cava, *RIJ* right internal jugular, *max.* maximum, *min.* minimum, *ML* mediolateral, *AP* anteroposterior, *diam.* diameter

measurements between patients. Moreover, our model-based approach partitioned trainee acquisition errors into systematic errors (consistent deficiencies of performance) and sporadic errors (inconsistent performance techniques from variable technique). Remediation of these two types of errors requires different approaches, and the output of the statistical model can be used, therefore, to focus further training on each trainee's deficiency (if any).

Thus, we found that clinical measurements obtained from point-of-care ultrasound images reflect image acquisition competence. Specifically, comparisons of four central vein diameters obtained from images acquired contemporaneously by two trainees and an instructor led to quantitative characterizations of each trainee's skills (Figs. 2 and 3) that were supported by qualitative assessments based on direct observations (Table 1). Acquisition deficiencies observed while trainee A was acquiring images, for example, mapped to both large systematic and large sporadic model-derived measurement errors. Because we were able to quantify the magnitude of trainee A's acquisition-level measurement errors in the metric used for diameter measurements (mm), and because those measurements follow a normal distribution [17], we can directly estimate how often images obtained by trainee A may be misleading if the underlying deficiencies are not remediated [9]. For example, maximum diameters obtained from trainee A's inferior vena cava images were systematically smaller than those obtained from the instructor's images by 1.8 mm (Fig. 2). This means that, in a typical population of spontaneously breathing patients with a mean inferior vena cava maximum diameter of 22 mm and standard deviation of 6 mm [25], 10% of images acquired by trainee A would underestimate central venous pressure. Trainee A would, therefore, misclassify 1 out of 10 patients with truly large inferior vena cava maximum diameters (greater than 20 mm) [23] as having normal-sized diameters (less than

Table 1 Mapping of instructor-observed technique deficiencies to model-derived acquisition-level errors

Instructor-observed acquisition technique deficiencies (trainee)[a]	Likely impact on vein dimensions depicted in ultrasound images (diameter types affected)	Model-derived acquisition-level error
Placing transducer		
Off-axis (A)	Smaller due to oblique plane (max, min)	Systematic
Full exhalation not recorded (A)	Not fully enlarged (all)	Systematic
Too much pressure (A)	Compressed (AP)	Systematic
Liver not included for acoustic enhancement (A, B)	Lumen edges indistinct (max, min)	Sporadic
Acoustic 'rib shadows' at target (A)	Lumen edges indistinct (max, min)	Sporadic
Not perpendicular to skin of the neck (A)	Lateral lumen edge indistinct (ML)	Sporadic
Not 'anchored' during patient movement (A)	Measurement target moving (all)	Sporadic
Confirming visualization		
Incomplete recovery after confirmatory compression (A)	Compressed (AP)	Systematic
Orientation landmarks not included (A, B)	Measurement target unknown (max, min)	Sporadic
Optimizing quality		
Far-field gain too high (A)	Smaller due to far wall artifacts (max, min, AP)	Systematic
Overall gain too high (A, B)	Lumen edges indistinct (all)	Sporadic
Target not centered on screen (B)	Lumen edges indistinct (all)	Sporadic

Max maximum diameter of inferior vena cava, *min* minimum maximum diameter of inferior vena cava, *AP* anteroposterior diameter of right internal jugular vein, *ML* mediolateral diameter of right internal jugular vein

[a] Instructor-observed errors related to positioning patients were not included because the instructor and trainees did not reposition patients between acquisitions

or equal to 20 mm). Such misclassifications during management of shock, for example, may lead to inappropriate prescriptions of further volume resuscitation for patients who already have high central venous pressures, possibly worsening their outcomes [26].

Current assessment methods for point-of-care ultrasound acquisition cannot directly quantify the clinical consequences of flawed techniques, because they do not use the actual clinical measurements obtained from the ultrasound images. Instead they use various subjective ratings of acquisition technique [27] and of ultrasound image quality [28]. These subjective ratings have little intrinsic value [2], serving as surrogates for the clinical measurements that ultimately matter most [29]. Summative assessments based on these methods, therefore, will remain subject to claims of arbitrariness, especially without sufficient evidence that such assessments are valid and well correlated with the clinical measurements [30]. We are aware of no subjective rating systems for acquisition of point-of-care ultrasound images that have been compared against contemporaneously acquired reference standards. This gap in validity of subjective assessments is particularly relevant to point-of-care ultrasound because images can appear to be high quality while still misrepresenting the actual in situ anthropometric dimensions. This often occurs, for example, when ultrasound images of cylindrical veins are acquired 'off-axis,' generating an oblique view of the vessel that falsely narrows the diameter [5]. In such cases the image may still appear high quality (easily detected edges and good image clarity), belying the flawed acquisition technique and the inaccuracy of the diameter measurement.

Subjective rating systems are also resource-intensive [31]. Raters must be trained and iteratively evaluated for inconsistencies [32]. Although we have not carried out a formal cost comparison, we expect that our method would be less expensive. Instructors simply acquire ultrasound images alongside candidate operators in a dozen participating patients (the sample size that we used in the current study). The only stipulations are that the acquisitions be contemporaneous and independent of each other, which means that (as in our study) ultrasound images be acquired in random order and out of view [12]. Point-of-care ultrasound programs can then focus resources on developing each operator's skills rather than building an infrastructures of trained raters to perform subjective assessments. Moreover, a similar quantitative assessment of image acquisition skill among instructors could be used to ensure competence and consistency among instructors.

Our study has several limitations. First, we neither collected patient characteristics (such as body habitus) nor incorporated these into our analysis; this potentially limits the generalizability of our findings [33]. Second, we assumed that the instructor's ultrasound images served as an adequate reference standard, but we did not confirm the accuracy of the measurements obtained from these images [34]. If an instructor and a trainee had a similar deficiency, it would go unnoticed. Third, we assumed that measurements obtained from ultrasound images were independent of who acquired them, because we did not incorporate the interaction term of image-by-interpreter in our multilevel models. However, because we removed all identifying information from the images when they were presented for interpretation in random order, measurement errors introduced by interpretations likely shared a common variance [35]. Fourth, as part of our training program we removed images that were not interpretable in group review (see Additional file 1: Table S1 and Figure S1). Future versions of our method could require trainees to do this independently. Last, we only studied one instructor and two trainees across 21 patients. However, we were not interested in generalizing the performance 'beyond the sample' to *other* trainees. The method that we developed is specifically focused on the competence of particular trainees—in our case, trainee A and trainee B—and their systematic and sporadic errors of image acquisition, which can then be remediated; we are not concerned with the population characteristics of all possible trainees. For this reason, we explicitly quantified trainee A's and trainee B's systematic and sporadic errors of acquisition by modeling them as 'fixed effects' and trainee-specific 'random coefficients', respectively [36]. On the other hand, we assumed that our patients were randomly selected from a wider population. Our small sample of patients is realistic, because real-world assessments will always be limited by time and cost constraints. Nonetheless, this small sample led to adequate statistical precision, as our a priori determination predicted.

Future work should aim to address these limitations by expanding our analysis to other representative samples of patients, trainees, and instructors. Strong support for our method would be a demonstration that intentional acquisition deficiencies cause specific model-derived acquisition-level measurement errors. This would then narrow remediation to possible deficiencies that have a causal link to those acquisition-level measurement errors. For example, we observed that measurements from trainee A's right internal jugular vein were consistently smaller than the instructor's, suggesting that trainee A was applying too much pressure with the ultrasound transducer (Table 1).

Many clinical decisions rely on clinical measurements, and first steps to improving these decisions require that measurement errors be identified [37]. We believe the quantitative, model-based method of assessment is widely applicable to any operator-dependent skill for which training is required. Like measurements derived from point-of-care ultrasound, many other clinical measurements are susceptible to errors from two distinct sources: the manual technique of acquiring a momentary rendition of a patient at some fixed time, and a cognitive technique that is later applied to interpret those renditions (Fig. 1). Wide-ranging examples include X-rays to measure joint angles, skin scrapings to identify infectious fungi, pressure tracings to estimate attributes of cardiac function, and electrocardiographic stress testing to identify the risk of coronary artery disease. Even routine blood tests are affected not only by the phlebotomists (how long was the tourniquet left in place before blood was drawn?), but also by the laboratory technicians (how long did blood samples sit idle before analysis?) [9]. Each facet of a clinical measurement has the potential to introduce measurement error.

Conclusions

Our method isolated the errors of the manual technique of acquisition in central vein point-of-care ultrasound. It may also be applied not only to other ultrasound applications beyond central veins but also more widely to assessments of any highly operator-dependent clinical measurements. The primary benefit of using clinical measurements, themselves, in the performance evaluation is that the assessment depends on the relevant performance of the operators, and the contribution of each operator to overall measurement error can be readily partitioned and remediated if deemed substantive.

Additional file

Additional file 1: Table S1. Components of training and how they contributed to competency assessment. **Figure S1.** Flow diagram of inferior vena cava and right internal jugular ultrasounds.

Abbreviations

CI: confidence interval; IVC: inferior vena cava; RIJ: right internal jugular; max.: maximum; min.: minimum; ML: mediolateral; AP: anteroposterior; diam.: diameter.

Authors' contributions

Concept or design BPL, CB, HLM, BR, JCL. Acquisition, analysis or interpretation of data BPL, AD, JCL. Drafted the article or revised it critically BPL, AD, CB, HLM, BR, JCL. Approved the version to be published BPL, AD, CB, HLM, BR, JCL. All authors read and approved the final manuscript.

Author details

[1] Medicine Service, White River Junction VA Medical Center, White River Junction, VT, USA. [2] Geisel School of Medicine at Dartmouth College, Hanover, NH, USA. [3] Department of Medicine, Dartmouth-Hitchcock Medical Center, Lebanon, NH, USA.

Acknowledgements

Not applicable.

References

1. Liebo MJ, Israel RL, Lillie EO, Smith MR, Rubenson DS, Topol EJ (2011) Is pocket mobile echocardiography the next-generation stethoscope? A cross-sectional comparison of rapidly acquired images with standard transthoracic echocardiography. Ann Intern Med 155:33–38
2. Kane MT (1994) Validating interpretive arguments for licensure and certification arguments. Eval Health Prof 17:133–159
3. Barnhart HX, Haber MJ, Lin LI (2007) An overview on assessing agreement with continuous measurements. J Biopharm Stat 17:529–569
4. Tartière D, Seguin P, Juhel C, Laviolle B, Mallédant Y (2009) Estimation of the diameter and cross-sectional area of the internal jugular veins in adult patients. Crit Care 13:R197
5. Tchernodrinski S, Artfield R (2015) Inferior vena cava. In: Soni NJ, Arntfield R, Kory P (eds) Point of care ultrasound. Elsevier Saunders, Philadelphia
6. Lucas BP, Candotti C, Margeta B, Evans AT, Mba B, Baru J, Asbury JK, Asmar A, Kumapley R, Patel M, Borkowsky S, Fung S, Charles-Damte M (2009) Diagnostic accuracy of hospitalist-performed hand-carried ultrasound echocardiography after a brief training program. J Hosp Med 4:340–349
7. Lucas BP, D'Addio A, Clark J, Block C, Manning H, Remillard B, Leiter JC - (2017) Reproducibility of point-of-care ultrasonography for central vein diameter measurement: separating image acquisition from interpretation. J Clin Ultrasound 45:488–496
8. Grant E, Rendano F, Sevinc E, Gammelgaard J, Holm HH, Grønvall S (1980) Normal inferior vena cava: caliber changes observed by dynamic ultrasound. AJR Am J Roentgenol 135:335–338
9. Fraser CG (2001) Biological variation: from principles to practice. AACC Press, Washington, DC
10. Molenberghs G, Laenen A, Vangeneugden T (2007) Estimating reliability and generalizability from hierarchical biomedical data. J Biopharm Stat 17:595–627
11. Hopkins WG (2000) Measures of reliability in sports medicine and science. Sports Med 30:1–15
12. Bartlett JW, Frost C (2008) Reliability, repeatability and reproducibility: analysis of measurement errors in continuous variables. Ultrasound Obstet Gynecol 31:466–475
13. Dunn G (1992) Design and analysis of reliability studies. Stat Method Med Res 1:123–157
14. Taylor JR (1997) An introduction to error analysis: the study of uncertainties in physical measurements, 2nd edn. University Science Books, Sausalito
15. Allen MJ, Yen WM (1979) Introduction to measurement theory. Waveland Press, Long Grove
16. Fraser CG, Petersen PH, Libeer JC, Ricos C (1997) Proposals for setting generally applicable quality goals solely based on biology. Ann Clin Biochem 34:8–12
17. Lyon M, Blaivas M, Brannam L (2005) Sonographic measurement of the inferior vena cava as a marker of blood loos. Am J Emerg Med 23:45–50
18. Browne WJ, Draper D (2006) A comparison of Bayesian and likelihood-based methods for fitting multilevel models. Bayesian Anal 1:473–514
19. Guldbrand Nielsen D, Jensen SL, O'Neill L (2015) Clinical assessment of transthoracic echocardiography skills: a generalizability study. BMC Med Educ 15:9
20. McGraw KO, Wong SP (1996) Forming inferences about some intraclass correlation coefficients. Psychol Methods 1:30–46
21. Leckie G, Charlton C (2013) runmlwin—A program to run the MLwiN multilevel modelling software from within Stata. J Stat Softw 52:1–40
22. Jang MJ, Lee Y, Lawson AB, Browne WJ (2007) A comparison of the hierarchical likelihood and Bayesian approaches to spatial epidemiological modelling. Environmetrics 18:809–821
23. Rudski LG, Lai WW, Afilalo J, Hua L, Handschumacher MD, Chandrasekaran K, Solomon SD, Louie EK, Schiller NB (2010) Guidelines for the echocardiographic assessment of the right heart in adults: a report from the American Society of Echocardiography. J Am Soc Echocardiogr 23:685–713
24. Keller AS, Melamed R, Malinchoc M, Reverly J, Tierney DM, Gajic O (2009) Diagnostic accuracy of simple ultrasound measurement to estimate central venous pressure in spontaneously breathing, critically ill patients. J Hosp Med 4:350–355
25. Tchernodrinski S, Lucas BP, Athavale A, Candotti C, Margeta B, Katz A, Kumapley R (2015) Inferior vena cava diameter change after intravenous furosemide in patients diagnosed with acute decompensated heart failure. J Clin Ultrasound 43:187–193
26. Malbrain ML, Marik PE, Witters I, Cordemans C, Kirkpatrick AW, Roberts DJ, Van Regenmortel N (2014) Fluid overload, de-resuscitation, and outcomes in critically ill or injured patients: a systematic review with suggestions for clinical practice. Anaesthesiol Intensive Ther 46:361–380
27. Bremer ML (2016) Relationship of sonographer credentialing to intersocietal accreditation commission echocardiography case study image quality. J Am Soc Echocardiogr 29:43–48
28. Bahner DP, Adkins EJ, Nagel R, Way D, Werman HA, Royall NA (2011) Brightness mode quality ultrasound imaging examination technique. J Ultrasound Med 30:1649–1655
29. Wass V, Van der Vleuten C, Shatzer J, Jones R (2001) Assessment of clinical competence. Lancet 357:945–949
30. Downing SM (2003) Validity: on the meaningful interpretation of assessment data. Med Educ 37:830–837
31. Lewiss RE, Pearl M, Nomura JT, Baty G, Bengiamin R, Duprey K, Stone M, Theodoro D, Akhtar S (2013) CORD-AEUS: consensus document for the emergency ultrasound milestone project. Acad Emerg Med 20:740–745
32. Gibbs V (2014) A proposed new clinical assessment framework for diagnostic medical ultrasound students. Ultrasound 22:113–117
33. Parker PC, Byass OR (2015) Successful implementation of a performance-related audit tool for sonographers. Ultrasound 23:97–102
34. Boulet JR, McKinley DW, Whelan GP, Hambleton RK (2003) Quality assurance methods for performance-based assessments. Adv Health Sci Educ Theory Pract 8:27–47
35. Haber M, Barnhart HX (2006) Coefficients of agreement for fixed observers. Stat Methods Med Res 15:255–271
36. Setodji CM, Shwartz M (2013) Fixed-effect or random-effect models: what are the key inference issues? Med Care 51:25–27
37. Harris EF, Smith RN (2009) Accounting for measurement error: a critical but often overlooked process. Arch Oral Biol 54:S107–S117

5

Management of cardiopulmonary assist devices in critically ill patients using point-of-care transthoracic echocardiography

Babar Fiza*, Michael Tang and Michael Maile

Abstract

Point-of-care transthoracic echocardiography is increasingly being utilized by the intensive care physicians in the management of hemodynamically unstable patients. However, its use in the management of critically ill patients requiring cardiopulmonary mechanical device support remains to be well described. In this case series, we present two case reports where point-of-care echocardiography was successfully used by the intensive care team in diagnosing and managing problems related to cardiopulmonary assist device malposition.

Introduction

Traditionally, echocardiography has been performed by cardiologists and cardiac anesthesiologists and, in some hospitals, by sonography technicians with interpretation by cardiologists. Over the past few years, the increasing availability, portability, and better image quality produced by ultrasound machines have resulted in an increased use of transthoracic echocardiogram (TTE) as a point-of-care (POC) ultrasound device. POC TTE is being widely adopted by emergency departments throughout the United States, where its utilization has been demonstrated to achieve great diagnostic capability [1]. In the operative room setting, focused TTE performed by anesthesiologists has been shown to alter management and provide new information in hemodynamically unstable patients [2]. POC echocardiography has even been used as a perioperative screening tool and successfully used in the management of critically ill patients [3, 4]. While the clinical use of POC cardiac ultrasonography continues to expand, this intricate skill requires appropriate education and training, including a comprehensive understanding of its scope and limitations [5].

To date, there are only a few published reports detailing its use in the critical care setting with regard to monitoring of patients with cardiovascular/cardiopulmonary assist devices [6–8]. In the following two case reports, we present the use of POC TTE by the intensive care physicians that resulted in immediate changes in the management of critically ill patients requiring cardiopulmonary mechanical device support.

Case one: Impella® repositioning

A 52-year-old male with history of chronic obstructive pulmonary disease (COPD), severe mitral regurgitation, severe tricuspid regurgitation, and non-ischemic cardiomyopathy (EF 25%) presented to an outside hospital with altered mental status and acute liver failure in the setting of cardiogenic shock. The patient's cardiac index was found to be 1.6 L/min at the time of presentation. Despite maximal medical therapy and subsequent placement of an intra-aortic balloon pump (IABP), there was little improvement in the patient's clinical status. Therefore, an Impella CP® was placed under fluoroscopic guidance in the cardiac catheterization lab. After placement of the Impella device, the patient's cardiac index improved to 2.4 L/min. An improvement in patient's mental status and liver function tests were also noted after placement of the Impella.

*Correspondence: babar@med.umich.edu
Department of Anesthesiology, University of Michigan Hospitals, 1500 East Medical Center Drive, Ann Arbor, MI 48109-5861, USA

The Impella CP® device is an axial flow type of temporary ventricular assist device that, typically, is placed in the femoral artery and positioned across the aortic valve. This allows it to withdraw blood from the left ventricle and eject it into the aorta. The device is placed percutaneously in patients with cardiogenic shock and provides more hemodynamic support than an IABP [9]. Its initial placement is guided by fluoroscopy or echocardiography to ensure that the inflow area is located approximately 3.5 cm below the aortic valve in the left ventricle and the outflow area is located above the aortic valve (Fig. 1). Typically, blood flows of 2.5–3.5 L/min are achieved through the catheter, which assists low native cardiac output states [10].

After undergoing placement of the Impella device, the patient was transferred to our cardiovascular intensive care unit (ICU) for evaluation of a left ventricular assist device placement. On arrival, the patient's hemodynamics were stable and urine was noted to be clear. The placement pressure waveform, a measure of pressure at the outflow of the Impella showed a waveform consistent with an aortic waveform. The motor current, showed good pulsatility, which also indicated correct placement. Next morning, the patient was found to have increasingly dark colored urine, raising concern for hemolysis. Placement waveform signals remained unchanged. A POC TTE performed by the intensive care team showed the Impella® tip to be approximately 5.9 cm below the aortic valve (previously 3.5 cm at the time of placement) in the parasternal long-axis view (Fig. 2). Laboratory workup obtained at this time was consistent with hemolysis and notable for an up-trending lactate dehydrogenase (LDH)

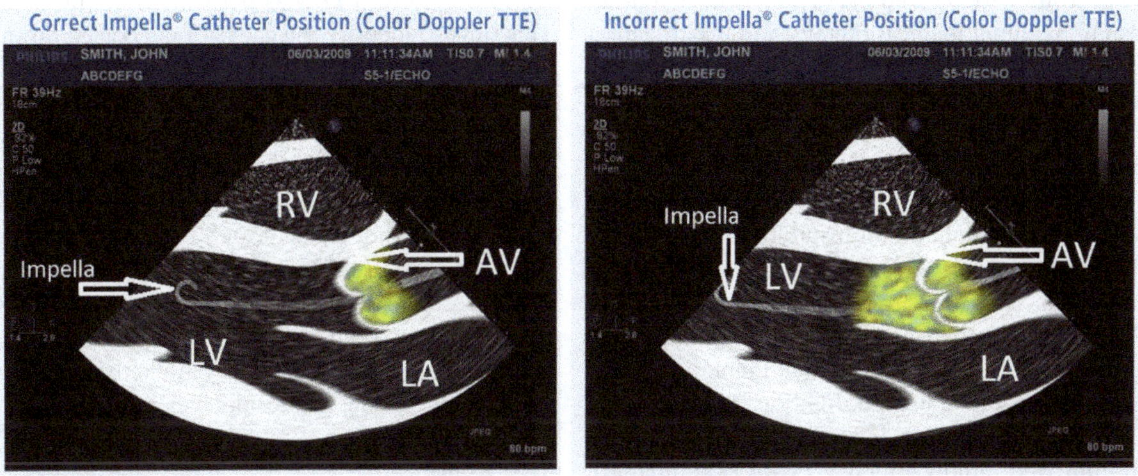

Fig. 1 Illustration showing incorrect and correct positioning of Impella® with color flow. Parasternal long-axis view on transthoracic echo (Illustration). In the incorrectly positioned Impella®, the outflow is seen below the aortic valve. The catheter is also located too deep in the left ventricle compared to a correctly placed catheter. *AV* aortic valve, *LV* left ventricle, *LA* left atrium, *RV* right ventricle. Image reproduced with permission from Abiomed Corporation

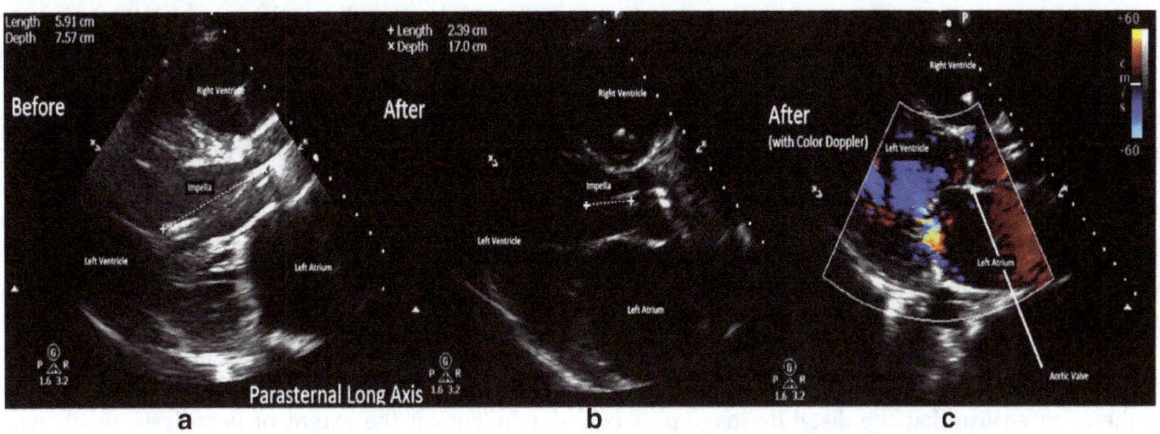

Fig. 2 Impella positioning visualized on the parasternal long-axis view on the TTE exam. **a** Images acquired at the time of improper positioning. The Impella® (hyperechoic structure) is located 5.9 cm beyond the aortic valve in the left ventricle. **b** Acquired after repositioning. Notice that the length of the Impella® in the left ventricle is now 2.4 cm beyond the aortic valve into the LV. **c** Acquired after repositioning with color Doppler. Flow at the outflow area can be visualized. The outflow area is now located above the aortic valve

and serum-free hemoglobin of 190.3 mg/dL (reference range 1–8 mg/dL for our institution). The cardiac surgery team was notified and subsequently withdrew the Impella by 3 cm. This resulted in resolution of hemolysis as evidenced by clearing of the urine and down-trending LDH and serum-free hemoglobin levels. A repeat POC TTE by the ICU team demonstrated that the catheter was in the correct position, and this was confirmed on color Doppler imaging (Fig. 2; Additional files 1, 2).

Case two: avalon veno-venous extracorporeal membrane oxygenation cannula malpositioning

A 67-year-old male with history of emphysema, chronic obstructive pulmonary disease, and hypertension presented to our ICU after undergoing a thoracoscopic bilateral lung volume reduction surgery. Postoperatively, the patient developed pneumonia and acute respiratory distress syndrome (ARDS) requiring mechanical ventilation. Despite maximal medical therapy and optimization of mechanical ventilator support, the patient's oxygenation worsened. On postoperative day seven, the patient's arterial blood gas analysis was notable for a PaO_2/FIO_2 ratio of 40. The patient was placed on pressure control mode of ventilation with inability to achieve greater than 150 mL of tidal volume on inspiratory pressures of 30 mmHg. The decision was made to place the patient on veno-venous extracorporeal membranous oxygenation (VV-ECMO) via the right internal jugular vein with the use of Avalon Elite Bicaval Dual Lumen catheter (MAQUET Holding B.V. and Co. KG, Rastatt, Germany) under direct fluoroscopic guidance. The patient's oxygenation improved rapidly after VV-ECMO cannulation. ECMO flow was set at 4.0 L/min, sweep at 1 L/min, and ventilation was continued in the same mode as prior to ECMO initiation. Arterial blood gas analysis at this time showed a pH of 7.38, [$PaCO_2$] 39, a PaO_2/FIO_2 ratio of 170, and a mixed venous oxygen saturation of 65%, indicating improved oxygenation.

VV-ECMO can be used as a salvage therapy for patients with severe or refractory hypoxia [11]. Multiple cannula configurations can be used to take blood from and return it to the venous system. The Avalon Elite Bicaval Dual Lumen Cannula® allows this to be accomplished using a single site. The inflow port of this particular catheter draws blood from both the superior and inferior vena cava. This blood flows into the oxygenator and is then returned through a reinfusion port, which is directed toward the tricuspid valve. Fluoroscopy or transesophageal echocardiography is utilized for proper placement of the catheter to ensure that the distal drainage port is located within the IVC, while the proximal drainage port lies in the superior vena cava [11–13].

On ECMO therapy day seven, the patient developed decreased flows, decreased inlet pressures, and chattering of the ECMO tubing. Chattering is vibration of the cannula and tubing that occurs when the drainage cannula abuts the wall of the blood vessel. Chattering most commonly occurs due to inadequate preload due to hypovolemia, or a process causing mechanical obstruction such as tamponade, tension pneumothorax, and abdominal compartment syndrome. Chattering can also occur independent of patient's volume status due to cannula malposition or excessive ECMO pump speeds. [14] Due to history of aggressive fluid diuresis in this patient, initially fluid boluses were administered to correct the chattering, but the patient continued to have problems with low circuit flows. This resulted in the deterioration in oxygenation with patient developing a pulse oximeter saturation of 80% and a mixed venous oxygen saturation of 43%. A POC TTE was performed by the ICU team at this time to identify the cause of decreased flows. On the POC TTE, the patient had normal right and left ventricular function and there was no pericardial effusion. On the subcostal inferior vena cava (IVC) view, it was noted that the catheter's distal tip had migrated into the hepatic vein. The Avalon® catheter was immediately withdrawn by 2–3 cm, and repeat POC TTE showed the cannula tip to be located in the inferior vena cava. Correct placement resulted in rapid improvement in ECMO flows and patient oxygenation with pulse oximeter saturation improving to 90% and mixed venous oxygenation saturation to 69% (Fig. 3; Additional files 3, 4, 5).

Discussion

These two cases illustrate the effective use of POC TTE in rapid diagnosis of clinical problems related to cardiopulmonary mechanical support devices. In the first case, POC echocardiography was used to diagnose Impella malposition. While hemolysis is a documented complication of the Impella device, the underlying mechanism can be related to either the shear stress of the device or improper positioning [15, 16]. The improper positioning of the device can lead to hemolysis as turbulent flow is generated when the outflow of the cannula is too close to the aortic valve or when the outflow of the device is partially below the aortic valve (Fig. 1). Given the different mechanisms that could lead to hemolysis in these patients, it is mandatory to check the cannula position before any therapeutic interventions are undertaken. Unlike the case of malposition, hemolysis related to shear stress would warrant either removal of the device, dependent on the extent of hemolysis, or change in the anticoagulation plan. Bedside TTE thus provides the clinician with the ability to quickly determine if cannula

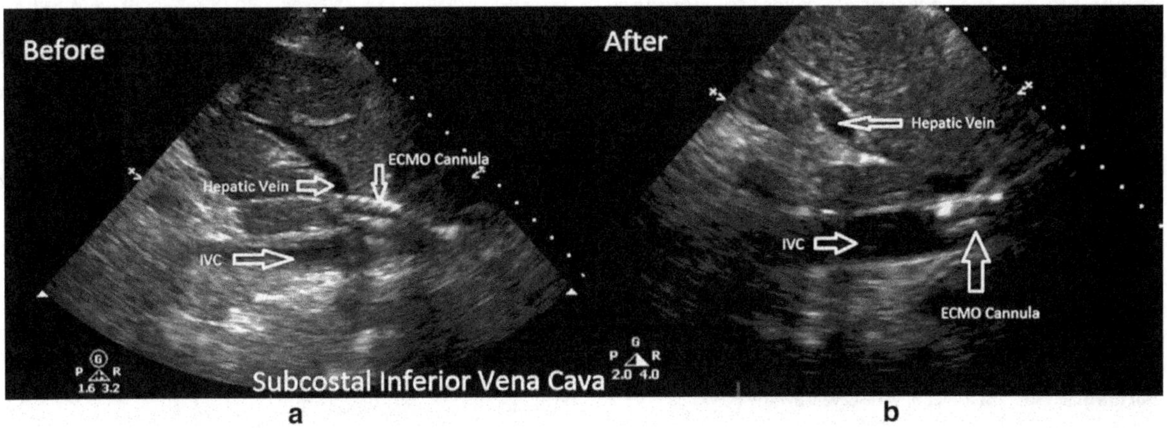

Fig. 3 Still Images taken from the subcostal inferior vena cava view on the TTE exam. **a** Image taken during low flows on the ECMO circuit. The ECMO cannula is visualized as a hyperechoic structure located in the hepatic vein. **b** Resolution of low flows on ECMO circuit after catheter repositioning. The ECMO cannula is now located in the lumen of the inferior vena cava. *IVC* inferior vena cava

malposition is the cause of hemolysis. The bedside availability of TTE for device placement is recommended by the European Expert Group although very few case reports in literature have described the utilization of bedside TTE for Impella device repositioning [17].

Case one also demonstrates the importance of real-time echocardiographic confirmation of device positioning even when device hemodynamic pressure signals do not display evidence of malposition. The Impella device is fitted with a display screen that continuously monitors device position using a waveform calculated from the pressure difference between the inlet and the outlet areas. Based on the changes in this waveform, a proximal or a distal migration of the device can be detected. As the distal pressures are monitored in an open area above the outlet port, migration of the device outlet area into the aortic valve is possible without a change in waveform [15]. We suspect this to be the case in our patient. In this case, even though the device console indicated appropriate device position, the device malposition was evident on the TTE exam.

The second case highlights the important role of bedside echocardiography in daily management of patients requiring VV-ECMO therapy. Traditionally, VV-ECMO support has been achieved via dual cannulation either through femoro-jugular or femoro-femoral venous cannulation. However, VV-ECMO support can now be achieved via single-vessel cannulation at the internal jugular vein with the use of Avalon Elite Bicaval Dual Lumen Cannula®. The advantages of this cannula include less recirculation, improved patient mobility, and decreased risk of infection. However, this catheter like other ECMO catheters when improperly positioned can lead to recirculation, arrhythmias, and a decrease in ECMO flows resulting in hypoxia [7, 8].

As highlighted by our case, echocardiography can assist in determining the cause of inadequate flows and allow clinicians to institute correct therapies. Due to underlying lung pathology, physicians treating these patients generally employ restrictive fluid strategy. This can result in a decrease in ECMO flows due to collapse of the IVC around the cannula. The collapse of the IVC around the catheter combined with signs of hypovolemia can be determined with real-time echocardiography and allow physicians to guide fluid therapy. However, ECMO catheter malpositioning can result in decreased flows as well, in which case the proper therapy would be to reposition the catheter in order to achieve adequate flows. As evidenced by this case, diagnosis of catheter malposition as the cause of decreased flows prevents excessive fluid administration that would otherwise risk worsening of pulmonary function due to volume overload. Additionally, cannula repositioning should always be performed under real-time fluoroscopy or echocardiography guidance as migration of the tip of the cannula into the right ventricle could lead to structural damage and poses risk of arrhythmias [7].

Conclusion

These two case studies show the effective use of POC TTE by the intensive care physicians to diagnose and manage problems arising from complications related to the use of cardiovascular assist devices. Routine imaging such as plain film X-rays can give us limited information and may not necessarily be sufficient to judge proper positioning. Point-of-care echocardiography proved to be invaluable in the presented cases to diagnose improper positioning, resulting in immediate changes in management.

Additional files

Additional file 1. Parasternal long-axis view obtained at time of improper positioning of the Impella®. The Impella® catheter is located 5.9 cm beyond the aortic valve in the left ventricle.

Additional file 2. Parasternal long-axis view obtained after repositioning. The Impella® is now located 2.4 cm beyond the aortic valve into the LV. On color Doppler interrogation flow at the outflow site is now located in the aorta.

Additional file 3. On subcostal inferior vena cava view the ECMO cannula is noted to be located in the hepatic vein.

Additional file 4. Subcostal inferior vena cava view after repositioning of the ECMO cannula. The cannula is now located within the IVC.

Additional file 5. Subcostal inferior vena cava view with color flow Doppler interrogation. Flow is seen in the hepatic vein and the ECMO cannula is located within the IVC.

Abbreviations

TTE: transthoracic echocardiography; POC: point of care; COPD: chronic obstructive pulmonary disease; IABP: intra-aortic balloon pump; EF: ejection fraction; cm: centimeter; ICU: Intensive Care Unit; LDH: lactate dehydrogenase; mg: milligram; dL: deciliter; AV: aortic valve; LV: left ventricle; LA: left atrium; RV: right ventricle; ARDS: acute respiratory distress syndrome; PaO_2: partial pressure of oxygen in arterial blood; FiO_2: fraction of inspired oxygen; mm Hg: millimeters of mercury; $PaCO_2$: partial pressure of carbon dioxide in arterial blood; VV-ECMO: veno-venous extracorporeal membranous oxygenation; ECMO: extracorporeal membrane oxygenation; IVC: inferior vena cava.

Authors' contributions

MT and BF have written the main portion of the manuscript. MM has reviewed and edited the manuscript. BF has been responsible for the discussion of the echo findings in each case and reviewing the imaging portion of the manuscript. All authors read and approved the final manuscript.

Acknowledgements

None.

References

1. Volpicelli G, Lamorte A, Tullio M, Cardinale L, Giraudo M, Stefanone V et al (2013) Point-of-care multiorgan ultrasonography for the evaluation of undifferentiated hypotension in the emergency department. Intensive Care Med 39(7):1290–1298. https://doi.org/10.1007/s00134-013-2919-7
2. Kratz T, Steinfeldt T, Exner M, Orto MCD, Timmesfeld N, Kratz C et al (2017) Impact of focused intraoperative transthoracic echocardiography by anesthesiologists on management in hemodynamically unstable high-risk non-cardiac surgery patients. J Cardiothorac Vasc Anesth 31(2):602–609. https://doi.org/10.1053/j.jvca.2016.11.002
3. Canty DJ, Royse CF, Kilpatrick D, Bowman L, Royse AG (2012) The impact of focused transthoracic echocardiography in the pre-operative clinic. Anaesthesia 67(6):618–625. https://doi.org/10.1111/j.1365-2044.2012.07074.x
4. Manasia AR, Nagaraj HM, Kodali RB, Croft LB, Oropello JM, Kohli-Seth R et al (2005) Feasibility and potential clinical utility of goal-directed transthoracic echocardiography performed by noncardiologist intensivists using a small hand-carried device (SonoHeart) in critically ill patients. J Cardiothorac Vasc Anesth 19(2):155–159. https://doi.org/10.1053/j.jvca.2005.01.023
5. Neskovic AN, Edvardsen T, Galderisi M, Garbi M, Gullace G et al (2014) Focus cardiac ultrasound: the European association of cardiovascular imaging viewpoint. Eur Heart Journal Cardiovascular Imaging 15(9):956–960
6. Uriel N, Morrison KA, Garan AR, Kato TS, Yuzefpolskaya M, Latif F et al (2012) Development of a novel echocardiography ramp test for speed optimization and diagnosis of device thrombosis in continuous-flow left ventricular assist devices. J Am Coll Cardiol 60(18):1764–1775. https://doi.org/10.1016/j.jacc.2012.07.052
7. Ratzlaff RA, Ripoll JG, Cushenbery KA, Lowman PE, Díaz-Gómez JL (2017) Transthoracic echocardiogram-guided avalon catheter repositioning. Anesth Analg 125(1):48–51. https://doi.org/10.1213/ANE.0000000000001909
8. Tanaka D, Pitcher HT, Cavarocchi N, Hirose H (2015) Migrated avalon veno-venous extracorporeal membrane oxygenation cannula: how to adjust without interruption of flow. J Card Surg 30(11):865–868. https://doi.org/10.1111/jocs.12629
9. Ouweneel DM et al (2017) Percutaneous mechanical circulatory support versus intra-aortic balloon pump in cardiogenic shock after acute myocardial infarction. J Am Coll Cardiol 69(3):278–287. https://doi.org/10.1016/j.jacc.2016.10.022
10. Rogers JG, Patel CB, Milano CA (2017) Mechanically assisted circulation. In: Fuster V, Harrington RA, Narula J, Eapen ZJ (eds) Hurst's the heart, 14e. McGraw-Hill Education, New York
11. Napolitano LM (2014) Extracorporeal Lung Support. In: Hall JB, Schmidt GA, Kress JP (eds) Principles of Critical Care, 4e. McGraw-Hill Education, New York
12. Platts David Gerard et al (2012) The role of echocardiography in the management of patients supported by extracorporeal membrane oxygenation. J Am Soc Echocardiogr 25(2):131–141. https://doi.org/10.1016/j.echo.2011.11.009
13. Trimlett RH, Cordingley JJ, Griffiths MJ et al (2011) A modified technique for insertion of dual lumen bicaval cannulae for venovenous extracorporeal membrane oxygenation. Intensive Care Med 37:1036–1037
14. Chung Mabel et al (2014) Monitoring of the adult patient on venoarterial extracorporeal membrane oxygenation. Sci World J 2014:1–10. https://doi.org/10.1155/2014/393258
15. Sibbald M, Džavík V (2012) Severe hemolysis associated with use of the Impella LP 2.5 mechanical assist device. Catheter Cardiovasc Interv 80(5):840–844. https://doi.org/10.1002/ccd.24280
16. Cardozo S, Ahmed T, Belgrave K (2015) Impella induced massive hemolysis: reemphasizing echocardiographic guidance for correct placement. Case Rep Cardiol 2015:1–3. https://doi.org/10.1155/2015/464135
17. Burzotta F, Trani C, Doshi SN, Townend J, van Geuns RJ, Hunziker P, Schiefer B, Karatolios K, Møller JE, Ribichini FL, Schäfer A, Henriques JPS (2015) Impella ventricular support in clinical practice: collaborative viewpoint from a European Expert User Group. Int J Cardiol 201(C):684–691. https://doi.org/10.1016/j.ijcard.2015.07.065

6

The role of Point-of-care ultrasound in the diagnosis and management of necrotizing soft tissue infections

Luís Magalhães[1*], Sara Raquel Pereira Martins[2] and Ramon Nogué[3]

Abstract

Background: Necrotizing soft tissue infections are associated with high morbidity and mortality, even when the correct treatment is initiated. The diagnosis of these conditions is hard and the most sensitive methods are time-consuming, expensive and not readily available. Point-of-care ultrasound can complement clinical evaluation to increase the diagnostic accuracy.

Case presentation: We bring a case of a woman, without comorbidities, who presented to the emergency department with signs of soft tissue infection. Bedside ultrasound showed subcutaneous tissue thickening, with fluid accumulation, and subcutaneous gas in the affected area. Based on the clinical suspicion and the ultrasound findings, the patient underwent prompt medical treatment and surgical debridement.

Conclusions: This case shows the utility of bedside ultrasound for the decision-making process in a disease where an early diagnosis is important. This information should always be used together with the clinical judgement, as it has a relative low sensitivity.

Keywords: Soft tissue infections, Ultrasonography, Emergency Medicine, Point-of-care testing, Diagnostic imaging

Background

Necrotizing soft tissue infections (NSTI) are a group of infections characterized by a fulminant destruction and necrosis of the skin and soft tissue and that is frequently associated with systemic illness [1]. Even when the correct treatment is initiated, this condition is associated with a high mortality and morbidity, with mortality rates between 25 and 50% [2–5]. The diagnosis of these conditions is hard, with studies showing high rates of misdiagnosis at presentation [6], mainly because the initial clinical manifestations can be underestimated. An early institution of appropriate treatment, which includes early surgical intervention and antibiotic therapy, improves the outcomes. The diagnosis is primarily clinical, consisting of pain and swelling with minimum skin involvement that progresses to induration and formation of bullae. To complement the clinical evaluation, computerized tomography (CT) is the most used method of diagnosis. However, CT can have some drawbacks, namely being a time-consuming and expensive method that is not readily available in all clinical practice contexts. Magnetic resonance imaging (MRI) has a higher sensitivity and specificity, but have the same problems of CT. Given the severity and time-dependency of this condition, surgical intervention should not be delayed when the degree of suspicion is high.

Ultrasonography is a widely used method for evaluating the soft tissue. In recent years, point-of-care ultrasound (POCUS) has gained a lot of visibility between the medical community as a complement to clinical evaluation, as a fifth pillar of the physical examination [7]. Incorporating this technique can improve diagnostic speed and accuracy. Its use is well established in different

*Correspondence: mag_luis@hotmail.com

[1] Hospital da Luz–Arrábida, Praceta de Henrique Moreira 150, 4400-346 Vila Nova de Gaia, Portugal

Full list of author information is available at the end of the article

areas, including the heart [8], lung [9], trauma [10], shock and even during cardiopulmonary resuscitation [11]. However, evaluation of the soft tissue performed by non-radiologists in the context of emergency is not so well established.

The purpose of this case is to demonstrate how POCUS can easily and quickly provide reliable additional information to the physical exam to support the diagnosis of NSTI and increase the confidence with which we stratify the severity of these patients and propose more invasive and expensive attitudes, such as CT or even surgical intervention.

Case presentation

We bring a case of a 54-year-old woman, without comorbidities, who presented to the emergency department with a 12-h redness and painful swelling in the left gluteal region. She denied trauma. At admission, she was afebrile (36.2 °C), with a normal blood pressure (109/65 mmHg), heart rate 89 bpm and mild peripheral oxygen desaturation (92% breathing room air), without other signs of respiratory distress. On the physical exam, she had a left gluteus induration with about 5 cm × 5 cm with redness in the surrounding area, as seen in Fig. 1a. There was no crepitus. The remaining physical exam was normal. Her initial labs were: hemoglobin 11.3 g/dL (*N* 13.5–17.5 g/dL), total white blood cell 6.550/μL (*N* 3.500–11.000/μL), 96% neutrophils (*N* 45–75%), platelets 164.000/μL (*N* 125.000–400.000/μL), creatinine 0.88 mg/dL (*N* 0.6–1.3 mg/dL), urea 51 mg/dL (*N* 22–52 mg/dL) and C-reactive protein 199.52 mg/dL (*N* < 5 mg/dL).

A bedside ultrasound scan using a linear probe was performed which showed subcutaneous tissue thickening, with a "cobblestone" appearance, hypoechoic foci of fluid accumulation in the subcutaneous space, as well as the presence of gas in the tissue (Fig. 2a), significantly different from the normal skin (Fig. 2b).

Even though the patient was initially stable, she was started on intravenous fluids and large spectrum antibiotics based on a high clinical suspicion for NSTI, supported with the ultrasound findings. After consultation with general surgery, considering the suggestive clinical and ultrasound findings, the presence of some alarming signs (tendentially low blood pressure, peripheral oxygen desaturation, elevated inflammatory parameters and rapid evolution of cutaneous inflammatory signs) and the time needed for the CT scan, unavailable at that moment, the patient underwent prompt surgical debridement to avoid delays in the treatment. In the procedure, the surgeon found necrotic tissue, purulent liquid and evidence of gas in the tissue, thus confirming the diagnosis. She was then transferred to the Intensive Care Unit, where, on the first day post-operative, evolved with septic shock, requiring vasopressor therapy. CT on day 2 showed no signs of additional complications (Fig. 3), namely enteric fistulas or bone involvement. She underwent one more major surgical debridement on day 3, as well as minor debridements and washouts, and was discharged 7 days later. Blood and tissue cultures were unable to identify the microorganism. Follow-up at 5 and 10 days after the discharge showed good evolution of the wound. The normalization of the image observed by ultrasonography gradually occurred after the fever, pain and the erythema

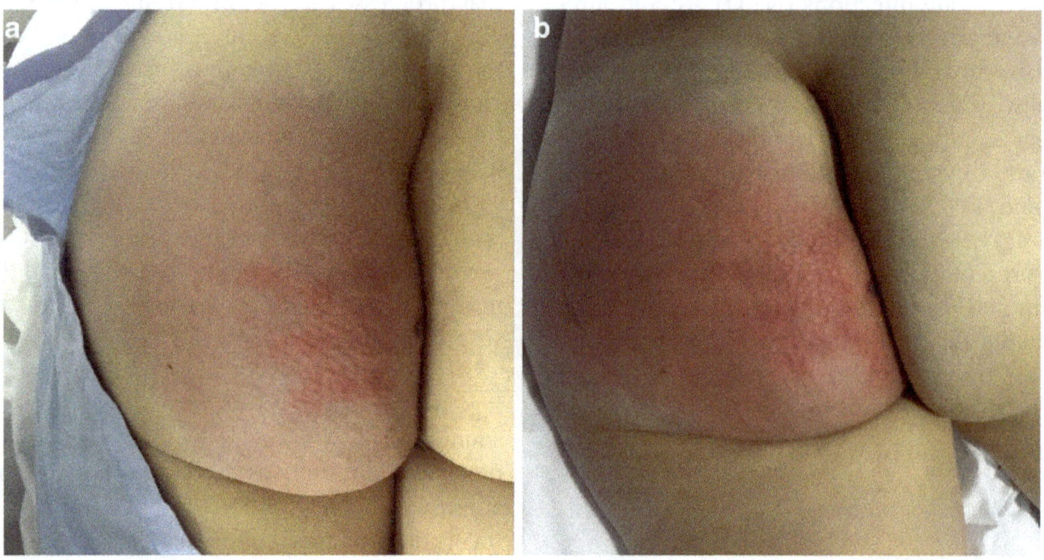

Fig. 1 Macroscopic aspect of the left gluteus with signs of cutaneous infection: **a** at admission and **b** 3 h after admission, showing rapid progression of the redness around a central area of induration

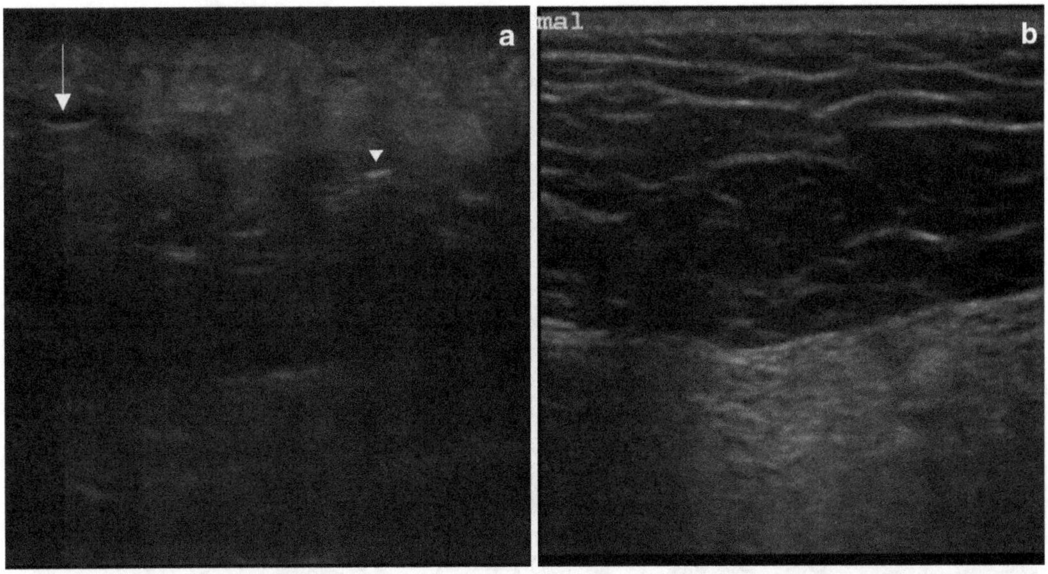

Fig. 2 Point-of-care ultrasound scan of the affected left gluteal soft tissue (**a**) and normal soft tissue on the contralateral side (**b**) using a 15–6 MHz linear probe. In the affected tissue, there is loss of the normal subcutaneous architecture, diffuse increased echogenicity, hypoechoic regions that correspond to little fluid accumulations (arrow) and an hyperechoic focus with posterior dirty acoustic shadowing, corresponding to gas in the soft tissue (arrowhead)

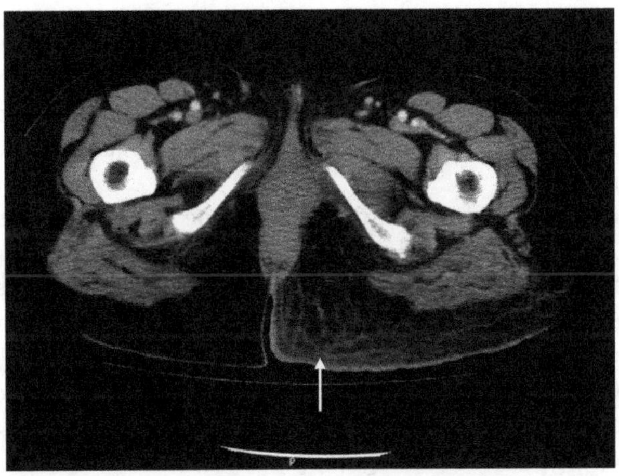

Fig. 3 Contrast CT scan of the lower limbs on day 2 after surgical debridement. Axial tomogram at the level of the proximal thigh showing abnormal enhancement of the subcutaneous and fascial layer of the left gluteal region (arrow)

was resolved (Fig. 4). The exam was normal at the 30-day post-discharge evaluation.

Discussion

As mentioned, NSTI are a group of diseases with high mortality and morbidity, even when the correct diagnosis and treatment is made on time. Unfortunately, this is not an easy diagnosis, as the initial manifestations can be mistaken with more frequent and less severe diseases like cellulitis, erysipelas, diabetes mellitus decompensation, gastroenteritis and others [6]. More specific clinical signs, like large hemorrhagic bullae, skin necrosis, fluctuance, crepitus, and sensory and motor deficits are late signs of this condition. Clinical criteria have been developed to increase the accuracy of the clinical evaluation, namely the LRINEC Score [12], but the sensitivity and specificity are still not ideal [13]. Gas on plain radiographs was only seen in 16.9% in one series [14]. POCUS can improve diagnose accuracy for NSTI when used in combination with clinical evaluation as it is increasingly available, fast and can be performed at the bedside. One study estimated a sensitivity of 88.2% and specificity of 93.3% for the diagnosis on patients with clinically suspected NSTI [15]. The main findings of NSTI by ultrasound are reflected in this case and can be summarized in [15–18]: loss of the normal tissue architecture to a "cobblestone" appearance, with irregularity and thickening of the fascia, abnormal fluid collections along the fascia, seen as hypoechogenic zones, and, in more advanced cases, the presence subcutaneous air, defined by hyperechogenic foci with a posterior dirty acoustic shadowing. Even in the absence of crepitus at physical examination or plain radiographs, POCUS can show evidence of gas in the soft tissue, indicative of advanced disease and a marker of worse prognosis. The presence of a thickened fascia can make it difficult to differentiate the underlying structures. Yet, there is always the possibility of comparing with another similar unaffected structure, usually the other limb. Ultrasound can also be helpful to

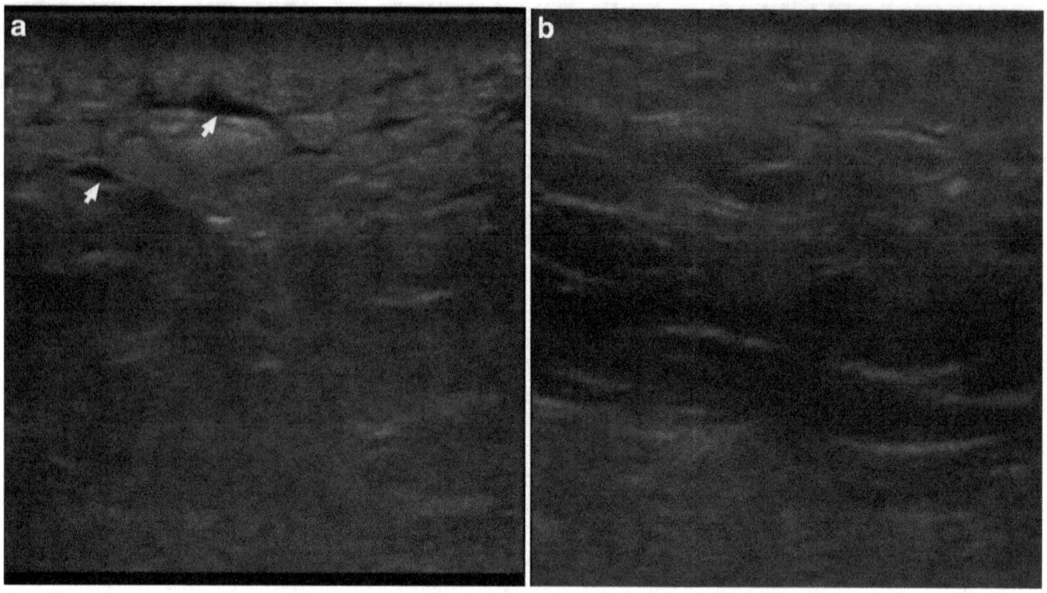

Fig. 4 Point-of-care ultrasound scan of the affected left gluteal soft tissue 4 days after admission (**a**) and 8 days after admission (**b**) using a 15–6 MHz linear probe. These images show the progression of the sonographic appearance of NSTI, initially with accumulation of fluid in the subcutaneous tissue (arrows), giving it a "cobblestone" appearance and a progressive return to the normal architecture of the subcutaneous tissue over time

guide fluid drainage if a collection is present and rule out deep vein thrombosis.

Contrary to plain radiographs and CT, ultrasound has no ionizing radiation and is also relatively cheap. These features allow the clinician to repeatedly monitor the evolution of the patient, searching for possible local or systemic complications.

Distinguishing NSTI from cellulitis (Fig. 5), the main alternative diagnosis, or other causes of soft-tissue edema using POCUS is not always possible, especially if it involves the deeper fascia, as a thickened fascia can appear in both cases [19]. Some ultrasound findings, including an irregularity of the fascia and an abnormal fluid collection along the fascial plane can help distinguish between the NSFI and cellulitis [16]. However, this evaluation is more difficult, strengthening the importance of taking the information obtained by POCUS together with the clinical evaluation and laboratory results.

Evaluation of deep structures can be difficult because of the hyperechogenic inflamed subcutaneous tissue that reflects most of the ultrasound beams. Also, as with other applications of POCUS, it is a user-dependent technique that requires some practice before being correctly used.

CT and MRI are still the most sensitive methods of diagnosis. CT is the most used imaging method to make the diagnosis, with a higher spacial resolution than ultrasound that allows the evaluation of deeper structures

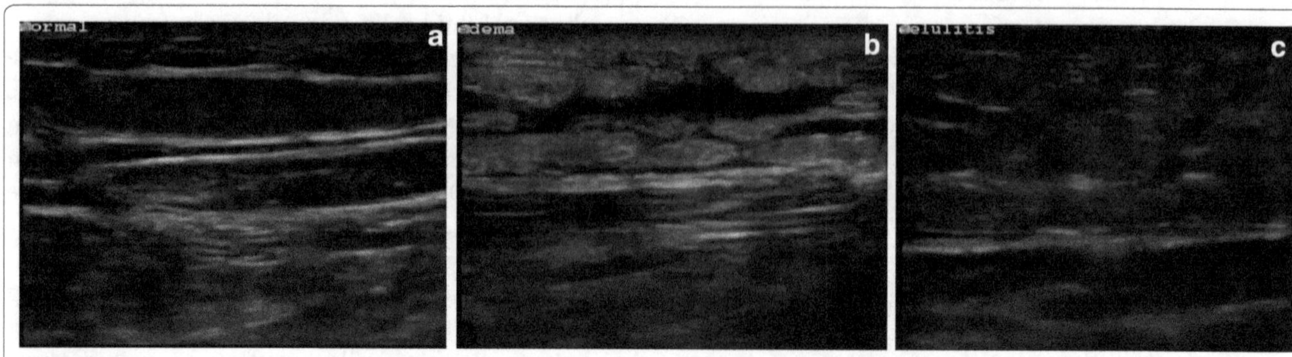

Fig. 5 Point-of-care ultrasound scan of a different patient showing normal soft tissue (**a**), peripheral edema (**b**) and cellulitis (**c**) using a 15–6 MHz linear probe

not accessible to ultrasound. It has a sensitivity of 80% in detecting NSTI [20]. MRI is the gold standard for the non-invasive diagnosis of NSTI, with sensitivity and specificity varying according the used criteria (presence of gas has a 100% specificity while extensive involvement of the intermuscular fasciae has a 100% sensitivity) [21]. However, these exams are less available, more time-consuming and expensive. The patient must also be transferred to the radiology department, which can lead to delays in the diagnosis and initiation of the therapy and lack of appropriate monitoring.

In this case, combining a high suggestive clinical evaluation and the documentation of the traditional signs observed in NSTI by POCUS, including the presence of gas in the tissue, allowed for a faster initiation of appropriate therapy and prompt surgical debridement, without having to transport the patient to a time-consuming exam like CT or MRI that could otherwise delay the diagnosis and the treatment. This case also shows complete remission of the ultrasound signs 1 month after the event.

Conclusion

This case shows the utility of bedside ultrasound for the decision-making process in a disease where an early diagnosis is important. This information should always be used together with the clinical judgement, as it has a low sensitivity.

Further studies are necessary to understand the implications of this exam in the treatment and prognosis of this disease and if a protocolized approach would be beneficial in this population.

Abbreviations

CT: computerized tomography; MRI: magnetic resonance imaging; NSTI: necrotizing soft tissue infections; POCUS: point-of-care ultrasound.

Acknowledgements

Not applicable.

Authors' contributions

LM was responsible for data collection, literature review and was a major contributor in writing the manuscript. SRPM was responsible for literature review and was a major contributor in writing the manuscript. RN critically revised the manuscript and contributed with important intellectual content. All authors read and approved the final manuscript.

Authors' information

RN: director of postgraduate training in Emergency Medicine and emergency and critical ultrasound at the University of Lleida School of Medicine in Spain. Coordinator for Spain's ultrasound training program in the Spanish Society of Emergency Medicine. Coordinator of WINFOCUS Spain. LM: Instructor of Ultrasound Life Support at REANIMA. SRPM: Instructor of Ultrasound Life Support at REANIMA.

Author details

[1] Hospital da Luz–Arrábida, Praceta de Henrique Moreira 150, 4400-346 Vila Nova de Gaia, Portugal. [2] Centro Hospitalar Universitário do Porto, Largo do Prof. Abel Salazar, 4099-001 Porto, Portugal. [3] Universitat de Lleida, Plaça de Víctor Siurana, 1, 25003 Lleida, Spain.

References

1. Stevens DL, Bryant AE (2017) Necrotizing soft-tissue infections. N Engl J Med 377(23):2253–2265
2. Yilmazlar T, Ozturk E, Alsoy A, Ozguc H (2007) Necrotizing soft tissue infections: APACHE II score, dissemination, and survival. World J Surg 31(9):1858–1862
3. Miller AT, Saadai P, Greenstein A, Divino CM (2008) Postprocedural necrotizing fasciitis: a 10-year retrospective review. Am Surg 74(5):405–409
4. Lee TC, Carrick MM, Scott BG, Hodges JC, Pham HQ (2007) Incidence and clinical characteristics of methicillin-resistant Staphylococcus aureus necrotizing fasciitis in a large urban hospital. Am J Surg 194(6):809–812 **(discussion 12-3)**
5. Childers BJ, Potyondy LD, Nachreiner R, Rogers FR, Childers ER, Oberg KC et al (2002) Necrotizing fasciitis: a fourteen-year retrospective study of 163 consecutive patients. Am Surg 68(2):109–116
6. Hefny AF, Eid HO, Al-Hussona M, Idris KM, Abu-Zidan FM (2007) Necrotizing fasciitis: a challenging diagnosis. Eur J Emerg Med 14(1):50–52
7. Narula J, Chandrashekhar Y, Braunwald E (2018) Time to add a fifth pillar to bedside physical examination: inspection, palpation, percussion, auscultation, and insonation. JAMA Cardiol 3(4):346–350
8. Jensen MB, Sloth E, Larsen KM, Schmidt MB (2004) Transthoracic echocardiography for cardiopulmonary monitoring in intensive care. Eur J Anaesthesiol 21(9):700–707
9. Volpicelli G, Elbarbary M, Blaivas M, Lichtenstein DA, Mathis G, Kirkpatrick AW et al (2012) International evidence-based recommendations for point-of-care lung ultrasound. Intensive Care Med 38(4):577–591
10. Scalea TM, Rodriguez A, Chiu WC, Brenneman FD, Fallon WF Jr, Kato K et al (1999) Focused Assessment with Sonography for Trauma (FAST): results from an international consensus conference. J Trauma 46(3):466–472
11. Seif D, Perera P, Mailhot T, Riley D, Mandavia D (2012) Bedside ultrasound in resuscitation and the rapid ultrasound in shock protocol. Crit Care Res Pract 2012:503254
12. Wong CH, Khin LW, Heng KS, Tan KC, Low CO (2004) The LRINEC (Laboratory Risk Indicator for Necrotizing Fasciitis) score: a tool for distinguishing necrotizing fasciitis from other soft tissue infections. Crit Care Med 32(7):1535–1541
13. Neeki MM, Dong F, Au C, Toy J, Khoshab N, Lee C et al (2017) Evaluating the laboratory risk indicator to differentiate cellulitis from necrotizing fasciitis in the Emergency Department. West J Emerg Med 18(4):684–689
14. Wong CH, Chang HC, Pasupathy S, Khin LW, Tan JL, Low CO (2003) Necrotizing fasciitis: clinical presentation, microbiology, and determinants of mortality. J Bone Joint Surg Am 85-A(8):1454–1460
15. Yen ZS, Wang HP, Ma HM, Chen SC, Chen WJ (2002) Ultrasonographic screening of clinically-suspected necrotizing fasciitis. Acad Emerg Med 9(12):1448–1451
16. Tsai CC, Lai CS, Yu ML, Chou CK, Lin SD (1996) Early diagnosis of necrotizing fasciitis by utilization of ultrasonography. Kaohsiung J Med Sci 12(4):235–240
17. Hanif MA, Bradley MJ (2008) Sonographic findings of necrotizing fasciitis in the breast. J Clin Ultrasound 36(8):517–519
18. Castleberg E, Jenson N, Dinh VA (2014) Diagnosis of necrotizing fasciitis with bedside ultrasound: the STAFF Exam. West J Emerg Med 15(1):111–113
19. Kuncir EJ, Tillou A, Hill CR, Petrone P, Kimbrell B, Asensio JA (2003) Necrotizing soft-tissue infections. Emerg Med Clin N Am 21(4):1075–1087
20. Wysoki MG, Santora TA, Shah RM, Friedman AC (1997) Necrotizing fasciitis: CT characteristics. Radiology 203(3):859–863
21. Malghem J, Lecouvet FE, Omoumi P, Maldague BE, Vande Berg BC (2013) Necrotizing fasciitis: contribution and limitations of diagnostic imaging. Joint Bone Spine 80(2):146–154

7

Quantifying systemic congestion with Point-of-care ultrasound: Development of the venous excess ultrasound grading system

William Beaubien-Souligny[1,2*], Philippe Rola[3], Korbin Haycock[4], Josée Bouchard[5], Yoan Lamarche[6], Rory Spiegel[7] and André Y. Denault[1,8]

Abstract

Background: Organ congestion is a mediator of adverse outcomes in critically ill patients. Point-Of-Care ultrasound (POCUS) is widely available and could enable clinicians to detect signs of venous congestion at the bedside. The aim of this study was to develop several grading system prototypes using POCUS and to determine their respective ability to predict acute kidney injury (AKI) after cardiac surgery. This is a post-hoc analysis of a single-center prospective study in 145 patients undergoing cardiac surgery for which repeated daily measurements of hepatic, portal, intra-renal vein Doppler and inferior vena cava (IVC) ultrasound were performed during the first 72 h after surgery. Five prototypes of venous excess ultrasound (VExUS) grading system combining multiple ultrasound markers were developed.

Results: The association between each score and AKI was assessed using time-dependant Cox models as well as conventional performance measures of diagnostic testing. A total of 706 ultrasound assessments were analyzed. We found that defining severe venous congestion as the presence of severe flow abnormalities in multiple Doppler patterns with a dilated IVC ($\geq$ 2 cm) showed the strongest association with the development of subsequent AKI compared with other combinations (HR: 3.69 CI 1.65–8.24 $p = 0.001$). The association remained significant after adjustment for baseline risk of AKI and vasopressor/inotropic support (HR: 2.82 CI 1.21–6.55 $p = 0.02$). Furthermore, this severe VExUS grade offered a useful positive likelihood ratio (+LR: 6.37 CI 2.19–18.50) when detected at ICU admission, which outperformed central venous pressure measurements.

Conclusions: The combination of multiple POCUS markers may identify clinically significant venous congestion.

Keywords: Acute kidney injury, Cardiac surgery, Point-Of-Care ultrasound, Venous congestion, Fluid balance

Background

Hemodynamic management in critically ill patients has traditionally focused on maintaining adequate cardiac output and arterial blood pressure by relying on fluid administration and vasopressor/inotropic support [1, 2]. However, organ perfusion is affected by other important factors [3, 4]. Among them, the venous pressure is often overlooked as a hemodynamic parameter that may be of critical importance. The development of clinically significant organ congestion is susceptible to occur in patients with right ventricular failure or pulmonary hypertension, and in patients with fluid overload. These contributors are likely to be synergistic in critically ill patients, particularly when renal dysfunction aggravates fluid retention. A reduction of the arteriovenous gradient across vital organs may hamper adequate perfusion [5]. This phenomenon may be worsened with the development of interstitial edema after prolonged elevation of capillary hydrostatic pressure in the context of a dysfunctional endothelial barrier [4]. In encapsulated organs such as the kidney and the brain, interstitial edema may result

*Correspondence: william.beaubien@gmail.com
[2] Division of Nephrology, Centre Hospitalier de l'Université de Montreal, 1000, Rue St-Denis, Montreal, QC H2X 0C1, Canada
Full list of author information is available at the end of the article

in a rapid elevation in interstitial pressure, which then decreases organ blood flow [6, 7]. Furthermore, interstitial edema is hypothesized to impair tissue oxygenation by increasing the diffusion distances within the interstitium [8].

An exceedingly challenging aspect of hemodynamic evaluation is determining what represents clinically significant venous hypertension. Central venous pressure (CVP) measurements performed in the intensive care unit (ICU) remain invasive and are subject to important measurement errors even among experienced operators [9]. Furthermore, while higher CVP has been associated with complications in multiple settings [10–12], it remains unclear what level of CVP is deleterious and may be considered a trigger for intervention [13]. Other metrics such as cumulative fluid balance, weight variations and physical examination for peripheral edema, each have important limitations and may not be proportional to systemic venous pressure [14–16].

Point-Of-Care ultrasound (POCUS) enables the clinician to visualize the vascular anatomy and assess blood velocity using Doppler imaging. Within any venous vascular system, the additional volume associated with congestive factors will eventually reach the upper limits of the systemic venous capacitance, causing a rapid rise in venous pressures. Several markers of the high pressures associated with this congestive process have been proposed including the assessment of large veins (vena cava, internal jugular) as well as detecting abnormal venous waveforms suggestive that the limit of the systemic venous compliance in the portal vein, hepatic veins and intra-renal veins [17]. All of these markers have been associated with adverse consequences of venous hypertension, both in acute and chronic settings [18–21]. However, they also all have significant limitations that may hamper their clinical usefulness when interpreted in isolation [22–24]. It is likely that considering a combination of these ultrasonographic features may increase the clinical usefulness of POCUS for the purpose of detecting significant venous congestion.

The primary objective of the exploratory study was to develop a prototypical Venous Excess Ultrasound (VExUS) grading system of the severity of venous congestion, and to validate its potential clinical value in predicting the occurrence of acute kidney injury (AKI) after cardiac surgery using existing data from a recent prospective cohort study. The secondary objective was to compare its clinical usefulness to CVP measurements.

Methods

Study design and participants

This is a post-hoc analysis of data collected during a prospective cohort study at a tertiary cardiac surgery center from August 2016 to July 2017 (NCT02831907) [21]. Written consent was obtained for all patients and the project was approved by the Montreal Heart Institute Ethics Committee (2016-1946).

Non-critically ill patients 18 years and older undergoing cardiac surgery with the use of cardiopulmonary bypass were eligible to participate. Complete inclusion and exclusion criteria have been previously described [21]. Notably, patients with critical illness, AKI or delirium before surgery were excluded as well as patients with conditions that may have interfered with portal Doppler assessment (cirrhosis, portal thrombosis) and patients with severe chronic kidney disease (estimated glomerular filtration rate < 15 mL/min per 1.73 m^2 calculated using the Modified Diet in Renal Disease formula [25]) or dialysis.

Ultrasound assessment

All patients underwent repeated POCUS assessment the day before surgery, at ICU admission after surgery and daily from post-operative days 1 to 3. Each ultrasound assessment consisted of hepatic vein Doppler, portal vein Doppler, intra-renal venous Doppler and inferior vena cava (IVC) ultrasound. The complete method for hepatic, portal and renal Doppler assessment has been previously published [21]. The assessments were performed with concurrent electrocardiogram tracing to adequately identify the hepatic waveform phases during the cardiac cycle. Inter-observer variability for identifying portal and intra-renal vein Doppler patterns were good, as previously reported [21].

The IVC diameter was measured in its intra-hepatic portion at 2 cm of the junction with the hepatic veins using a longitudinal view from a sub-xiphoid position [26]. When the sub-xiphoid window was not appropriate the probe was moved laterally to the right side of the body, over the liver, until an adequate view was achieved. The maximal diameter during the respiratory cycle was measured.

Development of VExUS grading system prototypes

Based on an original concept (P.R.), a multidisciplinary team composed of intensivists (A.D., P.R.), anesthesiologist (A.D.), emergency physicians (R.S., K.H.) and nephrologist (W.B.S) developed five VExUS grading system prototypes based on the severity of venous ultrasonographic markers (Fig. 1). For the hepatic vein Doppler, a systolic phase was of lesser amplitude than the diastolic phase but toward the liver was considered mild while the presence of a reversed systolic phase was considered severe [17, 27]. For the portal vein Doppler, a pulsatility fraction (PF) of 30–49% was considered mild while a PF > 50% was considered severe based on the previous

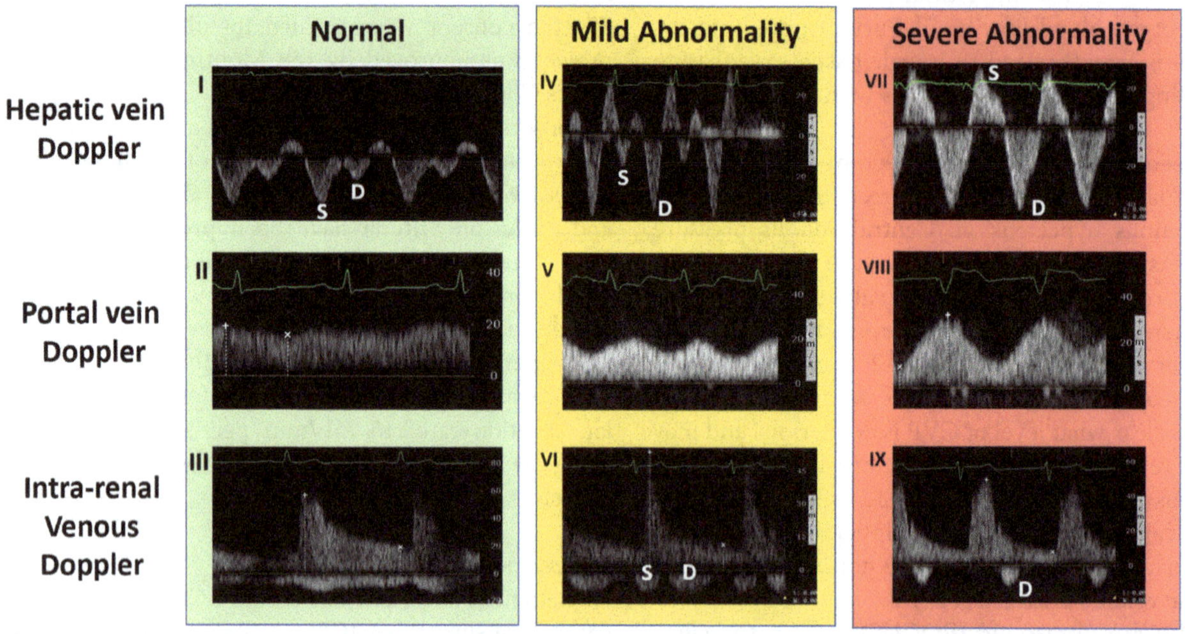

	VExUS A	VExUS B	VExUS C	VExUS D	VExUS E
Grade 0	IVC < 2 cm	IVC < 2 cm	IVC < 2 cm		
Grade 1	IVC ≥ 2 cm Normal patterns *(All three of: I, II, III)*	IVC ≥ 2 cm Normal patterns *(All three of: I, II, III)*	IVC ≥ 2 cm Normal patterns **or** mild abnormalitie(s) *(Any combination of: I, II, III, IV, V, VI)*	Normal patterns *(All three of: I, II, III)*	Normal patterns **or** mild abnormalitie(s) *(Any combination of: I, II, III, IV, V, VI)*
Grade 2: Mild congestion	IVC > 2 cm Mild abnormality in **at least one** pattern *(At least one of: IV, V, VI)*	IVC > 2 cm Mild **or** severe abnormality in **at least one** pattern *(At least one of: IV, V, VI, VII, VIII, IX)*	IVC > 2 cm Severe abnormalities in **at least one** pattern *(At least one of: VII, VIII, IX)*	Mild **or** severe abnormalities **in at least one** pattern *(At least one of: IV, V, VI, VII, VIII, IX)*	Severe abnormalities **in at least one** pattern *(At least one of: VII, VIII, IX)*
Grade 3: Severe congestion	IVC > 2 cm Severe abnormalities **in at least one** pattern *(At least one of: VII, VIII, IX)*	IVC > 2 cm Mild **or** severe abnormalities **in multiple** patterns *(At least two of: IV, V, VI, VII, VIII, IX)*	IVC > 2 cm Severe abnormalities **in multiple** patterns *(At least two of: VII, VIII, IX)*	Mild **or** severe abnormalities **in multiple** patterns *(At least two of: IV, V, VI, VII, VIII, IX)*	Severe abnormalities **in multiple** patterns *(At least two of: VII, VIII, IX)*

Fig. 1 The Venous Excess UltraSound (VExUS) grading system prototypes combining inferior vena cava (IVC) diameter and venous Doppler waveform of the portal, hepatic and interlobular renal veins. Hepatic Doppler is considered mildly abnormal when the systolic (S) component is lower in magnitude than the diastolic (D) component, but still toward the liver while it is considered severely abnormal when the S component is reversed (toward the heart). Portal Doppler is considered mildly abnormal when a variation in the velocities during the cardiac cycle of 30 to < 50% are observed, while is considered severely abnormal when a variation of ≥ 50% is seen. Intra-renal venous Doppler is considered mildly abnormal when it is discontinuous with a systolic (S) and diastolic (D) phase, while is it considered severely abnormal when it is discontinuous with only a diastolic phase seen during the cardiac cycle

studies [21, 28, 29]. For the intra-renal venous Doppler, a discontinuous pattern with a systolic and a diastolic phase was considered mild while a discontinuous pattern with only a diastolic phase was considered severe [18, 21]. The prototype grading systems were named VExUS "A" through "E" (Fig. 1) with multiple grades within each grading system. The VExUS score was determined for all patients and for all timepoints. Overall, echographic variables were > 95% complete within the dataset. In the case of a missing value for an echographic marker, the last known value for this marker for the patient (i.e., assessment performed the previous day) was imputed.

Clinical data collection

Demographic, baseline information, cumulative fluid balance information, hemodynamic parameters at the time of assessment and outcomes during hospitalization were all collected prospectively during the study as previously published [21]. The presence of left and right systolic ventricular dysfunction on trans-esophageal echocardiography performed by the attending anesthesiologist before cardiopulmonary bypass was also collected. Left ventricular dysfunction was defined as a left ventricular ejection fraction (LVEF) ≤ 40%, and right systolic ventricular dysfunction was defined by either tricuspid annular plane systolic excursion < 16 mm or right ventricular area of change < 35% [27]. Mean CVP measurements were obtained using a jugular central venous catheter. Measurements were noted before POCUS assessment at ICU admission and daily if the central line was still in place at the time of POCUS assessment. The mean CVP values were noted after verifying the position of the pressure transducer in relation with the patient. The height of the bed was adjusted if needed to insure proper positioning at the level of the right atrium (intersection between mid-axillary line and fourth intercostal space). N-terminal pro-beta natriuretic peptide (NT-pro-BNP) was also measured prospectively before surgery and on the morning of post-operative days 1, 2 and 3. The European System Operative Score Risk Evaluation score (EuroSCORE II) was calculated, as well as a validated risk score by Birnie et al. for the prediction of AKI in cardiac surgery patients based on pre-operative characteristics and validated for the Kidney Disease: Improving Global Outcomes (KDIGO) criteria [30]. During the post-operative period, AKI was defined by the KDIGO criteria as an increase of serum creatinine > 26 μmol/L within a 48-h period or 50% from baseline creatinine within a week from cardiac surgery [31]. Vasopressors (norepinephrine, vasopressin, dopamine) and inotrope (epinephrine, milrinone, dobutamine) use was noted at the time of ultrasound assessment. The vasopressor–inotrope score (VIS) was calculated to estimate the degree of pharmacologic support at the time of ultrasound assessment [32, 33]. The VIS was calculated using the following formula: VIS = dopamine dose (μg/kg/min) + dobutamine dose (μg/kg/min) + (100 * epinephrine dose (μg/kg/min)) + (10 * milrinone dose (μg/kg/min)) + (10,000 * vasopressin dose (U/kg/min)) + (100 * norepinephrine dose (μg/kg/min)) [32, 34].

Data analysis

Results are presented in number (%) for dichotomous variables and in mean ± standard deviation (SD) or median and interquartile range (IQR) for continuous variables, where appropriate. Comparisons between two groups for continuous variables were done using Student *t*-test or Mann–Whitney *U* test, as appropriate, and comparison between two groups for categorical variables was done using Chi squared test. The prevalence of each VExUS grade was presented as descriptive data for each timepoint. The association between the VExUS grades and the risk of new-onset of AKI was assessed using a Cox proportional hazards model with the VExUS grades considered as segmented time-dependent covariates. After identifying the VExUS grade most associated with AKI in univariable analysis, multivariable Cox regression was performed. A first model was constructed by including the pre-operative risk of AKI as performed by Birnie et al. [30] as an a priori covariate. This score included age, sex, body mass index, smoker status, New York Heart Association functional status, diabetes, peripheral vascular disease, chronic hypertension, hemoglobin level, renal function, recent coronary angiogram, triple vessel disease, operative priority and procedure type. In addition, a second model was created by adding the VIS as a segmented time-dependent covariate to the first model. As a sensitivity analysis, other multivariable models including CBP duration and cardiac output measured at the end of surgery were performed. Results are presented as hazard ratio (HR) with 95% confidence intervals (CI).

The sensitivity and specificity as well as the positive likelihood ratio (+LR) and the negative likelihood ratio (−LR) of the different VExUS grades assessed at ICU admission to predict AKI after cardiac surgery were presented. The same analysis was performed using different cut-offs of CVP (≥ 8, ≥ 10, ≥ 12 and ≥ 14 mmHg), as well as individual ultrasound findings included in the VExUS grading systems. The CVP cut-off used was chosen based on current literature and expert opinion [10, 11, 13, 35]. Results are presented with 95% CI. Leaf plots were created to visually compare the diagnostic performance of grade 3 of the VExUS C grading system and CVP ≥ 12 mmHg [36, 37]. Leaf plots were generated using an online tool [38]. As a supplementary analysis, specificity of grade 3 of the VExUS C grading system was compared to other variables using exact McNemar test for paired nominal data.

The association between the VExUS grading system prototypes and commonly used markers of venous congestion (cumulative fluid balance, NT-pro-BNP and CVP) and VIS was first assessed using generalized estimating equation models using a robust estimator for the covariance matrix and an exchangeable structure for the working correlation matrix was used. This type of analysis accounts for the repeated measures' design, implying that the sample was not independent. In addition to the VExUS grades, the time of assessment (4 timepoints: Day 0 to Day 3) was included as a factor in the analysis and the interaction between the studied variable and the time of ultrasound assessment was tested. We found multiple significant interactions ($p < 0.05$) with the time of assessment. Consequently, we presented the association for each timepoint and for each VExUS grade. The difference between the different grades was assessed using one-way ANOVA or Kruskall–Wallis test, where appropriate depending on the distribution of data. In the presence of a significant result ($p<0.05$), multiple post-hoc pairwise comparisons with Bonferroni correction were performed and significant results were presented. Statistical tests were performed in SPSS version 24 (IBM, Armonk, New York, USA).

Results

Complete data from all 145 participants included in the original prospective study were included in the analysis. Baseline characteristics of patients have been previously published [21] and a summary is available in Additional file 1: Table S1. The median age was 66 ± 13 years and the median risk of complications based on pre-operative characteristics according to the EuroSCORE II was 2.96% (1.70; 4.79%). Known heart failure with reduced ejection fraction (LVEF $\leq 40\%$) was present in 31 patients (21.4%) and stage III chronic kidney disease or higher (corresponding to an eGFR < 60 mL/min/1.73 m^2) was present in 37 patients (25.5%). At the start of the surgery before cardiopulmonary bypass, trans-esophageal echocardiography revealed low LVEF in 37 patients (25.5%) and systolic right ventricular dysfunction in 18 patients (12.4%). After surgery, 49 patients (33.8%) developed AKI but no patients received renal replacement therapy.

The complete distributions of all VExUS grades (0–3) according to candidate grading systems (A–E) during the peri-operative period are presented in Fig. 2. Severe venous congestion (Grade 3) was less often diagnosed with grading systems requiring the presence of severe flow abnormalities in multiple Doppler patterns (VExUS grading systems C and E) compared with grading systems requiring at least one severe Doppler finding (VExUS grading system A) or the combination of mild and severe Doppler findings (VExUS grading systems B or D). Compared with scores which did not consider IVC measurements (VExUS grading systems D and E), corresponding grading systems which included IVC measurements (VExUS grading systems B and C) identified less patients as having severe congestion (Grade 3). Before surgery, EuroSCORE II was different for all VExUS grading systems, with more severe VExUS grades being associated with a higher pre-operative risk assessment (Additional file 1: Table S2).

In the post-operative period, the presence of severe congestion (Grade 3) was associated with the development of subsequent AKI for all VExUS grading systems (Table 1). Severe congestion (Grade 3) defined by the VExUS C grading system was the most strongly associated with AKI (HR 3.69, CI 1.65–8.24, $p=0.001$). After adjustment for the baseline risk of AKI and pharmacologic support (VIS), severe congestion (Grade 3) defined by the VExUS C grading system remained associated with the subsequent development of AKI after surgery (HR 2.82, CI 1.21–6.55 $p=0.02$) (Table 2). Adjustment with cardiac output measured at the end of surgery and cardiopulmonary bypass duration yielded similar results (Additional file 1: Table S3). As for moderate congestion (Grade 2), only the VExUS C grading system was associated with the development of AKI (HR 2.65, CI 1.07–6.60 $p=0.036$).

While only considering the assessment performed at ICU admission after surgery, severe congestion (Grade 3) defined by the VExUS C grading system had a high specificity (96% CI 89–99%) but low sensitivity (27% CI 15–41%) for the development of subsequent AKI resulting in a moderate +LR of 6.37 (CI 2.19–18.5) which surpassed the performance of other grading systems (Table 3). All VExUS grading systems had a low sensitivity (<75%) resulting in poor −LR (>0.5). A low CVP cut-off (≥ 8 mmHg) had a moderately useful −LR of 0.49 (CI 0.28–0.86). However, none of the studied CVP cut-offs or individual ultrasound markers outperformed grade 3 of the VExUS C grading system with respect to the +LR. The performance of VExUS C grade 3 and CVP ≥ 12 mmHg is represented graphically in Fig. 3. The specificity of grade 3 of the VExUS C grading system was statistically better than all other candidate variables except severe portal vein pulsatility, severe alteration of intra-renal venous flow and VExUS E grade 3 (see Additional file 1: Table S4).

Other congestion markers including cumulative fluid balance, NT-pro-BNP and CVP were associated with severe congestion (Grade 3) in all studied VExUS grading systems (see Additional file 1: Table S5). However, a statistical interaction with the time of assessment is present in multiple analyses. For the VExUS C grading system, severe congestion (Grade 3) was associated with a greater cumulative fluid balance ($\beta=899$ CI 470; 1327 $p<0.001$) and a higher CVP ($\beta=2.4$ CI 0.70; 4.0 $p=0.004$) without statistical interaction with the time of assessment. While an interaction was present for the analysis involving NT-pro-BNP, a significant difference in NT-pro-BNP measurements among grades was also present at each studied timepoint was as shown in Fig. 4. Comparison for other VExUS grading systems yielded similar results (see Additional file 1: Tables S6 to S10).

Discussion

In this work, we aimed to investigate the performance of different venous congestion grading systems based on ultrasound markers to predict AKI after cardiac surgery. We found that severe congestion, defined as the presence of severe flow abnormalities in multiple Doppler patterns

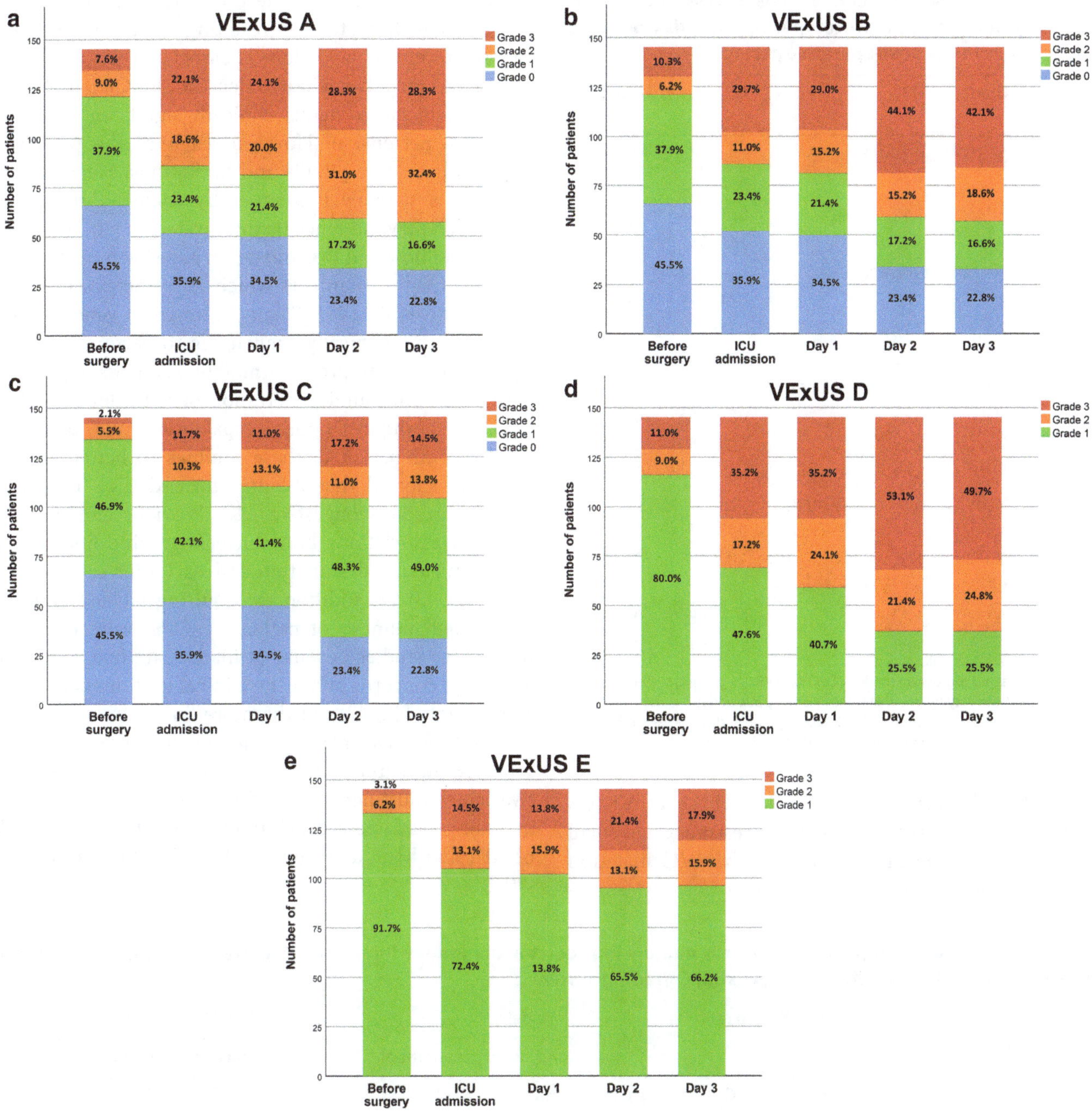

Fig. 2 Distribution of Venous Excess UltraSound (VExUS) grading system prototypes **a**, **b**, **c**, **d** and **e** in the perioperative period in 145 patients undergoing cardiac surgery

with a dilated IVC (VExUS grading system C—Grade 3), offered the strongest association with the development of subsequent AKI compared with other combinations of ultrasonographic features. Examples of VExUS C grading are presented in Fig. 5. Importantly, this association remained significant after adjustment with known risk factors for AKI as well as vasopressor–inotropic support after surgery, with a HR of 2.82. Furthermore, the presence of severe congestion defined by the VExUS C grading system at ICU admission after cardiac surgery offered a high specificity but low sensitivity to predict AKI resulting in a moderate +LR which outperformed the use of common CVP measurement cut-offs. Of note, IVC dilatation alone had poor diagnostic performance (Specificity 41%) suggesting that this commonly used ultrasound assessment in the ICU is not sufficient to

Table 1 Association between Venous Excess UltraSound (VExUS) grading system prototypes and the risk of acute kidney injury in the post-operative period

Grading system	Grade	HR	CI	*p* values
VExUS A	0	Reference category		
	1	1.10	0.44–2.73	0.84
	2	1.41	0.58–3.43	0.44
	3	3.21	1.55–6.67	0.002
VExUS B	0	Reference category		
	1	1.10	0.44–2.74	0.84
	2	2.11	0.85–2.74	0.11
	3	2.43	1.18–5.02	0.02
VExUS C	0	Reference category		
	1	1.25	0.58–2.66	0.57
	2	2.65	1.07–6.60	0.036
	3	3.69	1.65–8.24	0.001
VExUS D	0	Reference category		
	1	1.71	0.78–3.74	0.18
	2	1.95	1.02–3.75	0.045
VExUS E	0	Reference category		
	1	1.72	0.78–3.80	0.18
	2	2.68	1.41–5.12	0.003

Proportional hazard regression models (Cox) with VExUS grading systems considered as time varying covariates (i.e., VExUS grade at day 0 is used to predict acute kidney injury (AKI) at day 1, VExUS grade at day 1 is used for AKI at day 2 and so on). *HR* hazard ratio, *CI 95%* confidence intervals)

detect clinically significant congestion. However, VExUS grading systems that included IVC assessment had small improvement in specificity suggesting that IVC dilatation might be a useful to avoid false-positives.

While there is now a widespread agreement that systemic venous hypertension resulting from fluid overload and right ventricular failure is associated with multiorgan injury and adverse outcomes [39]. POCUS may enable the clinician to detect clinically significant systemic venous hypertension. However, each of the proposed markers has some pitfalls and limitations. Hepatic vein Doppler is strongly influenced by tricuspid regurgitation which may influence its interpretation [40]. Pulsatile portal vein flow and IVC dilatation have been reported in healthy athletic volunteers which raise the possibility of false-positives [24, 41]. Finally, intra-renal venous Doppler is more technically challenging to perform and has a greater chance to provide ambiguous results in patients with poor ultrasound penetration or with devices offering less-sensitive Doppler capabilities. We therefore used a combination of these findings to better predict AKI and showed that it outperformed CVP measurement to predict congestive AKI. Previous studies have reported associations between echographic findings of right ventricular dysfunction and AKI after cardiac surgery [42, 43]. In addition to requiring advanced training, a high number of patients (>25%) were excluded from these studies because of inadequate image quality. This raise concerns about the clinical usefulness of these assessments [42, 43]. Furthermore, in contrast to previous work, we performed a time-dependant analysis with repeated measurements. In addition, we performed multivariable adjustment for obvious potential confounders including validated scores summarizing the baseline risk of AKI and hemodynamic stability after cardiac surgery [30, 32].

Table 2 Multivariable proportional hazards models to predict acute kidney injury in 145 patients after cardiac surgery using the Venous EXcess UltraSound (VExUS) C grading system

	Crude hazard ratio			Model 1			Model 2		
				Adjusted hazard ratio[a]			Adjusted hazard ratio[b]		
	HR	CI	*p*	HR	CI	*p*	HR	CI	*p*
VExUS C Grade 0	Reference category			Reference category			Reference category		
VExUS C Grade 1	1.25	0.58–2.66	0.57	1.13	0.52–2.43	0.76	1.13	0.52–2.43	0.76
VExUS C Grade 2	2.65	1.07–6.60	0.036	2.31	0.92–5.80	0.074	2.32	0.92–5.83	0.073
VExUS C Grade 3	3.69	1.65–8.24	0.001	2.83	1.22–6.55	0.015	2.82	1.21–6.55	0.016
Pre-operative AKI risk score [30]	1.02	1.01–1.04	0.001	1.02	1.003–1.03	0.019	1.02	1.003–1.033	0.02
Vasopressor–inotrope score	1.01	0.99–1.03	0.51				1.001	0.98–1.03	0.93

Multivariable proportional hazard regression model (Cox) with the VExUS grade considered as a time-varying covariate (i.e., VExUS grade at day 0 is used to predict AKI at day 1, VExUS grade at day 1 is used for AKI at day 2 and so on). *HR* hazard ratio, *CI 95%* confidence intervals

[a] Variables included in the multivariate model were the VExUS C grade (segmented time-dependant) and pre-operative AKI risk score [30]

[b] Variables included in the multivariate model were the VExUS C grade (segmented time-dependant), vasopressor–inotrope score (segmented time-dependant) and pre-operative AKI risk score [30]

Table 3 Performance parameters of the different VExUS grading systems assessed at ICU admission to predict acute kidney injury in 145 patients after cardiac surgery

Grading system	Grade	Specificity (CI)	Sensitivity (CI)	+LR (CI)	– LR (CI)
VExUS A	1	41% (31–51%)	73% (59–85)	1.24 (0.98–1.57)	0.65 (0.40–1.07)
	2	67% (56–76%)	55% (40–69%)	1.65 (1.13–2.42)	0.67 (0.49–0.93)
	3	86% (78–92%)	39% (26–54%)	2.86 (1.54–5.30)	0.71 (0.56–0.89)
VExUS B	1	41% (31–51%)	73% (59–85%)	1.24 (0.98–1.57)	0.65 (0.40–1.07)
	2	67% (56–76%)	55% (40–69%)	1.65 (1.13–2.42)	0.67 (0.49–0.93)
	3	77% (67–85%)	43% (29–58%)	1.87 (1.15–3.05)	0.74 (0.58–0.95)
VExUS C	1	41% (31–51%)	73% (59–85%)	1.24 (0.98–1.57)	0.65 (0.40–1.07)
	2	87% (78–92%)	39% (26–54%)	2.86 (1.55–5.30)	0.71 (0.56–0.89)
	3	96% (89–99%)	27% (15–41%)	6.37 (2.19–18.5)	0.77 (0.65–0.91)
VExUS D	2	52% (42–62%)	61% (46–74%)	1.28 (0.94–1.73)	0.74 (0.51–1.08)
	3	70% (59–79%)	45% (31–60%)	1.49 (0.96–2.29)	0.79 (0.61–1.03)
VExUS E	2	79% (69–87%)	41% (27–56%)	1.96 (1.17–3.28)	0.75 (0.59–0.95)
	3	93% (85–97%)	29% (17–43%)	3.92 (1.69–9.07)	0.77 (0.64–0.92)
Portal Doppler only	Mild	73% (64–82%)	39% (25–52%)	1.46 (0.90–2.37)	0.83 (0.65–1.08)
	Severe	91% (86–97%)	27% (14–39%)	3.12 (1.39–7.01)	0.80 (0.67–0.96)
Hepatic vein Doppler only	Mild	56% (46–66%)	51% (37–65%)	1.16 (0.81–1.66)	0.88 (0.62–1.23)
	Severe	84% (76–91%)	34% (20–48%)	2.11 (1.15–3.89)	0.79 (0.63–0.98)
Renal Doppler only	Mild	80% (72–88%)	45% (31–59%)	2.27 (1.36–3.77)	0.69 (0.52–0.90)
	Severe	94% (89–99%)	25% (12–37%)	3.92 (1.57–9.81)	0.81 (0.68–0.95)
CVP	≥ 8 mmHg	48% (37–59%)	77% (61–88%)	1.47 (1.13–1.90)	0.49 (0.28–0.86)
	≥ 10 mmHg	66% (55–75%)	58% (42–73%)	1.71 (1.16–2.51)	0.64 (0.44–0.91)
	≥ 12 mmHg	83% (73–90%)	33% (20–49%)	1.91 (1.02–3.59)	0.81 (0.66–1.01)

CI confidence intervals, *CVP* central venous pressure, *+LR* positive likelihood ratio, *– LR* negative likelihood ratio

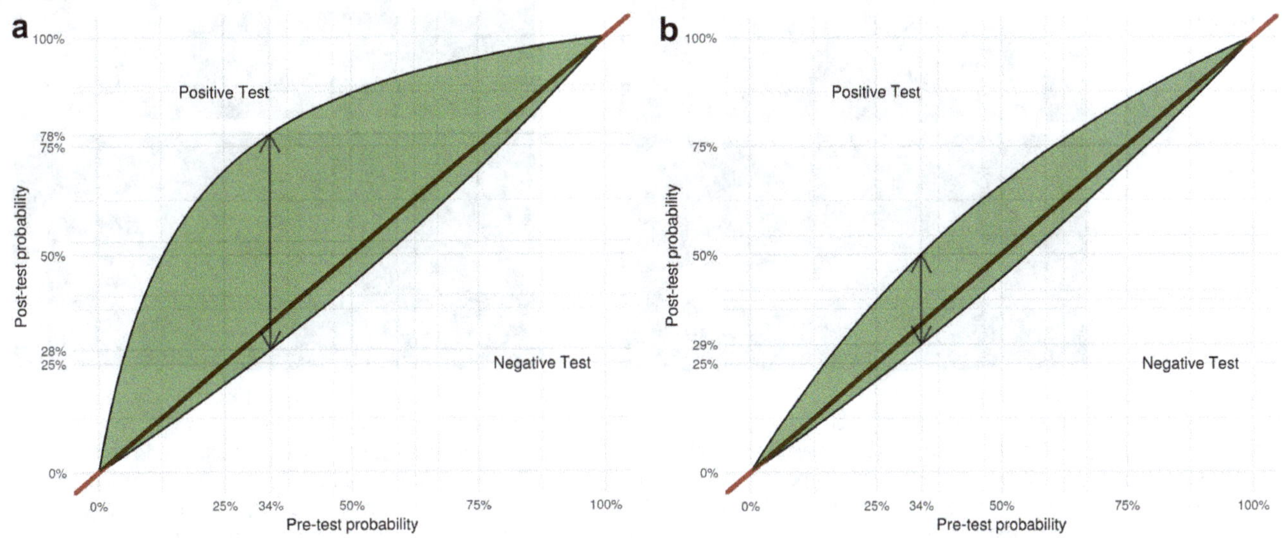

Fig. 3 Leaf plots displaying the relationship between the assumed pre-test probability (on the *x*-axis) and the post-test probability (on the *y*-axis) of acute kidney injury (AKI) for the following cut-off: **a** severe congestion (Grade 3) defined by the VExUS C grading system and **b** central venous pressure of ≥ 12 mmHg. The upper half part of the curve indicates the post-test probability in case of a positive result while the lower half indicated is for a negative test result. The dashed double-sided arrow indicated the test performance considering the incidence of acute kidney injury (pre-rest probability) within the studied cohort (33.8%)

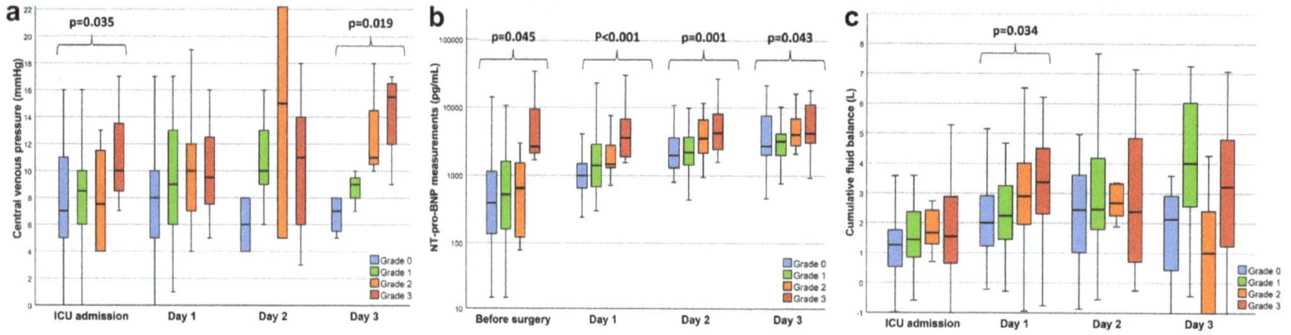

Fig. 4 Clinical parameters in relationship with the Venous Excess UltraSound (VExUS) grading system C during the peri-operative period. **a** Central venous pressure at the time of ultrasound assessment in relationship with VExUS C grading system. **b** N-terminal pro-beta natriuretic peptide (NT-pro-BNP) in relationship with VExUS C grading system. **c** Cumulative fluid balance in relationship with VExUS C grading system. Significant results ($p < 0.05$) are highlighted. Complete results of comparisons are presented in Additional file 1: Table S3

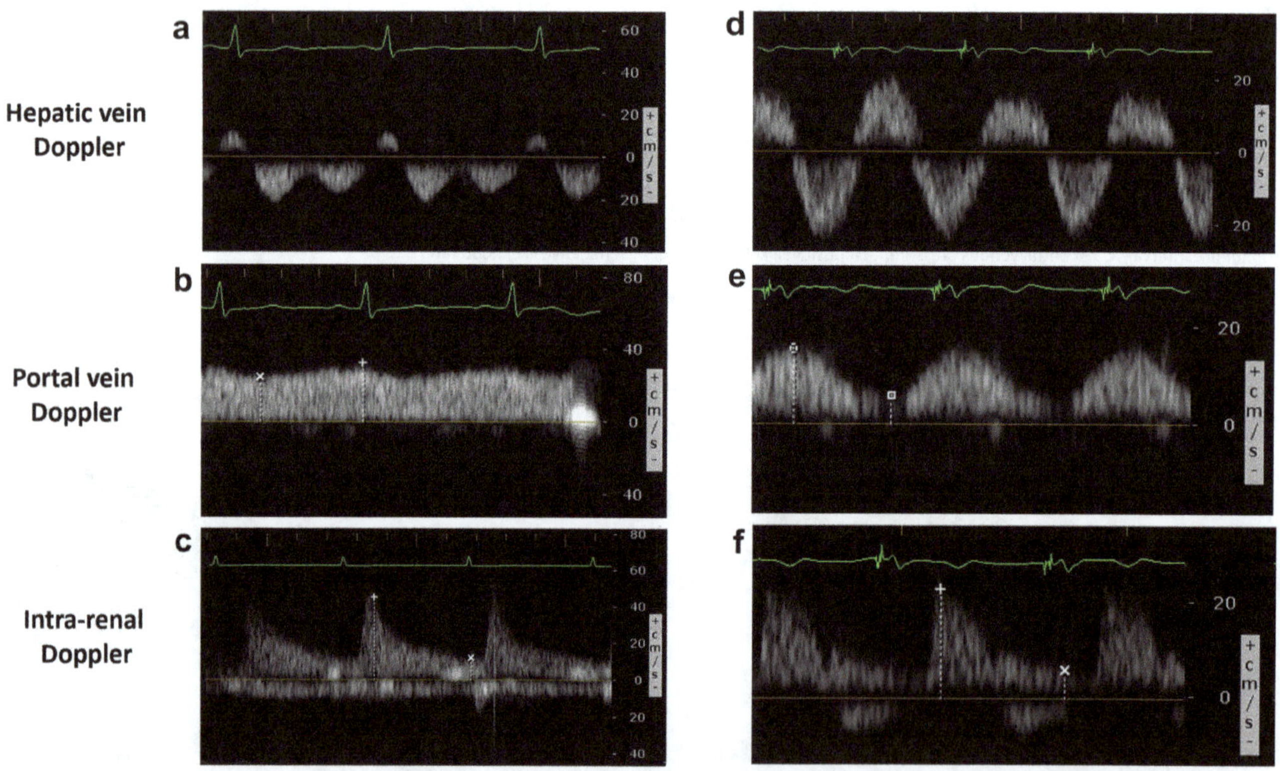

Fig. 5 Example of VExUS C grading system assessment in cardiac surgery. Patient #1: A 55-year-old woman undergoing tricuspid valve repair aortic valve replacement and mitral valve replacement known with chronic kidney disease (baseline eGFR = 35 mL/min/1.73 m^2) with left ventricular ejection fraction of 40% and a high risk of major complications (EuroSCORE II = 16.8%) presented the following ultrasound findings at ICU admission after surgery: **a** Normal hepatic triphasic pattern, **b** a non-pulsatile portal flow and **c** continuous intral-renal venous flow and an IVC diameter of > 2.1 cm (not shown) corresponding to Grade 1 of VExUS C grading system. The patient did not develop acute kidney injury, was extubated 2.2 h after ICU admission and was discharged from the ICU less than 24 h after surgery. Patient #2: A 70-year-old man undergoing mitral valve repair with a left ventricular ejection fraction of 50% and a moderate risk of major complication (EuroSCORE II = 1.54%) presented the following ultrasound findings at ICU admission after surgery complicated by right ventricular dysfunction after cardiopulmonary bypass: **d** Systolic reversal of the hepatic venous flow, **e** severe portal flow pulsatility and **f** severe alteration in intra-renal venous flow corresponding to Grade 3 of the VExUS C grading system. The patient developed severe acute kidney injury and delirium in the post-operative period

In the present work, the low sensitivity to predict AKI is not surprising since venous congestion is unlikely to be a contributive factor in all cases. A multitude of other factors, venous congestion being only one of them, may trigger AKI in the peri-operative period [44]. However, the positive likelihood ratio exhibited by VExUS C Grade 3 indicates that most patients (96%) with these ultrasound features at ICU admission will develop AKI in the post-operative period. A small proportion of patients did not develop AKI despite presenting signs of severe venous congestion. Clearly, the presence of severe congestion alone is not enough to perfectly predict organ failure. However, this may not be entirely unexpected as perfusion also depends on arterial flow. Damman et al. elegantly demonstrated in a cohort of acutely decompensated congestive heart failure patients that venous hypertension was particularly deleterious in patients with reduced cardiac output [45]. This finding is also consistent with early animal experiments in which only very high venous pressure ($\geq$25 mmHg) resulted in a decrease in the glomerular filtration rate when arterial blood flow was maintained [7, 46]. It is likely that the VExUS grading system, while being useful to assess the clinical importance of venous hypertension, will only give us partial information on how to guide intervention aimed at improving organ perfusion which could be complemented additional information related to arterial pefusion.

The present work has several limitations. First, we performed a relatively small single-center study including only cardiac surgery patients which limits the generalizability of the findings. Most importantly, the formation of interstitial edema also depends on vascular permeability which may be quite variable depending of the underlying disease. Consequently, caution should be taken when interpreting these finding in other clinical contexts. Furthermore, while the relationship between portal Doppler patterns and other echocardiographic variables during cardiac surgery has been previously described by our group [20] and others [47], we did not assess right ventricular function in this study which precludes us to determine if systolic right ventricular dysfunction was an important mechanism associated with severe VExUS grade in our cohort. Furthermore, because this analysis was based on retrospective data, other pertinent ultrasound features such as the respiratory collapsibility, 3-dimensional measurements of the IVC [48] or the evaluation of extra-vascular lung water could not be integrated in the VExUS grading systems. Finally, the confidence interval over the diagnostic performance parameters (sensitivity, specificity, +LR, −LR) is large due to the limited number of patients available in this cohort which also limits the power to detect significant differences in the performance of the studied grading systems. Consequently, we cannot definitely confirm based on the available data the superiority of the VExUS C grading system compared to the other candidate classifications or compared to individual findings.

Conclusions

In conclusion, we used existing data to propose a novel grading system for venous congestion, the Venous Excess UltraSound (VExUS) grading system based on the combination of multiple ultrasound findings. The presence of at least two severe alterations of hepatic vein, portal vein or intra-renal venous flow on pulse-wave Doppler ultrasound with an IVC of $\geq$2 cm of diameter at ICU admission after cardiac surgery indicates a high risk of post-operative AKI. Further studies should aim to validate this grading system in different clinical settings, confirm the optimal criteria for diagnostic performance and determine whether it could be used to personalize interventions to improve organ perfusion.

Supplementary information

Additional file 1. Quantifying systemic congestion with Point-Of-Care ultrasound: development of the Venous EXcess UltraSound (VExUS) grading system.

Abbreviations

AKI: Acute kidney injury; CI: Confidence interval; CVP: Central venous pressure; EuroSCORE II: European System Operative Score Risk Evaluation score; HR: Hazard ratio; KDIGO: Kidney disease: improving global outcomes; ICU: Intensive care unit; IQR: Interquartile range; IVC: Inferior vena cava; LR: Likelihood ratio; LVEF: Left ventricular ejection fraction; NT-Pro-BNP: N-terminal pro-beta natriuretic peptide; PF: Pulsatility fraction; POCUS: Point-Of-Care ultrasound; SD: Standard deviation; VExUS: Venous Excess Ultrasound; VIS: Vasopressor–inotrope score.

Acknowledgements

None.

Authors' contributions

WBS designed and conducted the study, performed data analysis and drafted the manuscript, PL, KH and RS contributed to the design of the study and reviewed the manuscript, JB and YL contributed to data analysis and reviewed the manuscript, AYD overviewed the conduct of the study, contributed to study design, to results interpretation and reviewed the manuscript. All authors read and approved the final manuscript.

Author details

[1] Department of Anesthesiology and Intensive Care, Montreal Heart Institute, Université de Montréal, Montreal, QC, Canada. [2] Division of Nephrology, Centre Hospitalier de l'Université de Montreal, 1000, Rue St-Denis, Montreal, QC H2X 0C1, Canada. [3] Division of Intensive Care, Santa Cabrini Hospital, Montreal, QC, Canada. [4] Department of Emergency Medicine, Loma Linda University School of Medicine, Loma Linda, CA 92354, USA. [5] Division of Nephrology, Hôpital Sacré-Cœur de Montréal, Montreal, QC, Canada. [6] Department of Surgery and Critical Care, Montreal Heart Institute, Université de Montréal, Montréal, QC, Canada. [7] Departments of Critical Care and Emergency Medicine, Washington Hospital Center, Georgetown University, Washington, DC, USA. [8] Division of Intensive Care, Centre Hospitalier de L'Université de Montreal, Montreal, QC, Canada.

References

1. Seymour CW, Rosengart MR (2015) Septic Shock: advances in diagnosis and treatment. JAMA 314:708–717
2. van Diepen S, Katz Jason N, Albert Nancy M, Henry Timothy D, Jacobs Alice K, Kapur Navin K, Kilic A, Menon V, Ohman EM, Sweitzer Nancy K, Thiele H, Washam Jeffrey B, Cohen Mauricio G (2017) Contemporary management of cardiogenic shock: a scientific statement from the American Heart Association. Circulation 136:e232–e268
3. Squara P, Hollenberg S, Payen D (2019) Reconsidering vasopressors for cardiogenic shock: everything should be made as simple as possible, but not simpler. Chest 156:392–401
4. De Backer D, Orbegozo Cortes D, Donadello K, Vincent J-L (2014) Pathophysiology of microcirculatory dysfunction and the pathogenesis of septic shock. Virulence 5:73–79
5. Saito S, Uchino S, Takinami M, Uezono S, Bellomo R (2016) Postoperative blood pressure deficit and acute kidney injury progression in vasopressor-dependent cardiovascular surgery patients. Crit Care 20:74
6. Cruces P, Salas C, Lillo P, Salomon T, Lillo F, Hurtado DE (2014) The renal compartment: a hydraulic view. Intensive Care Med Exp 2:26
7. Winton FR (1931) The influence of venous pressure on the isolated mammalian kidney. J Physiol 72:49–61
8. Lim HS (2016) Cardiogenic shock: failure of oxygen delivery and oxygen utilization. Clin Cardiol 39:477–483
9. Figg KK, Nemergut EC (2009) Error in central venous pressure measurement. Anesth Analg 108:1209–1211
10. Chen KP, Cavender S, Lee J, Feng M, Mark RG, Celi LA, Mukamal KJ, Danziger J (2016) Peripheral edema, central venous pressure, and risk of AKI in critical illness. Clin J Am Soc Nephrol 11:602–608
11. Boyd JH, Forbes J, Nakada TA, Walley KR, Russell JA (2011) Fluid resuscitation in septic shock: a positive fluid balance and elevated central venous pressure are associated with increased mortality. Crit Care Med 39:259–265
12. Li DK, Wang XT, Liu DW (2017) Association between elevated central venous pressure and outcomes in critically ill patients. Ann Intensive Care 7:83
13. De Backer D, Vincent J-L (2018) Should we measure the central venous pressure to guide fluid management? Ten answers to 10 questions. Crit Care 22:43
14. Perren A, Markmann M, Merlani G, Marone C, Merlani P (2011) Fluid balance in critically ill patients. Should we really rely on it? Minerva Anestesiol 77:802–811
15. Flentje KM, Knight CL, Stromfeldt I, Chakrabarti A, Friedman ND (2018) Recording patient bodyweight in hospitals: are we doing well enough? Intern Med J 48:124–128
16. Cook DJ, Simel DL (1996) The rational clinical examination. Does this patient have abnormal central venous pressure? JAMA 275:630–634
17. Beaubien-Souligny W, Bouchard J, Desjardins G, Lamarche Y, Liszkowski M, Robillard P, Denault A (2017) Extracardiac signs of fluid overload in the critically ill cardiac patient: a focused evaluation using bedside ultrasound. Can J Cardiol 33:88–100
18. Iida N, Seo Y, Sai S, Machino-Ohtsuka T, Yamamoto M, Ishizu T, Kawakami Y, Aonuma K (2016) Clinical implications of intrarenal hemodynamic evaluation by Doppler ultrasonography in heart failure. JACC Heart Fail 4:674–682
19. Ikeda Y, Ishii S, Yazaki M, Fujita T, Iida Y, Kaida T, Nabeta T, Nakatani E, Maekawa E, Yanagisawa T, Koitabashi T, Inomata T, Ako J (2018) Portal congestion and intestinal edema in hospitalized patients with heart failure. Heart Vessels 33:740–751
20. Eljaiek R, Cavayas YA, Rodrigue E, Desjardins G, Lamarche Y, Toupin F, Denault AY, Beaubien-Souligny W (2019) High postoperative portal venous flow pulsatility indicates right ventricular dysfunction and predicts complications in cardiac surgery patients. Br J Anaesth 122:206–214
21. Beaubien-Souligny W, Benkreira A, Robillard P, Bouabdallaoui N, Chasse M, Desjardins G, Lamarche Y, White M, Bouchard J, Denault A (2018) Alterations in portal vein flow and intrarenal venous flow are associated with acute kidney injury after cardiac surgery: a prospective observational cohort study. J Am Heart Assoc 7:e009961
22. Goldhammer E, Mesnick N, Abinader EG, Sagiv M (1999) Dilated inferior vena cava: a common echocardiographic finding in highly trained elite athletes. J Am Soc Echocardiogr 12:988–993
23. Hedman K, Nylander E, Henriksson J, Bjarnegard N, Brudin L, Tamas E (2016) Echocardiographic characterization of the inferior vena cava in trained and untrained females. Ultrasound Med Biol 42:2794–2802
24. Gallix BP, Taourel P, Dauzat M, Bruel JM, Lafortune M (1997) Flow pulsatility in the portal venous system: a study of Doppler sonography in healthy adults. AJR Am J Roentgenol 169:141–144
25. Levey AS, Coresh J, Greene T, Stevens LA, Zhang YL, Hendriksen S, Kusek JW, Van Lente F, Epidemiology Chronic Kidney Disease (2006) Using standardized serum creatinine values in the modification of diet in renal disease study equation for estimating glomerular filtration rate. Ann Intern Med 145:247–254
26. Wallace DJ, Allison M, Stone MB (2010) Inferior vena cava percentage collapse during respiration is affected by the sampling location: an ultrasound study in healthy volunteers. Acad Emerg Med 17:96–99
27. Rudski LG, Lai WW, Afilalo J, Hua L, Handschumacher MD, Chandrasekaran K, Solomon SD, Louie EK, Schiller NB (2010) Guidelines for the echocardiographic assessment of the right heart in adults: a report from the American Society of Echocardiography endorsed by the European Association of Echocardiography, a registered branch of the European Society of Cardiology, and the Canadian Society of Echocardiography. J Am Soc Echocardiogr 23:685–713 **(quiz 786-688)**
28. Denault AY, Beaubien-Souligny W, Elmi-Sarabi M, Eljaiek R, El-Hamamsy I, Lamarche Y, Chronopoulos A, Lambert J, Bouchard J, Desjardins G (2017) Clinical significance of portal hypertension diagnosed with bedside ultrasound after cardiac surgery. Anesth Analg 124:1109–1115
29. Benkreira A, Beaubien-Souligny W, Mailhot T, Bouabdallaoui N, Robillard P, Desjardins G, Lamarche Y, Cossette S, Denault A (2019) Portal hypertension is associated with congestive encephalopathy and delirium after cardiac surgery. Can J Cardiol 35:1134–1141
30. Birnie K, Verheyden V, Pagano D, Bhabra M, Tilling K, Sterne JA, Murphy GJ, Collaborators UAiCS (2014) Predictive models for kidney disease: improving global outcomes (KDIGO) defined acute kidney injury in UK cardiac surgery. Crit Care 18:606
31. Kellum JA, Lameire N, Aspelin P, Barsoum RS, Burdmann EA, Goldstein SL, Herzog CA, Joannidis M, Kribben A, Levey AS, MacLeod AM (2013) Kidney disease: improving global outcomes (KDIGO) CKD Work Group. KDIGO 2012 clinical practice guideline for the evaluation and management of chronic kidney disease. Kidney inter Suppl 3:1–150
32. Koponen T, Karttunen J, Musialowicz T, Pietilainen L, Uusaro A, Lahtinen P (2019) Vasoactive-inotropic score and the prediction of morbidity and mortality after cardiac surgery. Br J Anaesth 122:428–436
33. Gaies MG, Gurney JG, Yen AH, Napoli ML, Gajarski RJ, Ohye RG, Charpie JR, Hirsch JC (2010) Vasoactive-inotropic score as a predictor of morbidity and mortality in infants after cardiopulmonary bypass. Pediatr Crit Care Med 11:234–238
34. McIntosh AM, Tong S, Deakyne SJ, Davidson JA, Scott HF (2017) Validation of the vasoactive-inotropic score in pediatric sepsis. Pediatr Crit Care Med 18:750–757
35. Legrand M, Dupuis C, Simon C, Gayat E, Mateo J, Lukaszewicz AC, Payen D (2013) Association between systemic hemodynamics and septic acute kidney injury in critically ill patients: a retrospective observational study. Crit Care 17:R278
36. Zampieri FG, Einav S (2019) When will less monitoring and diagnostic testing benefit the patient more? Intensive Care Med 45(10):1447–1450
37. Coulthard MG, Coulthard T (2019) The leaf plot: a novel way of presenting the value of tests. Br J Gen Pract 69:205–206
38. Saxhaug L (2019) Leaf plot. In: Editor (ed)^(eds) Book Leaf plot. City, pp. Leaf plot generator
39. Prowle JR, Echeverri JE, Ligabo EV, Ronco C, Bellomo R (2010) Fluid balance and acute kidney injury. Nat Rev Nephrol 6:107–115
40. Scheinfeld MH, Bilali A, Koenigsberg M (2009) Understanding the spectral Doppler waveform of the hepatic veins in health and disease. Radiographics 29:2081–2098
41. Mordi I, Manian U, Bagur R, Tzemos N (2019) Diagnosis and follow-up of idiopathic dilatation of inferior vena cava. Echocardiography 36:831–836
42. Yockelson SR, Heitner SB, Click S, Geleto G, Treggiari MM, Hutchens MP (2019) Right ventricular systolic performance determined by 2D speckle-tracking echocardiography and acute kidney injury after cardiac surgery. J Cardiothorac Vasc Anesth 33:725–731

43. Guinot PG, Abou-Arab O, Longrois D, Dupont H (2015) Right ventricular systolic dysfunction and vena cava dilatation precede alteration of renal function in adult patients undergoing cardiac surgery: an observational study. Eur J Anaesthesiol 32:535–542
44. Thiele RH, Isbell JM, Rosner MH (2015) AKI associated with cardiac surgery. Clin J Am Soc Nephrol 10:500–514
45. Damman K, Navis G, Smilde TD, Voors AA, van der Bij W, van Veldhuisen DJ, Hillege HL (2007) Decreased cardiac output, venous congestion and the association with renal impairment in patients with cardiac dysfunction. Eur J Heart Fail 9:872–878
46. Firth JD, Raine AE, Ledingham JG (1988) Raised venous pressure: a direct cause of renal sodium retention in oedema? Lancet 1:1033–1035
47. Singh NG, Kumar KN, Nagaraja PS, Manjunatha N (2020) Portal venous pulsatility fraction, a novel transesophageal echocardiographic marker for right ventricular dysfunction in cardiac surgical patients. Ann Card Anaesth 23:39–42
48. Huguet R, Fard D, d'Humieres T, Brault-Meslin O, Faivre L, Nahory L, Dubois-Rande JL, Ternacle J, Oliver L, Lim P (2018) Three-dimensional inferior vena cava for assessing central venous pressure in patients with cardiogenic shock. J Am Soc Echocardiogr 31:1034–1043

8

The development of a provincial multidisciplinary framework of consensus-based standards for Point-of-care Ultrasound at the University of Saskatchewan

Paul Olszynski[1*], Daniel J. Kim[2], Irene W. Y. Ma[3], Michelle Clunie[4], Peggy Lambos[5], Tom Guzowski[6], Matthew Butz[7] and Brent Thoma[1]

Abstract

Objectives: The development and adoption of Point-of-Care Ultrasound (POCUS) across disciplines have created challenges and opportunities in implementing training and utilization standards. Within the context of a large, geographically disparate province, we sought to develop a multidisciplinary POCUS framework outlining consensus-based standards.

Methods: A core working group of local POCUS leaders from Anesthesia, Emergency Medicine, Family Medicine, Intensive Care, Internal Medicine, Pediatrics, and Trauma, in collaboration with western Canadian colleagues, developed a list of key domains for the framework along with a range of potential standards for each area. The members of the working group and the registrants for a multidisciplinary Roundtable discussion at the University of Saskatchewan's annual POCUS conference (SASKSONO19, Saskatoon, Saskatchewan, March 2nd, 2019) were invited to complete a survey on POCUS standards for each domain. The survey results were presented to and discussed by participants at the Roundtable discussion at SASKSONO19 who reached consensus on modified standards for each domain. The modified standards were considered for endorsement by all conference attendees using an audience-response system.

Results: The working group proposed standards in eight domains: scope of use, credentialing and privileges, documentation, quality assurance, leadership and governance, teaching, research, and equipment maintenance. Consensus on modified standards was achieved in the 18 participant Roundtable. Each standard was then endorsed by >90% of conference respondents.

Conclusion: The resulting framework will inform the utilization of POCUS within Saskatchewan. Both this process and its outcomes could inform the development of multidisciplinary POCUS standards within other jurisdictions.

Keywords: Point of Care Ultrasound, Framework, Standards, Multidisciplinary, Consensus, Quality assurance

*Correspondence: p.olszynski@usask.ca
[1] Department of Emergency Medicine, University of Saskatchewan, Saskatoon, Canada
Full list of author information is available at the end of the article

Introduction

Point of Care Ultrasound (POCUS) is defined as "diagnostic or procedural guidance ultrasound that is performed by a clinician during a patient encounter to help guide the evaluation and management of that patient." [1] It can impact a range of patient-related outcomes including diagnostic accuracy [2–6], time to diagnosis [7, 8], time to definitive management [8–10], procedural safety [11–16], decreased complications [15, 16], morbidity [17, 18], and mortality [19]. Several disciplines have developed guidelines and standards for the use of POCUS in clinical practice [12, 13, 20–25]. These POCUS standards offer guidance for evidence-based application, general training requirements, documentation standards, quality assurance, and equipment maintenance. As more healthcare disciplines adopt POCUS, it will be increasingly common for healthcare providers to exchange POCUS findings during transitions in care.

POCUS is used by a wide range of disciplines. While individual applications and specific uses of POCUS vary between disciplines, domains such as scope of use, training, and governance are similar and amenable to forming a common standard [26]. Multidisciplinary POCUS collaboration and consensus on standards may help ensure consistent patient care and support optimal POCUS training within our clinical context. The establishment of a common framework of standards for POCUS users may also increase the quality of POCUS scans and improve communication regarding patient findings. Given that some disciplines have more extensive experience in the integration of POCUS into clinical practice, we anticipate that the creation of a multidisciplinary, mutually agreed upon POCUS framework will facilitate the spread of best practices between disciplines.

We sought to develop and build consensus around a local multidisciplinary framework of consensus-based POCUS standards. We believe that this process could be utilized by other institutions and/or health associations to develop their own set of multidisciplinary POCUS standards.

Methods

Collectively, we developed an iterative, four-part process to draft and build consensus around a multidisciplinary framework of POCUS standards (Fig. 1). Our process was informed in part by similar consensus-based processes carried out by colleagues in other fields [27, 28]. A Research Ethics Board exemption was sought and obtained from the University of Saskatchewan's Research Ethics Board (BEH 957). Participation in any of the aspects of the framework process was voluntary and consent was implied through participation.

First, a working group of local POCUS leaders from Anesthesia, Critical Care, Emergency Medicine, Family

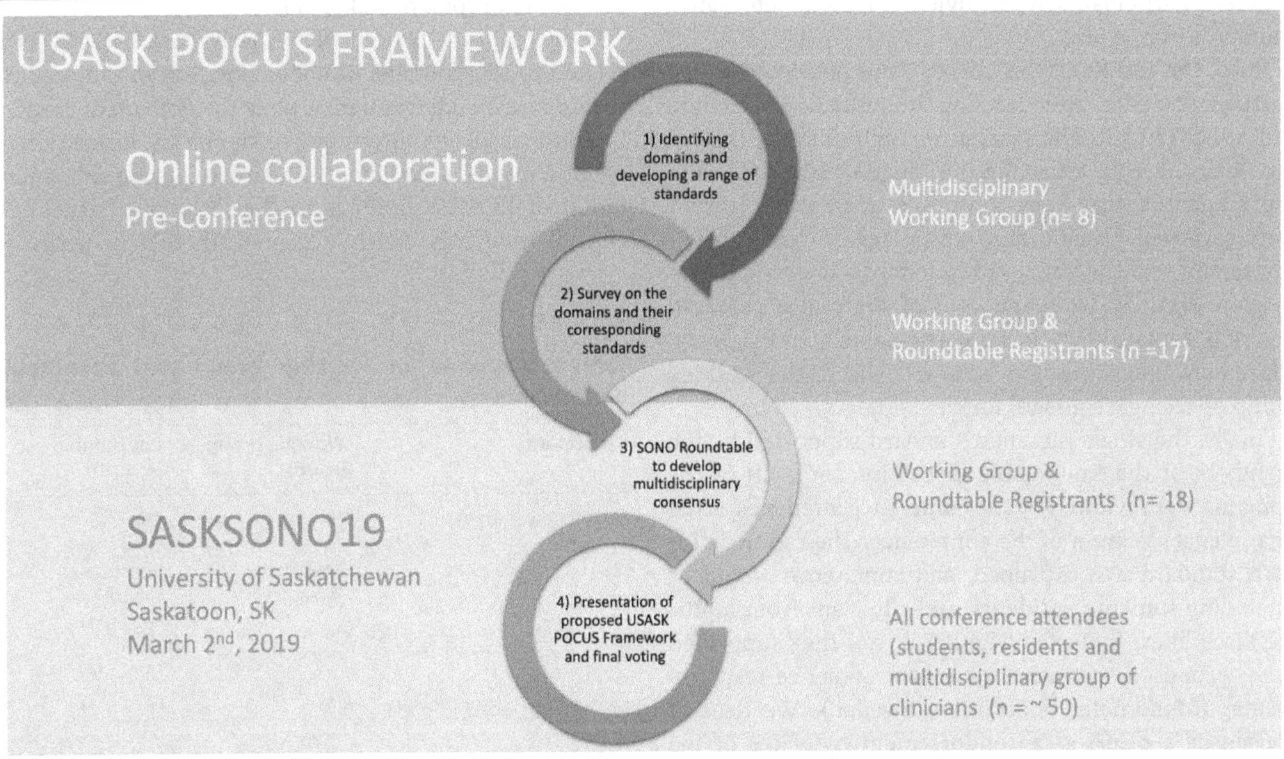

Fig. 1 Four-part process to draft and build consensus around a multidisciplinary framework of POCUS standards

Medicine, Internal Medicine, Pediatrics, and Trauma was identified based upon their leadership roles in the adoption of POCUS within their discipline in Saskatchewan and subsequently invited to participate via email invitations. The expertise within this group was buttressed through collaboration with western Canadian POCUS leaders that had been invited to present at the University of Saskatchewan's annual POCUS Conference (SASKSONO19, Saskatoon, Saskatchewan, March 2nd, 2019). We reviewed other previously published domain-specific POCUS guidelines to develop a list of key domains for a multidisciplinary framework [12, 13, 20–25]. Once the domains had been determined, a range of potential standards for each domain was proposed by one working group member (PO). These potential standards were disseminated to the working group who reviewed and edited them until it was felt that they represented a reasonable possible standard that could be considered (Additional file 1: Appendix S1).

Second, members of the working group along with the registrants for a Roundtable discussion at SASKSONO19 were invited to complete a survey of the aforementioned proposed standards. Roundtable participants were required to be clinicians who use POCUS regularly in their practice. The survey was hosted on Google Forms (Google, Mountain View, CA) and asked each participant to indicate their preferred standard from the range of potential standards developed for each domain. 'Other' was also an option within each domain and, when selected, participants were invited to input alternative standards in free text.

Third, the results of this survey were presented to the participants who attended the Roundtable discussion at SASKSONO19. The results for each domain, including both the vote totals for the range of standards and the standards that were proposed within the survey were reviewed. Where there was a lack of clear consensus on one of the proposed standards, a detailed discussion occurred with the goal of drafting a standard for each domain that all the participants could support. Ultimately, consensus was achieved within the working group on a single standard for each domain.

Finally, the single modified standard supported by the members of the Roundtable discussion for each of the domains was reviewed by the conference attendees at the final plenary session of the conference. The rationale for each standard was explained, and conference attendees (including students, residents, and clinicians from multiple disciplines) indicated whether or not they supported each proposed standard using an audience-response system (Mentimeter, Stockholm, Sweden). We defined consensus a priori as an endorsement by >80% of the respondents in each of our iterative consensus process (working group members, roundtable participants and conference attendees).

Results

The eight working group participants developed a list of nine domains to be addressed in the framework (scope of use, credentialing and privileges, documentation, quality assurance, leadership and governance, teaching, research, and equipment maintenance) and proposed three potential standards for each (Additional file 1: Appendix S1).

The survey of the potential standards sent to the working group members and Roundtable registrants was completed by 17 clinicians (Table 1). Survey results (Table 2) revealed unanimous agreement in some domains (e.g., Scope of Use: The appropriate application of POCUS should be defined by individual disciplines and be used whenever supported by reasonable evidence) whereas there were a range of opinions and suggestions on other domains (e.g., Documentation standards). The standards that were suggested for each domain are outlined in Additional file 2: Appendix S2.

The survey results (Table 2) were presented to the 18 attendees at the Roundtable discussion (Table 1). For each domain, informal consensus was sought and obtained on one of the initial proposed standards or a new standard drafted within the session. Several items within the framework generated significant discussion at the Roundtable, likely stemming from the variable stages of development and utilization of POCUS by the multidisciplinary group of stakeholders.

Image capture proved particularly controversial as it related to the domains of documentation in the medical record and quality assurance while the domain of credentials and privileges also required significant discussion to reach consensus. While a standard requiring documentation of POCUS findings in the form of a structured clinical note was widely accepted, there was extensive

Table 1 Discipline of working group and roundtable participants

Participants	Working group ($n=8$)		Roundtable ($n=18$)	
Saskatchewan-based	EM	3	EM	7
	IM	1	IM	1
	Anesthesia	1	Anesthesia	3
	Pediatrics	1	Critical care	1
			Pediatrics	1
			FM	3
			NP acute care	1
Invited from out-of-province	EM	1	EM	1
	IM	1		

EM emergency medicine, *IM* internal medicine, *FM* family medicine, *NP* nurse practitioner

Table 2 Results of the pre-conference survey of the potential standards[a] for each domain in order of preference

Domain	Preferred option[a]	Support ($n=17$) (%)
Scope of use	1. The appropriate application of POCUS should be defined by individual specialties/disciplines and be used whenever supported by reasonable evidence	100
Credentials and privileges	1. Departments should define specific credentials that are required to receive privileges to use POCUS	35
	2. No credentials or additional privileges should be required for the use of POCUS; its use should be up to the clinician similar to any other aspect of the clinical assessment	25
	3. Any additional training required (and associated privileges) to use POCUS should be determined on a case-by-case basis by each department	18
Documentation	1. POCUS findings should be documented, and images captured when they play a significant role in patient care decisions	59
	2. POCUS findings should be documented, and all images should be captured for inclusion in the patient's medical record	25
	3. POCUS should be documented in the same way as physical exam findings as part of the overall clinical assessment	18
Quality assurance	1. An audit of POCUS should be coordinated by any groups utilizing POCUS. Review of images, when available, is strongly encouraged	88
	2. POCUS use should include image capture and all images must be reviewed for quality assurance purposes. (12%)	12
Leadership and governance	1. Multidisciplinary committee with representatives from each specialty/discipline using POCUS	59
	2. Each specialty/discipline oversees its own use (41%)	41
Teaching	1. POCUS education can be provided by those with privileges recognized by their department	41
	2. POCUS education can be provided only by those with specific credentials as determined by a multidisciplinary POCUS committee	35
	3. POCUS education can be provided by clinicians without specific credentials	6
Research	1. Concerted and coordinated efforts to maximize research productivity to help propel USASK as a leader in POCUS research	59
	2. Clinical and educational/training research should be encouraged within each department	41
Equipment support and maintenance	1. Universal standards for POCUS equipment support and maintenance should be coordinated centrally within SHA	59
	2. Standards for POCUS equipment support and maintenance standards should be coordinated by each institution within SHA	41

[a] Only potential standards which received at least one vote in support are included. The full set of potential standards is included in the survey in Additional file 1: Appendix S1

Roundtable discussion on the capture, storage, and accessibility of POCUS images as they relate to the domains of documentation and quality assurance. Those in favor of image capture saw it as a best practice that should be regularly used at major teaching/training institutions to facilitate indirect supervision of trainee scans as well as quality assurance [29]. Further, it was felt that the ability to share images and/or videos in real time would add value to patient care in cases where a consultant could review pertinent POCUS findings in real time. It was highlighted that in some cases, this may make the difference between a patient staying at a regional site or being transferred to a referral centre. On the other hand, some participants countered that in certain instances image capture seemed an unreasonable requirement.

Rural and regional stakeholders noted that it was not feasible nor cost-effective to implement image capture middleware in every rural centre using POCUS at this time.

It was highlighted that practice audits can be performed by comparing the clinical notes of the POCUS findings with consultative images when these are available. Ultimately, consensus on documentation was reached along with the understanding that the advancement of POCUS technology, and the evolution of POCUS as a distinct imaging modality [21] with its own criteria for image capture, would guide further iterations of the framework.

The consensus built among this group paved the way for broad agreement among the conference attendees. Table 3 outlines the standards endorsed in the plenary session along with the results of the vote totals. Consensus (defined a priori as >80% agreement) was reached for the standards under each of the domains.

Table 3 Consensus domains and plenary session support for each of the standards within the multidisciplinary POCUS framework

Domain	Standard	Support[a]
1. Scope of use	The appropriate application of POCUS should be defined by individual disciplines and be used whenever supported by reasonable evidence	46/48 96%
2. Credentials and privileges	Disciplines should define specific and evolving required credentials that must be met for their providers to receive and maintain privileges to use POCUS. These credentials should be consistent with national standards	49/50 98%
3. Documentation in the medical record	POCUS findings should be documented in the patient chart, much like the physical exam findings as part of the overall clinical assessment. When image capture is available, select POCUS images should be archived and available to support the patient's ongoing care. When image capture is not available, departments should develop a system to track POCUS to support quality assurance and the patient's ongoing care	47/49 96%
4. Quality assurance	An audit of POCUS should be coordinated by any groups utilizing POCUS. Review of images, when available, is strongly encouraged. The details of this process should be determined by each discipline	45/49 92%
5. Leadership and governance	Each discipline should oversee its own use of POCUS. A multidisciplinary committee with representatives from each discipline should be formed to collaborate and promote best practices	47/50 94%
6. Teaching	Formal POCUS education and assessment can be provided by those with credentials recognized by their discipline	50/52 96%
7. Research	Clinical and educational research should be encouraged within each department. There should be a concerted effort to coordinate research between disciplines to maximize research productivity to help propel the University of Saskatchewan as a leader in POCUS research	50/53 94%
8. Equipment support and maintenance	Standards for POCUS equipment support and maintenance standards should be coordinated by each discipline as per current best practices and safety guidelines	47/52 90%

[a] Not all conference attendees responded to each of the polls

Discussion

We have developed a consensus-based multidisciplinary POCUS framework outlining standards for eight domains: scope of use, credentialing and privileges, documentation, quality assurance, leadership and governance, teaching, research, and equipment maintenance. Consensus on modified standards was achieved in the 18 participant Roundtable and endorsed by >90% of respondents at the conference.

We anticipate that this framework will be used in two ways. Locally, our working group will present our findings to our Health Association's Provincial Practitioner Advisory Committee as a next step in establishing minimum standards. We expect that these standards will inform the local adoption of discipline-specific guidelines that meet or exceed the requirements we have outlined (our Department of Emergency Medicine has already begun this process). More broadly, we anticipate that our process could be used by health professionals in other jurisdictions to develop their own multidisciplinary framework in a similar consensus-building manner.

Our working group sought to develop a multidisciplinary framework that was both provincial and institutional in application. Foundational to our approach was an understanding that, as per the American Medical Association resolution 802, training and education standards for the use of ultrasound imaging be developed by each physician's respective specialty [30]. Building from this, our goal was to develop a common framework upon which POCUS will continue to thrive within our institution. Other consensus processes described in the literature have been either specialty specific, hospital-based [26], or part of a broader clinical or billing protocol issued by a provincial College [31]. Notably, the Canadian Association of Radiologists recently published a position statement written exclusively by radiologists with no evidence of input from the POCUS community or any other discipline [32]. We believe our process is more pragmatic and has greater legitimacy in that we utilized a collaborative and consensus-based approach that incorporated the perspectives of multiple disciplines and clinical environments.

One area of discussion which was not anticipated within the pre-developed domains was the question of which instances and images (when captured on a middleware platform) should then be exported to the patient's permanent medical record. While all agreed that, when possible, scans that significantly impacted medical-decision making should be documented with images and/or video, questions remain regarding the necessity of recording procedural scans (e.g., central venous catheter placement). In addition, it would seem appropriate to consult patients about their preference as well. A subsequent review of the literature on this topic provided limited guidance. Local audits within the department of Emergency Medicine, comparing the written findings with consultative imaging, have revealed a concordance rate in excess of 90% and demonstrated appropriate application and integration of POCUS [33]. As such, there were concerns that the adoption of an image capture requirement would potentially and unjustifiably delay the uptake of POCUS by providers and for patients with the least access to advanced imaging. Further, given the vast range of POCUS applications, several participants suggested that a "one size fits all" approach is likely not appropriate. It was noted that POCUS findings land along a spectrum of clinical meaning and utility, at one end serving as an extension of the physical exam (consider POCUS for jugular venous pressure or interstitial lung syndrome) and the other performing as diagnostic imaging (consider POCUS for intrauterine pregnancy or lower extremity deep venous thrombosis). This spectrum of utility and impact will need to be kept under consideration as image capture standards evolve. As this was not addressed in our current framework, image capture for the patients' permanent record will need to be determined by both discipline-specific experts as well as our colleagues on the receiving end of transitions in care.

Limitations

The process of developing the multidisciplinary framework had several limitations. Despite efforts to recruit representatives from all disciplines using POCUS in our province, specialties including Neonatal Critical Care and Physiatry were not involved. Further, although we did have working group representatives from three western Canadian provinces, the majority of our experts were based in one province. Therefore, applicability of our POCUS standards to other jurisdictions will need to be decided on a case-by-case basis. Additionally, we did not grade the strength of each recommendation, as this was not part of our protocol. A significant outstanding question regarding when image capture needs to be used was raised during the Roundtable discussion, but was not addressed through this process. Finally, we believe our multidisciplinary approach would be enriched by having input from colleagues who have traditionally interpreted diagnostic ultrasonography in the fields of cardiology, obstetrics/gynecology, and medical imaging. These specialties were invited to participate in our working group, but unfortunately, there was no response to the invitation.

The adoption of provincial standards will be an iterative process, with members of our working group dedicated to ongoing discussions with our health authority as well as with other colleagues. We plan to reconvene the Roundtable annually at each SASKSONO event to address current standards and evolving issues.

Conclusion

In conclusion, our multidisciplinary POCUS framework provides a provincial standard upon which each discipline utilizing POCUS can build. It represents one of many initiatives to ensure high-quality use of POCUS that accounts for its use across many different clinical settings (including pre-hospital, the emergency department, the operating room, critical care unit, surgical and medical wards, and outpatient clinics). Locally, it will inform the implementation and utilization of POCUS within the University of Saskatchewan and the Saskatchewan Health Authority. More broadly, this process and its outcomes could be used as a template for the development of multidisciplinary POCUS standards within other jurisdictions.

Supplementary information

Additional file 1. USASK POCUS Framework survey.

Additional file 2. Survey results (comprehensive).

Acknowledgements

In collaboration with the SASKSONO19 Sono-Roundtable attendees/participants: Faisal Al-Sani, Robert Appleton, Rachit Batta, Kex Cau, Joann Kawchuk, Malcolm Lucy, Dalmar Lynds, Brady Murphy, Quinten Paterson, Rob Peverseff, James Prunell, James Stempien, Krista Wempe, and Rob Woods.

We also thank the attendees of SASKSONO19 for their participation in the audience poll-response system that provided feedback on the proposed standards.

Authors' contributions

PO and BT contributed to the conception and design of the study, the acquisition of data, the analysis and/or interpretation of data, the drafting of the manuscript, revising the manuscript critically for important intellectual content, and approval of the version of the manuscript to be published. DK contributed to the design of the study, the acquisition of data, the analysis and/or interpretation of data, the drafting of the manuscript, revising the manuscript critically for important intellectual content, and approval of the version of the manuscript to be published. IM contributed to the design of the study, data acquisition and interpretation, the analysis and/or interpretation of data, revised manuscript critically for intellectual content, and approved final manuscript. MC contributed to the design of the study, the acquisition of data, the analysis and/or interpretation of data, revising the manuscript critically for important intellectual content, and approval of the version of the manuscript to be published. PL, TG and MB contributed to the acquisition of data, revising the manuscript critically for important intellectual content, and approval of the version of the manuscript to be published. All authors read and approved the final manuscript.

Author details

[1] Department of Emergency Medicine, University of Saskatchewan, Saskatoon, Canada. [2] Department of Emergency Medicine, University of British Columbia, Vancouver, Canada. [3] Department of Medicine, University of Calgary, Calgary, Canada. [4] Department of Anesthesia and Perioperative Medicine, University of Saskatchewan, Saskatoon, Canada. [5] Department of Pediatrics, University of Saskatchewan, Prince Albert, Canada. [6] Department of Internal Medicine, University of Saskatchewan, Saskatoon, Canada. [7] Department of Family Medicine, University of Saskatchewan, Regina, Canada.

References

1. Moore CL, Copel JA (2011) Point-of-Care Ultrasonography. N Engl J Med 364(8):749–757. https://doi.org/10.1056/NEJMra0909487
2. Rubano E, Mehta N, Caputo W, Paladino L, Sinert R (2013) Systematic review: emergency department bedside ultrasonography for diagnosing suspected abdominal aortic aneurysm. Acad Emerg Med 20(2):128–138. https://doi.org/10.1111/acem.12080

3. Burnside PR, Brown MD, Kline JA (2008) Systematic review of emergency physician–performed ultrasonography for lower-extremity deep vein thrombosis. Acad Emerg Med 15(6):493–498. https://doi.org/10.1111/j.1553-2712.2008.00101.x
4. Long L, Zhao H-T, Zhang Z-Y, Wang G-Y, Zhao H-L (2017) Lung ultrasound for the diagnosis of pneumonia in adults. Medicine (Baltimore) 96(3):e5713. https://doi.org/10.1097/MD.0000000000005713
5. Subramaniam S, Bober J, Chao J, Zehtabchi S (2016) Point-of-care Ultrasound for diagnosis of abscess in skin and soft tissue infections. Acad Emerg Med 23(11):1298–1306. https://doi.org/10.1111/acem.13049
6. Nishijima DK, Simel DL, Wisner DH, Holmes JF (2012) Does this adult patient have a blunt intra-abdominal injury? JAMA 307(14):1517. https://doi.org/10.1001/jama.2012.422
7. Plummer D, Clinton J, Matthew B (1998) Emergency department ultrasound improves time to diagnosis and survival of ruptured abdominal aortic aneurysm. Acad Emerg Med 5:417
8. Rodgerson JD, Heegaard WG, Plummer D, Hicks J, Clinton J, Sterner S (2001) Emergency department right upper quadrant ultrasound is associated with a reduced time to diagnosis and treatment of ruptured ectopic pregnancies. Acad Emerg Med 8(4):331–336
9. Plummer D, Brunette D, Asinger R, Ruiz E (1992) Emergency department echocardiography improves outcome in penetrating cardiac injury. Ann Emerg Med 21(6):709–712
10. Melniker LA, Leibner E, McKenney MG, Lopez P, Briggs WM, Mancuso CA (2006) Randomized controlled clinical trial of point-of-care, limited ultrasonography for trauma in the emergency department: the first sonography outcomes assessment program trial. Ann Emerg Med 48(3):227–235. https://doi.org/10.1016/j.annemergmed.2006.01.008
11. Practice Guidelines for Central Venous Access (2012) A report by the american society of anesthesiologists task force on central venous access. Anesthesiology 116(3):539–573. https://doi.org/10.1097/ALN.0b013e31823c9569
12. Soni NJ, Schnobrich D, Mathews BK et al (2019) Point-of-care ultrasound for hospitalists: a position statement of the society of hospital medicine. J Hosp Med. https://doi.org/10.12788/jhm.3079
13. Ma IWY, Arishenkoff S, Wiseman J et al (2017) Internal medicine point-of-care ultrasound curriculum: consensus recommendations from the canadian internal medicine ultrasound (CIMUS) group. J Gen Intern Med 32(9):1052–1057. https://doi.org/10.1007/s11606-017-4071-5
14. Cho J, Jensen TP, Reierson K et al (2019) Recommendations on the use of ultrasound guidance for adult abdominal paracentesis: a position statement of the society of hospital medicine. J Hosp Med 14:E7–E15. https://doi.org/10.12788/jhm.3095
15. Latteri S, Malaguarnera G, Mannino M et al (2017) Ultrasound as point of care in management of polytrauma and its complication. J Ultrasound 20(2):171–177. https://doi.org/10.1007/s40477-017-0252-7
16. Peabody CR, Mandavia D (2017) Deep needle procedures: improving safety with ultrasound visualization. J Patient Saf 13(2):103–108. https://doi.org/10.1097/PTS.0000000000000110
17. Mateer JR, Valley VT, Aiman EJ, Phelan MB, Thoma ME, Kefer MP (1996) Outcome analysis of a protocol including bedside endovaginal sonography in patients at risk for ectopic pregnancy. Ann Emerg Med 27(3):283–289
18. Mitchell D, Leng A, Gardiner S et al (2016) Using point-of-care bedside ultrasound for volume assessment in early shock: an outcome study. Chest 149(4):A148. https://doi.org/10.1016/j.chest.2016.02.154
19. Hans SS, Huang RR (2003) Results of 101 ruptured abdominal aortic aneurysm repairs from a single surgical practice. Arch Surg 138(8):898. https://doi.org/10.1001/archsurg.138.8.898
20. McCormick TJ, Miller EC, Chen R, Naik VN (2018) Acquiring and maintaining point-of-care ultrasound (POCUS) competence for anesthesiologists. Can J Anesth Can d'anesthésie 65(4):427–436. https://doi.org/10.1007/s12630-018-1049-7
21. Guidelines Ultrasound (2017) Emergency, point-of-care and clinical ultrasound guidelines in medicine. Ann Emerg Med 69(5):e27–e54. https://doi.org/10.1016/j.annemergmed.2016.08.457
22. Contra Costa Family Medicine Residency Program. Recommended Curriculum Guidelines for Family Medicine Residents Point of Care Ultrasound. Martinez, CA; 2016. https://www.aafp.org/dam/AAFP/documents/medical_education_residency/program_directors/Reprint290D_POCUS.pdf. Accessed 2 Apr 2019
23. Arntfield R, Millington S, Ainsworth C et al (2014) Canadian recommendations for critical care ultrasound training and competency. Can Respir J 21(6):341–345. https://doi.org/10.1155/2014/216591
24. Shefrin AE, Warkentine F, Constantine E et al (2019) Consensus core point-of-care ultrasound applications for pediatric emergency medicine training. AEM Educ Train. https://doi.org/10.1002/aet2.10332
25. Henneberry RJ, Hanson A, Healey A et al (2012) Use of point of care sonography by emergency physicians. CJEM 14(02):106–112. https://doi.org/10.2310/8000.CAEPPS
26. Mathews B, Zwank M (2017) Hospital medicine point of care ultrasound credentialing: an example protocol. J Hosp Med 12(9):767–772. https://doi.org/10.12788/jhm.2809
27. Woods RA, Artz JD, Carrière B et al (2017) CAEP 2016 academic symposium on education scholarship: training our future clinician educators in emergency medicine. Can J Emerg Med 19(S1):S1–S8. https://doi.org/10.1017/CEM.2017.41
28. Humphrey-Murto S, Varpio L, Gonsalves C, Wood TJ (2017) Using consensus group methods such as Delphi and Nominal Group in medical education research. Med Teach 39(1):14–19. https://doi.org/10.1080/0142159X.2017.1245856
29. Lewis D, Rang L, Kim D et al (2019) Recommendations for the use of point-of-care ultrasound (POCUS) by emergency physicians in Canada. CJEM. https://doi.org/10.1017/cem.2019.392
30. American Medical Association. Privileging for Ultrasound Imaging H-230.960. https://policysearch.ama-assn.org/policyfinder/detail/Ultrasoundimaging?uri=%2FAMADoc%2FHOD.xml-0-1591.xml. Published 2010. Accessed 22 Aug 2019
31. College of Physicians and Surgeons of Alberta. Diagnostic Imaging Modality Application for Physician Approval Ultrasound Restricted Approval; 2019. http://www.cpsa.ca/wp-content/uploads/2017/02/US-Restricted.02142017.pdf. Accessed 19 Aug 2019
32. Chawla TP, Cresswell M, Dhillon S et al (2019) Canadian association of radiologists position statement on point-of-care ultrasound. Can Assoc Radiol J 70(3):219–225. https://doi.org/10.1016/j.carj.2019.06.001
33. Denton C, Iradukunda D, Trickovic J, Turnquist A, Olszynski P. ED Ultrasound in Saskatoon: a quality assurance study; 2019. https://sasksonic.files.wordpress.com/2019/03/wecoc-edus-poster.pdf. Accessed 30 Mar 2019

9

Barriers to learning and using Point-of-care ultrasound: A survey of practicing internists in six North American institutions

Jonathan Wong[1], Steven Montague[2], Paul Wallace[3], Kay Negishi[4], Andrew Liteplo[5], Jennifer Ringrose[6], Renee Dversdal[7], Brian Buchanan[8], Janeve Desy[6] and Irene W. Y. Ma[6*]

Abstract

Background: Point-of-care ultrasound (POCUS) is increasingly used in internal medicine, but a lack of trained faculty continues to limit the spread of POCUS education. Using a framework based on organizational change theories, this study sought to identify barriers and enablers for hospital-based practicing internists to learn and use POCUS in clinical practice.

Methods: We invited practicing internists at six North American institutions to participate in an electronic survey on their opinions regarding 39 barriers and enablers.

Results: Of the 342 participants invited, 170 participated (response rate 49.3%). The top barriers were lack of training (79%), lack of handheld ultrasound devices (78%), lack of direct supervision (65%), lack of time to perform POCUS during rounds (65%), and lack of quality assurance processes (53%). The majority of participants (55%) disagreed or strongly disagreed with the statement "*My institution provides funding for POCUS training.*" In general, participants' attitudes towards POCUS were favourable, and future career opportunities and the potential for billing were not considered significant factors by our participants in the decision to learn or use POCUS.

Conclusions: This survey confirms the perceived importance of POCUS to practicing internists. To assist in closing faculty development gap, interventions should address training, supervision, quality assurance processes, availability of handheld devices, as well as dedicated time to perform POCUS during clinical care.

Keywords: Ultrasonography, Internal medicine, Continuing medical education, Barriers

Background

The use of point-of-care ultrasound (POCUS) is increasing in internal medicine (IM), not only for the guidance of bedside procedures [1–3], but also for bedside assessments of medical patients to answer focused clinical questions [4, 5]. In 2018, the American College of Physicians (ACP) officially acknowledged the important role of POCUS to improve diagnostic timeliness and care of the medical patient [6]. Following this acknowledgement from the ACP, the Society of Hospital Medicine issued a similar position statement highlighting their support for the use of POCUS by hospitalists [5]. Nationally and internationally, POCUS is increasingly incorporated in IM residency training programs over the last decade [7–11]. Recognizing the importance of POCUS in medical education, the Alliance of Academic Internal Medicine supports the integration of POCUS across the training continuum [12]. Despite the growing appetite for POCUS training, progress in expanding POCUS in IM has been slow. A major obstacle to the expansion of POCUS training is a lack of skilled faculty, and previous studies have cited limited time, money and resources as

*Correspondence: ima@ucalgary.ca
[6] Department of Medicine, Division of General Internal Medicine, Cumming School of Medicine, University of Calgary, 3330 Hospital Dr NW, Calgary, AB T2N 4N1, Canada
Full list of author information is available at the end of the article

the key barriers to faculty adoption of POCUS [7, 11, 13–18]. A more nuanced understanding of perceived faculty barriers is needed, however, to allow for more targeted interventions.

Faculty adoption of POCUS requires significant behavioural change. Encouraging behavioural change is complex; it involves not only the individual practitioner in question (his/her motivation, aptitude, and attitudes), but also requires support within the organizational environment, such as proper leadership, policies, economics, and social and structural infrastructures [19–24]. It follows that any intervention to achieve system-level behavioural change will require a comprehensive, evidence-based strategy to identify and resolve barriers to POCUS adoption.

In this multi-centre survey study, we sought to identify IM faculty barriers and enablers to learning and using POCUS in clinical practice. Using a holistic approach based on organization change theories [19–21], we sought to explore both individual, as well as organizational barriers and enablers. The information obtained from this study will provide a deeper understanding of the barriers that IM faculty encounter to using POCUS to care for hospitalized patients.

Methods

Participants

In this multi-centre survey study, IM physicians caring for hospitalized patients were invited to complete an online survey. Six centres were chosen based on convenience, where site investigators indicated a reasonable likelihood of achieving an approximate target response rate of 40% or greater. The six study sites involved in this study were three centres in Canada (the University of Calgary in Calgary, Alberta; the University of Alberta in Edmonton, Alberta; Queen's University in Kingston, Ontario) and three centres in the United States (Oregon Health & Science University in Portland, Oregon; Massachusetts General Hospital in Boston, Massachusetts; and the University of Pennsylvania in Philadelphia, Pennsylvania). Only consenting physicians were included. Physicians in Canadian centres were all internists or general internists certified by the Royal College of Physicians and Surgeons of Canada, with or without additional subspecialty certifications, and attended on hospital-based general medical teaching wards. Physicians in the United States were all board certified internists (or board eligible if in their first year of practice) who worked as hospitalists in their institutions. We excluded IM physicians practicing exclusively in an ambulatory care setting. Each study site sought and obtained local research ethics board approval for this study. The central coordinating site's ethics approval was obtained from the Conjoint Health Research Ethics Board from the University of Calgary (Protocol REB 18-1498).

Survey development

After reviewing key principles of organizational change theories [19–21], an online draft survey was developed by co-investigator (JW) and principal investigator (IM). The survey covered items on (1) demographics; (2) baseline POCUS experience; (3) individual barriers including emotional, clinical, financial factors; (4) group or social barriers; and (5) systemic or environmental barriers. This initial draft survey contained 11 questions regarding baseline demographics and POCUS experience information and 40 items on barriers and enablers. For each barrier and enabler, participants were asked to rate their agreement with the item on a 5-point Likert scale (from strongly disagree to strongly agree). The draft survey was piloted by 10 physician volunteers with a range in experience and knowledge of POCUS. These individuals were not part of the final participant pool. We sought their input on survey flow, wording, acceptability, administrative ease, question quality, and missing items. The survey was then revised based on their feedback. The final survey contained questions on baseline demographic and POCUS experience, and 39 items on barriers and enablers.

Between January and April 2019, participants were invited via email by the site investigator to complete the anonymized online survey administered using SurveyMonkey Inc. (San Mateo, California, USA).

Statistical analysis

Standard descriptive statistics (mean, standard deviation, median, interquartile range) were calculated using SAS version 9.4 (SAS Institute Inc., Cary, NC, USA).

Results

Of the 342 participants invited to complete the survey, 184 (53.8%) responded. Of these, 14 were excluded (declined consent $n=3$; consented but did not complete the survey $n=11$), resulting in a final pool of 170 participants (response rate 49.7%). Baseline characteristics of the participants are presented in Table 1.

Clinical and procedural use

Participants reported using POCUS infrequently during clinical assessments of their patients (used on only a median of 5% of their patients, interquartile range 0–11%, range 0–90%). The majority of participants performed paracentesis in their practice ($n=126$, 74%), whilst only a minority performed thoracentesis and central venous catheterization ($n=77$, 45% and $n=66$, 39%, respectively). For those who performed procedures, ultrasound

Table 1 Baseline characteristics of 170 participants who completed the survey

Baseline characteristics	N (%)
Sex	
Male	95 (56)
Female	74 (44)
Age	
< 35 years	51 (30)
35–44 years	59 (41)
45–54 years	37 (22)
55–64 years	9 (5)
65 years or older	4 (2)
Years in clinical practice	
1–4 years	71 (42)
5–10 years	45 (26)
11–20 years	28 (16)
21 years or more	26 (15)
Prior point-of-care (POCUS) ultrasound training[a]	
No prior training	32 (19)
Self-learned (textbooks, YouTube, websites)	64 (38)
Bedside teaching (supervised scanning)	54 (38)
Didactic lecture(s)	55 (32)
< 1 day workshop/course	48 (28)
1–3 day workshop/course	61 (36)
Dedicated POCUS elective during training	17 (10)
POCUS-specific certifications	8 (5)
POCUS fellowship	4 (2)

Not every participant answered every question

[a] Participants were able to choose more than one response

was used for guidance *usually* or *always* for the majority of the participants (60/66 = 90% for central venous catheterization, 101/126 = 80% for paracentesis, and 63/77 = 82% for thoracentesis). A minority *never* used ultrasound for guidance when performing central venous catheterization (3/66 = 5%), paracentesis (7/126 = 6%), and thoracentesis (6/77 = 8%).

Barriers to using POCUS

Figure 1 outlines the results on the 39 barriers and enablers. The top 5 barriers were

1. Need for more training: 135/170, 79% agreed or strongly agreed with *"I would use POCUS more if I had more training."*
2. Lack of handheld ultrasound device: 132/170, 78% agreed or strongly agreed with *"I would use POCUS more if I was provided with a handheld device."*
3. Lack of direct supervision: 110/168, 65% agreed or strongly agreed with *"I would use POCUS more if I had direct supervision as I apply it to my patient care."*
4. Lack of time to perform POCUS during rounds: 111/170, 65% agreed or strongly agreed with *"I would use POCUS more if I had more time to perform it during rounds."*
5. Lack of quality assurance processes: 89/168, 53% agreed or strongly agreed with *"I would use POCUS more if my images could be archived and reviewed later by a qualified expert."*

The 5 *least* important barriers appeared to be related to attitude regarding POCUS:

1. Irrelevance to internal medicine: 8/170, 5% agreed or strongly agreed with *"In general, I think POCUS is irrelevant to the practice of internal medicine,"* whilst 153/170, 90% disagreed or strongly disagreed with the statement.
2. POCUS is a fad: 7/170, 4% agreed or strongly agreed with *"I think POCUS is a fad that will pass with time,"* whilst 139/170, 82% disagreed or strongly disagreed.
3. Irrelevant to participant's practice: 13/170, 8% agreed or strongly agreed with *"I think POCUS is irrelevant to my specific clinical practice,"* whilst 147/170, 86% disagreed or strongly disagreed.
4. Loss of physical examination skills: 10/170, 6% agreed or strongly agreed with *"I worry I will lose my physical examination skills if I use POCUS,"* whilst 135/170, 79% disagreed or strongly disagreed.
5. Patient harm: 10/170, 6% agreed or strongly agreed with *"In general, I worry that POCUS use by internists will harm medical patients,"* whilst 141/170, 83% disagreed or strongly disagreed.

Enablers to using POCUS

Consistent with the lack of barriers regarding attitude against POCUS, data were triangulated with participants reporting an overall positive attitude towards the use of POCUS (e.g. high interest in learning more about POCUS, belief that POCUS is a useful adjunct to the traditional physical examination, Fig. 1, Table 2). The work environment (e.g. colleague attitudes, availability of POCUS experts) was overall seen as favourable to POCUS adoption. In general, participants reported a lack of funding for POCUS training, with 92/166 (55%) disagreed or strongly disagreed with the statement *"My institution provides funding for POCUS training."* Future career opportunities and the potential for billing were not considered significant enablers by our participants (Fig. 1).

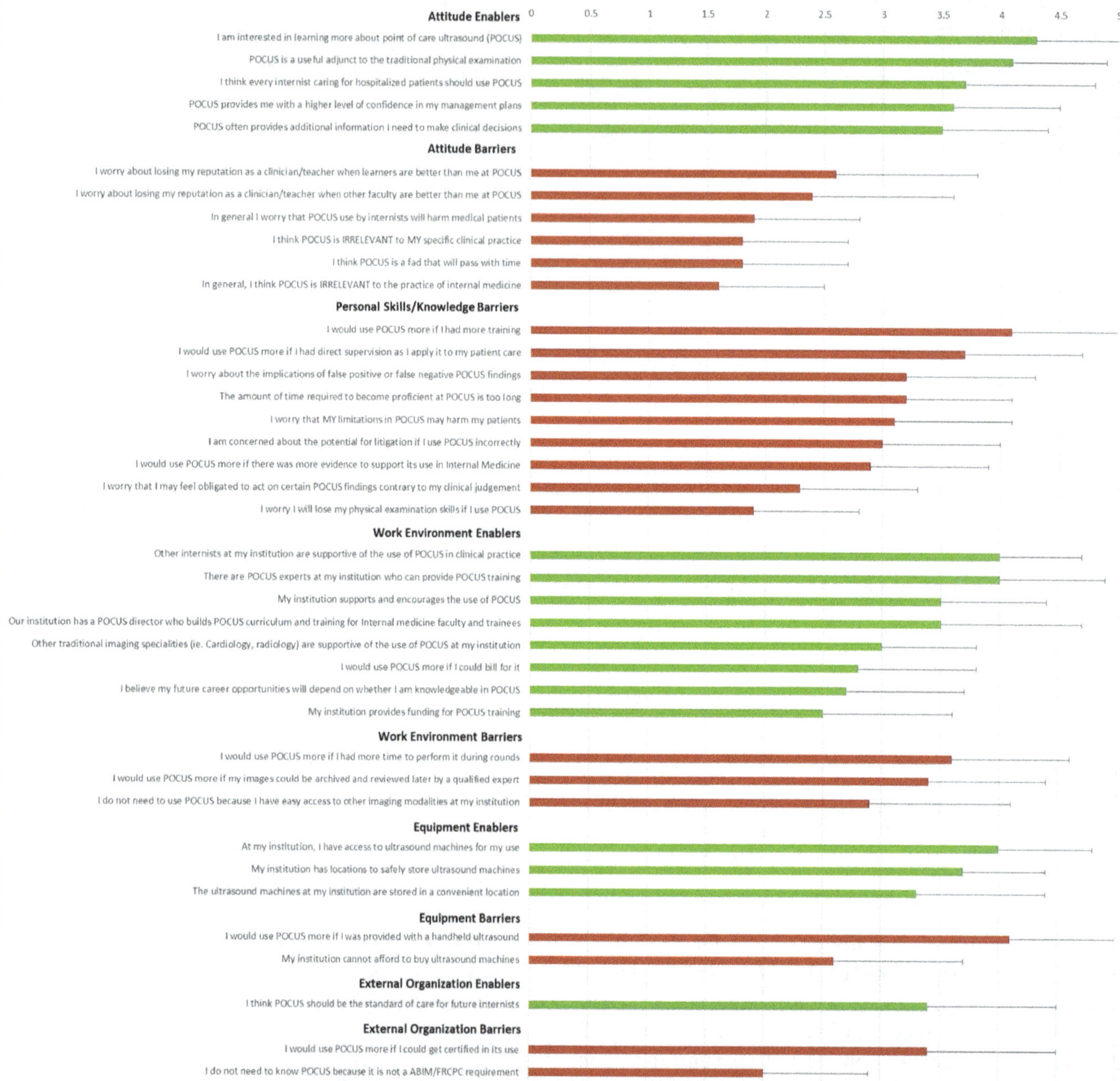

Fig. 1 Barriers and enablers, presented in the descending order of agreement within each category. Barrier (red) and enablers (green) were rated on a 5-point Likert scale, where 1 = strongly disagree and 5 = strongly agree

Discussion

In this multi-centre survey of six North American academic institutions' practicing internists who look after hospitalized patients, several findings emerged. First, whilst POCUS is commonly used for procedural guidance, its frequency of use in the general clinical assessments was only done on a median of 5% of patients. Second, general attitudes towards POCUS were positive, including high interest in learning POCUS and an overall positive belief about the utility of POCUS. Third, practicing internists reported a number of barriers, including the lack of training, supervision, quality assurance processes (archiving and review of images), handheld devices, and time to perform POCUS during rounds. Whilst there was only moderate concern regarding the use of POCUS potentially resulting in patient harm, participants did not particularly feel that POCUS findings will compel them to act contrary to their clinical judgement, or that they may lose their physical examination skills if they used POCUS. Further, external factors such as career opportunities and billing opportunities were not considered significant enabling factors. Overall, our results suggest that

Table 2 Barriers and enablers, in the descending order of agreement

Attitude enablers	Mean (SD)[a]
I am interested in learning more about point-of-care ultrasound (POCUS)	4.3 (1.0)
POCUS is a useful adjunct to the traditional physical examination	4.1. (0.8)
I think every internist caring for hospitalized patients should use POCUS	3.7 (1.1)
POCUS provides me with a higher level of confidence in my management plans	3.6 (0.9)
POCUS often provides additional information I need to make clinical decisions	3.5 (0.9)
Attitude barriers	
I worry about losing my reputation as a clinician/teacher when learners are better than me at POCUS	2.6 (1.2)
I worry about losing my reputation as a clinician/teacher when other faculties are better than me at POCUS	2.4 (1.2)
In general I worry that POCUS use by internists will harm medical patients	1.9 (0.9)
I think POCUS is IRRELEVANT to MY specific clinical practice	1.8 (0.9)
I think POCUS is a fad that will pass with time	1.8 (0.9)
In general, I think POCUS is IRRELEVANT to the practice of internal medicine	1.6 (0.9)
Personal/general skills/knowledge barriers	
I would use POCUS more if I had more training	4.1 (0.9)
I would use POCUS more if I had direct supervision as I apply it to my patient care	3.7 (1.0)
I worry about the implications of false-positive or false-negative POCUS findings	3.2 (1.1)
The amount of time required to become proficient at POCUS is too long	3.2 (0.9)
I worry that MY limitations in POCUS may harm my patients	3.1 (1.0)
I am concerned about the potential for litigation if I use POCUS incorrectly	3.0 (1.0)
I would use POCUS more if there was more evidence to support its use in Internal Medicine	2.9 (1.0)
I worry that I may feel obligated to act on certain POCUS findings contrary to my clinical judgement	2.3 (1.0)
I worry I will lose my physical examination skills if I use POCUS	1.9 (0.9)
Work environment enablers	
Other internists at my institution are supportive of the use of POCUS in clinical practice	4.0 (0.7)
There are POCUS experts at my institution who can provide POCUS training	4.0 (0.9)
My institution supports and encourages the use of POCUS	3.5 (0.9)
Our institution has a POCUS director who builds POCUS curriculum and training for Internal medicine faculty and trainees	3.5 (1.2)
Other traditional imaging specialities (i.e. Cardiology, radiology) are supportive of the use of POCUS at my institution	3.0 (0.8)
I would use POCUS more if I could bill for it	2.8 (1.0)
I believe my future career opportunities will depend on whether I am knowledgeable in POCUS	2.7 (1.0)
My institution provides funding for POCUS training	2.5 (1.1)
Work environment barriers	
I would use POCUS more if I had more time to perform it during rounds	3.6 (1.0)
I would use POCUS more if my images could be archived and reviewed later by a qualified expert	3.4 (1.0)
I do not need to use POCUS because I have easy access to other imaging modalities (i.e. Chest X-rays, diagnostic ultrasound, CT, MRI, echocardiography, etc.) at my institution	2.9 (1.2)
Equipment-related enablers	
At my institution, I have access to ultrasound machines for my use	4.0 (0.8)
My institution has locations to safely store ultrasound machines	3.7 (0.7)
The ultrasound machines at my institution are stored in a convenient location	3.3 (1.1)
Equipment-related barriers	
I would use POCUS more if I was provided with a handheld ultrasound	4.1 (1.0)
My institution cannot afford to buy ultrasound machines	2.6 (1.1)
External organization-related enablers	
I think POCUS should be the standard of care for future internists	3.4 (1.1)

Table 2 (continued)

External organization-related barriers	
I would use POCUS more if I could get certified in its use	3.4 (1.1)
I do not need to know POCUS because it is not a ABIM/FRCPC requirement	2.0 (0.9)

[a] Rated on a 5-point Likert scale, where 1 = strongly disagree and 5 = strongly agree

the practicing internists at these six academic centres have limited personal, attitudinal, work environment, or externally related barriers to using POCUS but significant skill and knowledge-based barriers may be limiting POCUS use. Whilst access to machines did not seem to be a barrier at their institutions, participants did feel that provision of a handheld ultrasound would facilitate increased use.

Our results are consistent with prior survey studies on barriers in using POCUS in practicing physicians. For example, personal and general attitude to the use of POCUS has been favourable in prior studies [7, 11, 13, 14, 17, 25, 26]. However, unlike other studies where time, equipment, and funding were the primary barriers [7, 11, 16–18], our study participants were more concerned with their own lack of training, supervision, and the lack of quality assurance processes. This concern with lack of training and supervision has also been suggested in other studies [14, 15, 25, 26]. Last, in one study of neonatal and pediatric critical care specialists, over 40% of participants were concerned with both liability issues and resistance from imaging specialists [16]. These two issues were only of moderate importance to our survey participants.

Our study has several limitations. First is the issue of generalizability. The academic centres in our study all have a designated internal medicine POCUS champion, a marker of higher quality POCUS education [27], as well as availability of machines and supportive work environment and colleagues. As such, our results may not apply to practitioners in POCUS-naïve settings. Indeed, a prior study found that attitudes of critical care fellowship program directors differed between programs that had an ultrasound machine, compared with programs that did not [13]. Second, our overall response rate was only 49%. Whilst five of our six sites achieved our target of greater than 40% response rate, one site achieved only 33%. Nonetheless, our response rate is typical of studies of this kind; in a systematic review of 68 surveys, a mean response rate of 39.6% was reported [28]. Third, despite an attempt to more comprehensively explore barriers, a complete catalogue of all barriers is not possible. Fourth, whilst statistics convey central tendencies, for each barrier and enabler, the responses ranged from 1 to 5 (from *strongly disagree* to *strongly agree*), with the exception of 2 items: "*I do not need to know POCUS because it is not a ABIM/FRCPC requirement*" (range 1–4); "*Other internists at my institution are supportive of the use of POCUS in clinical practice*" (range 2–5). The implication of these observed ranges is that despite our reported results, in our study population are individuals whose attitude towards POCUS was very negative, who felt very strongly that POCUS is a fad that will pass with time, and who still would not use POCUS if they had more training and supervision. The usual interventions to effect behavioural change may be less effective on these individuals. Finally, our online survey was administered anonymously; despite the absence of identical responses in surveys, we cannot exclude the possibility that some individuals may have responded more than once.

Conclusions

In conclusion, in our multi-centre survey of practicing hospital-based internists who look after hospitalized patients, lack of training, supervision, quality assurance processes (archiving and review of images), handheld devices, and time to perform POCUS during rounds were the key barriers to using POCUS. Personal attitudes about the utility of POCUS, current lack of requirement by external organizations for the practice of internal medicine, and inability to bill were not considered important barriers by our participants. Future studies should systematically address barriers to POCUS use.

Abbreviations

ACP: American College of Physicians; IM: Internal medicine; POCUS: Point-of-care ultrasound.

Acknowledgements

We wish to thank all our colleagues who participated in this survey.

Authors' contributions

JW and IWM contributed to the conception and design of the work, acquisition, analysis, and interpretation of data, and drafted and revised the work. SM, PW, KN, AL, JR, RD, BB, and JD contributed to the acquisition and interpretation of data and revised it critically for important intellectual content. All authors read and approved the manuscript.

Author details

[1] Department of Medicine, University of Alberta, Edmonton, AB, Canada.
[2] Department of Medicine, Queen's University, Kingston, ON, Canada.

[3] Department of Medicine, University of Pennsylvania, Philadelphia, PA, USA. [4] Department of Medicine, Massachusetts General Hospital, Boston, MA, USA. [5] Department of Emergency Medicine, Massachusetts General Hospital, Boston, MA, USA. [6] Department of Medicine, Division of General Internal Medicine, Cumming School of Medicine, University of Calgary, 3330 Hospital Dr NW, Calgary, AB T2N 4N1, Canada. [7] Department of Medicine, Oregon Health & Science University, Portland, OR, USA. [8] Department of Critical Care, University of Alberta, Edmonton, AB, Canada.

References

1. Cho J, Jensen TP, Rierson K, Matthews BK, Bhagra A, Franco-Sadud R, Grikis L, Mader M, Dancel R, Lucas BP et al (2019) Recommendations on the use of ultrasound guidance for adult abdominal Pparacentesis: a position statement of the Society of Hospital Medicine. J Hosp Med 14:E7–E15
2. Dancel R, Schnobrich D, Puri N, Franco-Sadud R, Cho J, Grikis L, Lucas BP, El-Barbary M, Soni NJ (2018) Recommendations on the use of ultrasound guidance for adult thoracentesis: a position statement of the Society of Hospital Medicine. J Hosp Med 13(2):126–135
3. National Institute for Health and Clinical Excellence (NICE). Technology Appraisal No 49: guidance on the use of ultrasound locating devices for placing central venous catheters. http://www.nice.org.uk/Guidance/TA49/Guidance/pdf/English. Accessed 18 Nov 2019
4. Liu RB, Donroe JH, McNamara RL, Forman HP, Moore CL (2017) The practice and implications of finding fluid during point-of-care ultrasonography: a review. JAMA Intern Med 177(12):1818–1825
5. Soni NJ, Schnobrich D, Matthews BK, Tierny DM, Jensen TP, Dancel R, Cho J, Dversdal RK, Mints G, Bhagra A et al (2019) Point-of-care ultrasound for hospitalists: a position statement of the society of hospital medicine. J Hosp Med 14:E1–E6
6. American College of Physicians. ACP statement in support of point-of-care ultrasound in internal medicine. https://www.acponline.org/meetings-courses/focused-topics/point-of-care-ultrasound/acp-statement-in-support-of-point-of-care-ultrasound-in-internal-medicine. Accessed 18 Nov 2019
7. Schnobrich DJ, Gladding S, Olson APJ, Duran-Nelson A (2013) Point-of-care ultrasound in internal medicine: a national survey of educational leadership. J Grad Med Educ 5(3):498–502
8. Ma IWY, Arishenkoff S, Wiseman J, Desy J, Ailon J, Martin L, Otremba M, Halman S, Willemot P, Blouw M et al (2017) Internal Medicine Point-of-Care Ultrasound Curriculum: Consensus Recommendations from the Canadian Internal Medicine Ultrasound (CIMUS) Group. J Gen Intern Med 32(9):1052–1057
9. Ma IWY, Cogliati C, Bosch FH, Tonelli de Oliveira AC, Arienti V, Blans MJ, Chan B, Bhagra A (2018) Point-of-care ultrasound for internal medicine: an international perspective. South Med J 111(7):439–443
10. LoPresti CM, Schnobrich DJ, Dversdal RK, Schembri F (2019) A road map for point-of-care ultrasound training in internal medicine residency. Ultrasound J 11(1):10
11. Ailon J, Nadjafi M, Mourad O, Cavalcanti R (2016) Point-of-care ultrasound as a competency for general internists: a survey of internal medicine training programs in Canada. Can Med Educ J 7(2):e51–e69
12. LoPresti CM, Jensen TP, Dversdal RK, Astiz DJ (2019) Point of care ultrasound for internal medicine residency training: a position statement from the alliance of academic internal medicine. Am J Med 132(11):1356–1360
13. Eisen LA, Leung S, Gallagher AE, Kvetan V (2010) Barriers to ultrasound training in critical care medicine fellowships: a survey of program directors. Crit Care Med 38(10):1978–1983
14. Mosier JM, Malo J, Stolz LA, Bloom JW, Reyes NA, Snyder LS, Adhikari S (2014) Critical care ultrasound training: a survey of US fellowship directors. J Crit Care 29(4):645–649
15. Hall J, Holman H, Bornemann P, Barreto T, Henderson D, Bennett K, Chamberlain J, Maurer DM (2015) Point of care ultrasound in family medicine residency programs: a CERA study. Fam Med 47(9):706–711
16. Nguyen J, Amirnovin R, Ramanathan R, Noori S (2016) The state of point-of-care ultrasonography use and training in neonatal–perinatal medicine and pediatric critical care medicine fellowship programs. J Perinatol 36(11):972
17. Micks T, Braganza D, Peng S, McCarthy P, Sue K, Doran P, Hall J, Holman H, O'Keefe D, Rogers P (2018) Canadian national survey of point-of-care ultrasound training in family medicine residency programs. Can Fam Physician 64(10):e462–e467
18. Mok D, Schwarz SKW, Rondi K (2017) Point-of-care ultrasonography in Canadian anesthesiology residency programs: a national survey of program directors. Can J Anesth 64(10):1023–1036
19. Burke WW (2018) Organization change: theory and practice, 5th edn. Sage Publications, Thousand Oaks
20. Kotter JP (2012) Leading change. Harvard Business Review Press, Boston
21. HBR's 10 Must Reads (2011) On change management. Harvard Business School Publishing Corporation, Boston
22. Cabana MD, Rand CS, Powe NR, Wu AW, Wilson MH, Abboud PA, Rubin HR (1999) Why don't physicians follow clinical practice guidelines? A framework for improvement. JAMA 282(15):1458–1465
23. Grol R, Grimshaw J (2003) From best evidence to best practice: effective implementation of change in patients' care. Lancet 362(9391):1225–1230
24. Grimshaw JM, Shirran L, Thomas R, Mowatt G, Fraser C, Bero L, Grilli R, Harvey E, Oxman A, O'Brien MA (2001) Changing provider behavior: an overview of systematic reviews of interventions. Med Care 39(8Supple 2):II2–II45
25. Smallwood N, Matsa R, Lawrenson P, Messenger J, Walden A (2015) A UK wide survey on attitudes to point of care ultrasound training amongst clinicians working on the Acute Medical Unit. Acute Med 14(4):159–164
26. Peh WM, Kang ML (2018) A pilot survey on an understanding of point of care bedside ultrasound (POCUS) among medical doctors in internal medicine: exposure, perceptions, interest and barriers to training. Proc Singapore Healthcare 27(2):85–95
27. Ambasta A, Balan M, Mayette M, Goffi A, Mulvagh S, Buchanan B, Montague S, Ruzycki S, Ma IW (2019) Education Indicators for Internal Medicine Point-of-Care Ultrasound: a Consensus Report from the Canadian Internal Medicine Ultrasound (CIMUS) Group. J Gen Intern Med 34(10):2123–2129
28. Cook C, Heath F, Thompson RL (2000) A meta-analysis of response rates in web- or internet-based surveys. Educ Psychol Meas 60(6):821–836

10

Role of point-of-care ultrasound during the COVID-19 pandemic: our recommendations in the management of dialytic patients

Ana Luisa Silveira Vieira[1*], José Muniz Pazeli Júnior[2] and Marcus Gomes Bastos[3,4]

Abstract

COVID-19 is a viral disease due to the infection of the novel Corona virus SARS-CoV-2, that has rapidly spread in many countries until the World Health Organization declared the pandemic from March 11, 2020. Elderly patients and those affected by hypertension, diabetes mellitus, and chronic pulmonary and cardiovascular conditions are more susceptible to present more severe forms of COVID-19. These conditions are often represented in dialytic renal end-stage patients. Moreover, dialysis patients are more vulnerable to infection due to suppression of the immune system. Growing evidences, although still supported by few publications, are showing the potential utility of ultrasound in patients with COVID-19. In this review, we share our experience in using point-of-care ultrasound, particularly lung ultrasound, to indicate the probability of COVID-19 in patients with end-stage renal disease treated by hemodialysis. We also propose recommendations for the application of lung ultrasound, focused echocardiography and inferior vena cava ultrasound in the management of patients in hemodialysis.

Keywords: COVID-19, SARS-CoV-2, Dialysis, COVID-19 pandemic, Ultrasound

Introduction

The world is currently facing a pandemic disease caused by a novel coronavirus (SARS-CoV-2) and called COVID-19 (COronaVIrus Disease-19, described in 2019). This viral infection showed rapid dissemination and potential harm due to complications in the respiratory system characterized by a severe form of pneumonia with respiratory failure. Only a minority of patients are at risk of developing the severe form of the disease, but the extremely high number of infected patients is causing a surge that is creating a serious crisis even in the most advanced medical organizations [1]. The big challenge is to recognize, efficiently and quickly, those patients with COVID-19 pneumonia who need isolation, hospitalization and intensive care management.

The Chinese experience shows that clinical symptoms at presentation are not able to predict the severity of the disease and that transmission is frequent from asymptomatic infected subjects [2]. Chest radiography, despite its wide availability and low cost, has low diagnostic sensitivity for pneumonia in cases of COVID-19 [3]. On the other hand, lung computed tomography (CT) is considered to be the best image modality for early identification of pulmonary involvement in patients infected with SARS-CoV-2 [1]. In a recent study, the sensitivity of CT was reported to be superior to reverse transcription polymerase chain reaction (RT-PCR) (98% vs. 71%, respectively, $p < 0.001$) in the diagnosis of COVID-19 [4]. However, a role of CT imaging in the diagnosis of COVID-19 is ambiguous and this latter study has been heavily criticized [5]. Moreover, it is difficult to imagine

*Correspondence: analuisasvieira@gmail.com
[1] Department of Nephrology, Santa Casa de Misericórdia de Barbacena and University of Medicine of Barbacena Department of Point of Care Ultrasound, Minas Gerais, Brazil
Full list of author information is available at the end of the article

a scenario where CT is systematically performed in all suspected cases of COVID-19 because of costs, time consumption, exposure to radiation, possibility of cross-infections, and even non-availability in scarce resource areas.

Patients with end-stage renal disease (ESRD) are at increased risk of infection with SARS-CoV-2 virus. Reports from health services around the world have indicated that patients with diabetes mellitus and hypertension, two of the main causes of ESRD worldwide, and also advanced age and cardiovascular complications, two frequent accompanying conditions in dialysis patients, are more susceptible to SARS-CoV-2 infection and more prone to develop severe COVID-19 pneumonia, eventually requiring intensive care treatment [2, 6, 7]. Moreover, the logistical characteristics of hemodialytic procedures, performed three times a week in closed areas to group of patients, are at increased risk of disease transmission [8]. So far, epidemiological data in patients on ambulatorial hemodialysis with COVID-19 are limited. During the outbreak in a hemodialysis unit of Wuhan, it was reported that 37 out of 230 patients (16.1%) and 4 out of 33 staff personal (12.1%) were diagnosed with COVID-19 [7]. During the 33 days of follow-up, seven of those patients died.

Lung ultrasound (LUS) shows superior sensitivity when compared to X-ray in patients with acute respiratory failure [9]. Moreover, LUS has been experienced during the Chinese outbreak of COVID-19 [3, 10]. Nonetheless, LUS may be a more feasible and practical alternative since it can be quickly done at the bedside, is repeatable and reduces the possibility of cross-infections. In Italy, LUS has been proposed as an alternative to CT for suspected cases of COVID-19 [11–14].

Based on our experience and supported by the existing literature, we suggest the use of LUS in dialysis patients to allow the early recognition of the disease as well as to indicate the severity of pulmonary involvement, allowing a safer allocation of dialysis patients during the COVID-19 pandemic.

The special role of LUS during the COVID-19 pandemic

The role of LUS to evaluate several respiratory conditions is nowadays widely documented [9]. The lesions observed in CT scan of patients with COVID-19 are generally peripheral and subpleural, perhaps due to the fact that SARS-CoV-2 is a novel virus with an average diameter of only about 120 nm, which allows it to be easily inhaled down to the peripheric airways and alveoli without immune barrier [10].

LUS is an image method that classically allows the evaluation of the pulmonary periphery which makes it an excellent technique in the assessment of COVID-19. The same physician in charge of the patient can obtain pulmonary images by LUS performed at bedside, thus minimizing the number of health professionals potentially exposed to the virus. This is a crucial point, considering that data from Italy and Spain, two of countries with the highest rate of COVID-19, show that approximately 9 to 12% of health workers became infected and were quarantined [15].

The technology of modern ultrasound machines (portable and ultra-portable) currently available has many favorable characteristics. The easy portability at the bedside, the long battery life and the possibility to be connected to smartphones and tablets make them suitable even in remote areas. The small dimension is also a favorable characteristic to allow an easy procedure for disinfection, which is crucial in the context of the current pandemic. The application of LUS by portable machines allows the examination without the need to move the patient to radiology facilities, which would increase the risk of cross-infections. Another important advantage of modern technology is connectivity that allows the possibility of image sharing through social media and other internet systems, making telemedicine a possible help to local medical staffs. However, not always handheld machines are available in the medical units. LUS is becoming critical in the front door of this COVID-19 outbreak. Thus, any ultrasound machine should be used based on the availability. Carriable ultrasound machines can be dedicated to specific areas where patients suspected for COVID-19 are examined. Anyway, we recommend an accurate disinfection of the probes after each exam using alcohol solutions to avoid contamination. In case of use of the ultrasound machine during invasive procedures at risk of aerosol dispersion, we also recommend using transparent covers on the keyboard and a full disinfection of the screen and other parts at the end of the maneuver.

Basic principles of LUS

LUS is a relatively new technique that has been used increasingly since the pioneering work of Lichtenstein and Axler, published in the early 90s [16]. Nowadays, LUS is frequently used in the emergency departments and intensive care units in the diagnosis of several lung diseases [17]. More recently, nephrologists also discovered LUS as a great tool to evaluate their dialytic patients [18, 19].

The images obtained with LUS most of the time are not anatomical. They are based on artifacts generated by the interaction of the ultrasound beam with the acoustic interface between the tissues of the chest wall and the air in the alveoli distributed in the pulmonary surface. Indeed, LUS can only study lung diseases that abut the pleura [16, 20]. Patients can be examined either in supine/semi-recumbent (with arm abducted over the head) or in sitting position, as similarly done during the standard physical examination [21]. Each hemithorax is generally divided into three areas: anterior (between parasternal and anterior axillary lines), lateral (between anterior and posterior axillary lines) (Fig. 1) and posterior (between posterior axillary line and the spine) (Fig. 2). Each area is further divided into superior and inferior [9]. In the case of critical care patients who cannot collaborate and lie down in the supine position, the dorsal region of both lungs can be assessed by slightly moving the patient in lateral decubitus [22]. The lungs can be scanned using a high-frequency probe (linear) or by a low-frequency probe (convex, microconvex and phased array). The higher the frequency, the greater is the image resolution, even though penetration is reduced. On the other hand, low-frequency transducers can reach greater depths, but at the expense of a lower image resolution. In the context of this pandemic, we recommend using a probe with a large surface of emission and a technique for LUS that allows a quick examination of the whole chest surface. Also, the probe should transmit at a low frequency to allow enough penetration and evaluate pleural surface and vertical artifacts at the same time. This description corresponds to the convex probe. The transducer should be positioned longitudinally to the chest and perpendicular to the ribs. On occasion, the probe can be turned to obtain an oblique scan along the intercostal space to visualize more in detail the LUS pattern in a wider portion of the pleural surface. LUS allows a dynamic examination in real time and the transducer must be handled

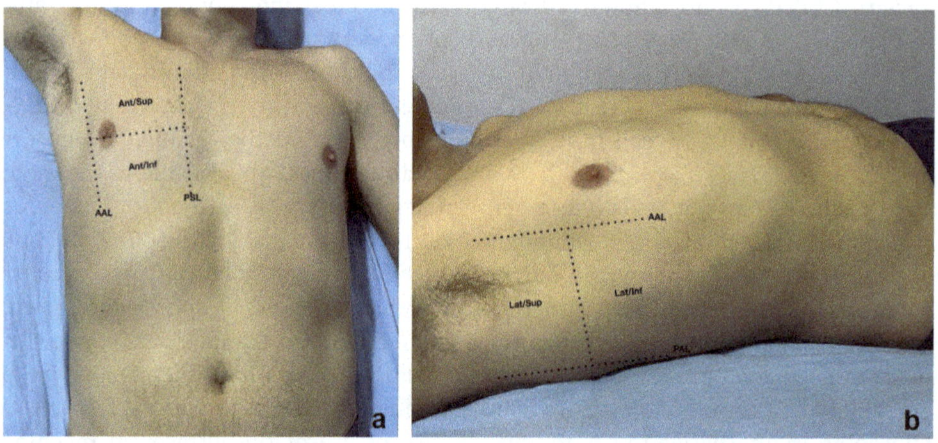

Fig. 1 Anterior and lateral chest. **a** Anterior chest is delimited by parasternal line (PSL) and anterior axillary line (AAL) and divided in superior (ant/sup) and inferior (ant/inf). **b** Lateral chest is delimited by anterior axillary line (AAL) and posterior axillary line (PAL) and divided in superior (lat/sup) and inferior (lat/inf)

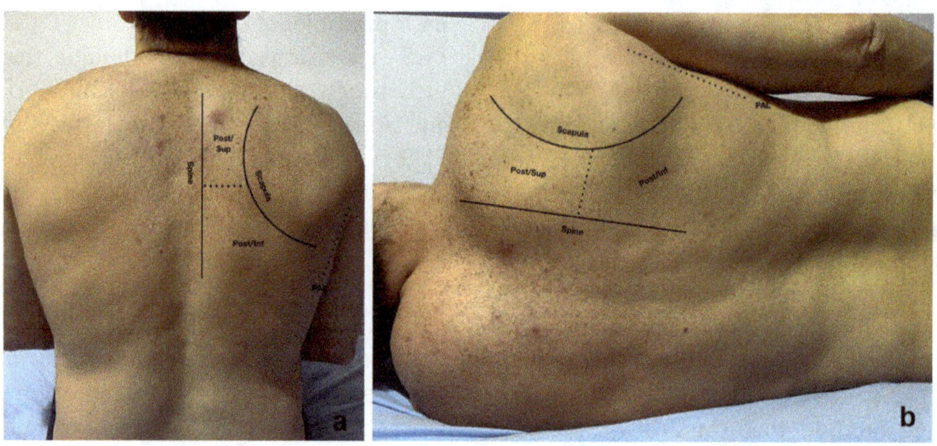

Fig. 2 Posterior chest in sitting and lateral decubitus positions. Posterior chest is delimited by the spine and posterior axillary line (PAL) and divided in superior (post/sup) and inferior (post/inf). **a** Patient in sitting position. **b** Patient in lateral decubitus position

with continuous slow movements of tilting, sliding and rotating to optimize the image. During the insonation, it is also helpful to adjust the image gain and depth (around 8 to 10 cm) and position the focus (when available) at the level of the pleural line. As LUS is based on artifacts, it is important to disable the "Multi Beam", "Tissue Harmonic Imaging" features and filters that optimize the real images and decrease artifacts [20].

Lung patterns

LUS is a technique mainly based on the visualization of artifacts originating by the acoustic mismatch between tissue and air in the surface of the lung [12]. Normally, in the periphery of the lung, there is basically alveoli-filled with air. When the ultrasound beam encounters the interface between two structures with opposite values of acoustic impedance, it is completely reflected back to the transducer. Thus, during the chest insonation, the ultrasound beam will pass through skin, subcutaneous tissue, muscles, until it reaches the pleura. This latter corresponds to the interface where the maximum acoustic tissue/air mismatch is encountered and will be visualized as an echoic horizontal linear artifact, the pleural line. Below the pleural line, the examiner may see echoes that reproduce the pleural line at regular equidistant intervals echoing more times the distance between the probe and the pleura. These horizontal artifacts, indicated as A-lines, are visualized when the lung is well aerated (Fig. 3) (Additional file 1) [23].

Accumulation of subpleural interstitial exudate, transudate, collagen, and blood causes loss of aeration and changes the air–liquid balance. Also, the fibrotic thickenings of the interlobular septa create a similar deaeration. In these pathologic conditions, the pulmonary surface will not be a strong reflector of the ultrasound beams. The first grade of loss of aeration causes a partial penetration of the ultrasound creating vertical artifacts on the images displayed on the screen. Nowadays, these artifacts are called B-lines [12]. B-lines are defined as discrete laser-like vertical hyperechoic reverberation artifacts that arise from the pleural line, extend to the bottom of the screen without fading, and move synchronously with lung sliding [24] (Fig. 4) (Additional file 2). When the accumulation of fluid raises, the B-lines proportionally increase in number and intensity until tend to coalesce, originating a pattern called white lung [23] (Fig. 5) (Additional file 3). In this progression, the final step of loss of aeration and increase in density gives the pattern of a consolidated lung parenchyma [21] (Fig. 6) (Additional file 4).

How to interpret the findings of LUS in dialytic patients suspicious for COVID-19

LUS allows a first screening of patients admitted at the dialysis unit presenting symptoms that raise suspicion of COVID-19. It can help triaging between low-risk patients

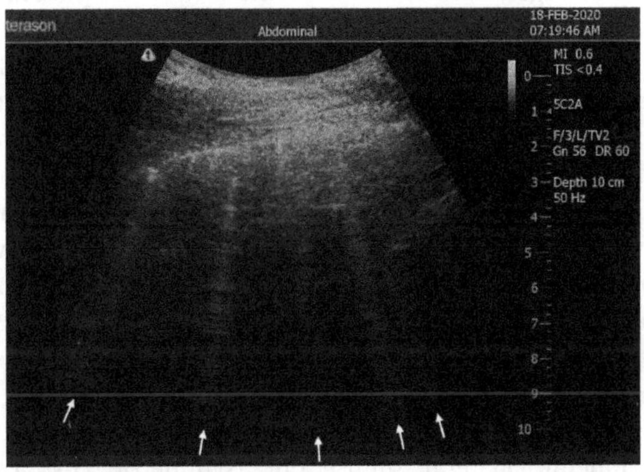

Fig. 4 Sonographic appearance of B-lines in oblique view. White arrows indicate multiple B-lines

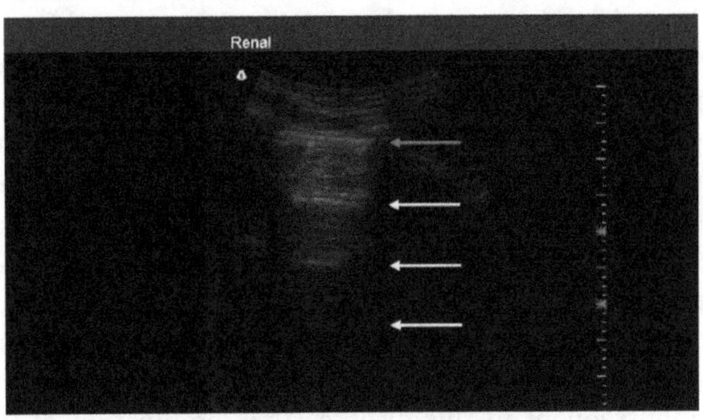

Fig. 3 Sonographic appearance of an aerated lung scan in longitudinal view. Red arrow indicates pleural line; white arrows indicate A-lines

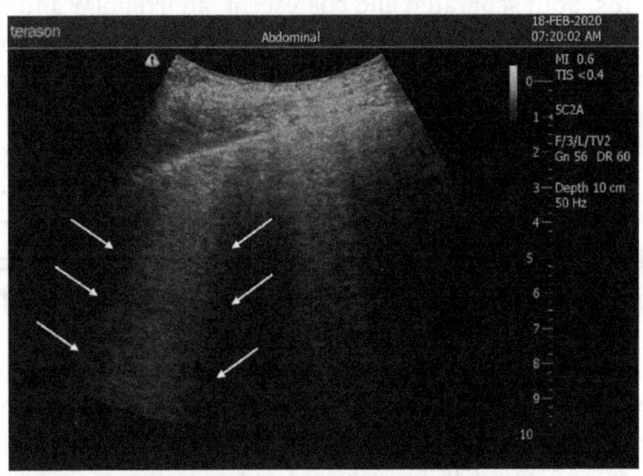

Fig. 5 Sonographic appearance of coalescent B-lines. White arrows indicate area with coalescent B-lines, called white lung

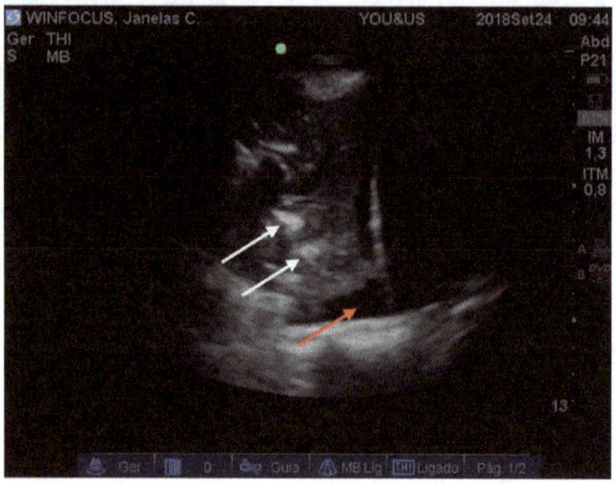

Fig. 6 Sonographic features of lung consolidation. The echo-texture of lung becomes similar to the liver. White arrows indicate air bronchograms. Red arrow indicates pleural effusion

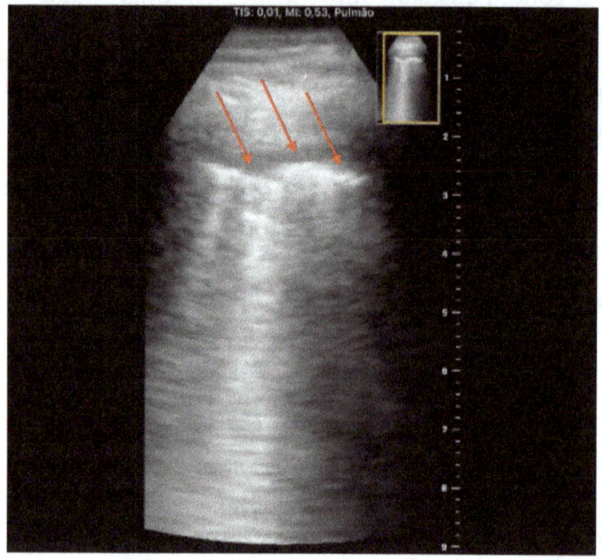

Fig. 7 Sonographic appearance of pleural irregularities in a COVID-19 patient. Red arrows indicate fragmented and irregular pleural line

(patients clinically stable who do not present pathologic LUS changes) and those who show signs of pneumonia and high risk for severe forms of the disease. Thus, LUS allows us to diagnose pneumonia in COVID-19 and differentiate the severity of the disease at presentation, useful to select who requires hospitalization and limit unnecessary nosocomial exposure. However, it is important to highlight that in case of abnormal LUS pattern suggestive of viral pneumonia, ruling out alternative conditions may represent a challenge. Indeed, B-lines and consolidations are not enough specific and cannot easily differentiate hydrostatic/cardiogenic edema or other pathologic conditions [14].

The interstitial pneumonia in COVID-19 is typically peripheral, bilateral, diffuse but asymmetric [14]. For this reason, the LUS exam in the suspected patient must be performed all over the chest surface [10]. The typical patterns detected by LUS in patients with COVID-19 pneumonia are characterized by B-lines in different forms, both separated and coalescent, an irregular and/or fragmented pleural line, peripheral small consolidations, and large consolidations with dynamic air bronchograms [3] (Fig. 7) (Additional file 5). These patterns are usually intercalated with "spared areas" (A-lines) [13]. A large pleural effusion is not a common finding [3]. Detection of the typical signs, described above combined in a pattern with a typical bilateral and patchy distribution, raises the high probability of the presence of the disease in a symptomatic patient.

However, in dialytic patients the interpretation of the artifacts is more challenging, due to the fact that these frequently are affected by cardiovascular complications and quite frequently present a status of hypervolemia [25]. It is especially critical to differentiate the characteristics of the B-lines in dialytic patients admitted with dyspnea, since these artifacts are the most frequent findings in COVID-19 pneumonia and also typically found in hypervolemic patients with lung congestion. B-lines due to hypervolemia are symmetrically distributed in both lungs and initially well separated. The symmetric distribution is gravity related and the anterior superior areas are the last part of the lung to be involved in the process of progression of the severity of lung congestion. Thus, correlation of the severity of the B-lines representation and the severity of the symptoms of the patient becomes critical. Furthermore, the pleural line is usually diffusely regular, and lung consolidations are not detected. Another differential characteristic is that the pleural effusion is a common finding in hypervolemia. On the other hand, although B-lines due to COVID-19 are also typically bilateral, they have a different distribution. In pneumonia during the course of COVID-19, it is typical the visualization of clusters of B-lines, both in separated and coalescent forms. Moreover, other authors described an intense "shining band-form artifact spreading down from a large portion of a regular pleura, often appearing and disappearing with an on–off effect in the context of a normal A-lines lung pattern visible on the background" [14] (Fig. 8). This sign has been called "light beam" artifact (Additional file 6). This band may also originate from an irregular pleural line or from small subpleural consolidations. The "light beam" is not only observed in COVID-19 pneumonia but it is highly frequent in this disease. The combination of the light beam with the other artifacts in clusters alternating abruptly with spared A-lines areas, with the typical

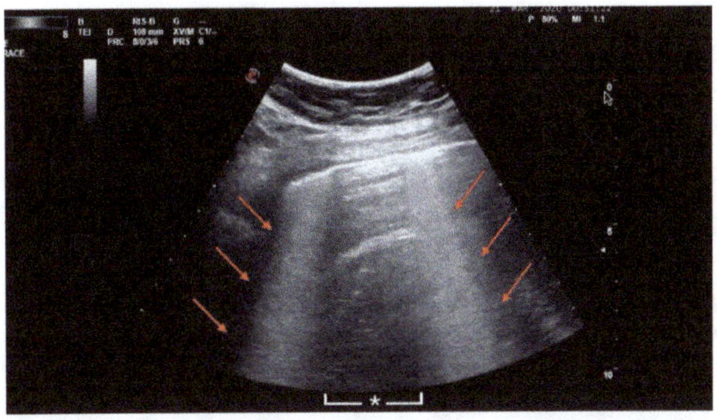

Fig. 8 Sonographic appearance of "light beam" artifact. Red arrows indicate band-form signs arising from a large portion of a regular pleural, called "light beam". The asterisk indicates the spared area (A-lines). Image kindly provided by Dr. Giovanni Volpicelli

patchy distribution, gives the specificity to LUS for the diagnosis of COVID-19 pneumonia [13, 14]. This is particularly effective when LUS is applied in patients presenting with the typical symptoms of COVID-19, in this specific moment of outbreak with a high prevalence of the disease.

If the B-lines pattern that can be observed by LUS in dialytic patients does not fully respect the typical characteristics of a COVID-19 pneumonia and cannot allow a definitive conclusion, we suggest to extend the ultrasound scan to the heart and the inferior vena cava (IVC). ESRD patients frequently present cardiovascular complications, giving combined or separated diastolic and systolic dysfunctions. These dysfunctions frequently are associated and even favor hypervolemia, and may easily result in pulmonary congestion [26]. Fluid congestion of the pulmonary interstitium is represented with high sensitivity by multiple and diffuse B-lines at LUS. Not only LUS is highly sensitive in the detection of pulmonary congestion, but also it can indicate the effectiveness of a treatment that reduces the congestion. Thus, if monitoring the patients during the dialysis session the number of B-lines decreases after the ultrafiltration, it is a reliable indicator that the origin of the LUS pattern is hypervolemia and not the infection [27].

The ultrasound evaluation of the diameter and the respiro-phasic change of IVC can also be helpful in a scenario where differential interpretation of B-lines is a challenge. A collapsing or close to collapsing IVC before the dialysis session is not compatible with a condition of hypervolemia. On the other hand, a plethoric IVC shortly after dialysis implies a still filled intravascular space. However, the ultrasound examination of the IVC poses always the necessity to consider possible confounding factors. It is essential to consider the clinical settings. For instance, there are situations when the decrease of IVC diameter is not related to progression to hypovolemia, but may be linked to increased abdominal pressure, an abnormal inspiratory effort, and others. At the same time, situations revealing increase in the IVC diameter may be not necessarily related to hypervolemia, like it is observed in some specific cardiac conditions determining an obstacle to the venous return or in pulmonary conditions with alveolar hyperinflation, and so on [28].

Using ultrasound in dialysis patients during COVID-19 pandemic

As seen previously in this article, it is clear that dialysis patients are at a greater risk of developing the most severe forms of COVID-19, in addition to being potential vectors of the disease; since due to the specificities of their treatment, they cannot fully adhere to the social distancing, recommended by the World Health Organization [29].

Based on current evidence and our experience with point-of-care ultrasound in nephrology, we suggest the following recommendations in the management of dialytic patients during the pandemic (Fig. 9):

1. The creation of different allocations, whenever possible, for patients who arrive and leave the clinic, thus reducing contacts between patients;
2. Immediate supply of surgical masks as soon as patients arrive to the unit for the dialysis session. The mask must be kept by the patient for the entire stay in the clinic. During triage, a health professional, also wearing a surgical mask, should investigate about any suspected symptom of COVID-19 infection, such as fever, cough and dyspnea, and possibility of any contact with confirmed cases of COVID-19 or permanence in areas with diffuse presence of the disease. In addition, the temperature must be checked using an infrared thermometer, minimizing contacts with the patient;
3. If the patient is asymptomatic and does not confirm any contact with confirmed cases, the patient can be referred to his/her dialysis session, as usual;
4. If the patient is asymptomatic but confirms any contact with positive COVID-19 cases or provenience from an area of strong epidemic, he/she should preferably be referred to an isolated room dedicated to suspected cases, where patients remain separated with a minimum distance of 1.82 m [8]. In this room, particular care should be reserved to allow isolation from contact and protection of the dialysis personnel, who should wear full protective gear such as waterproof disposable gown, cap, gloves, face shield, and at least N95 face mask, and proceed with more rigorous cleaning and disinfection. Complementary tests

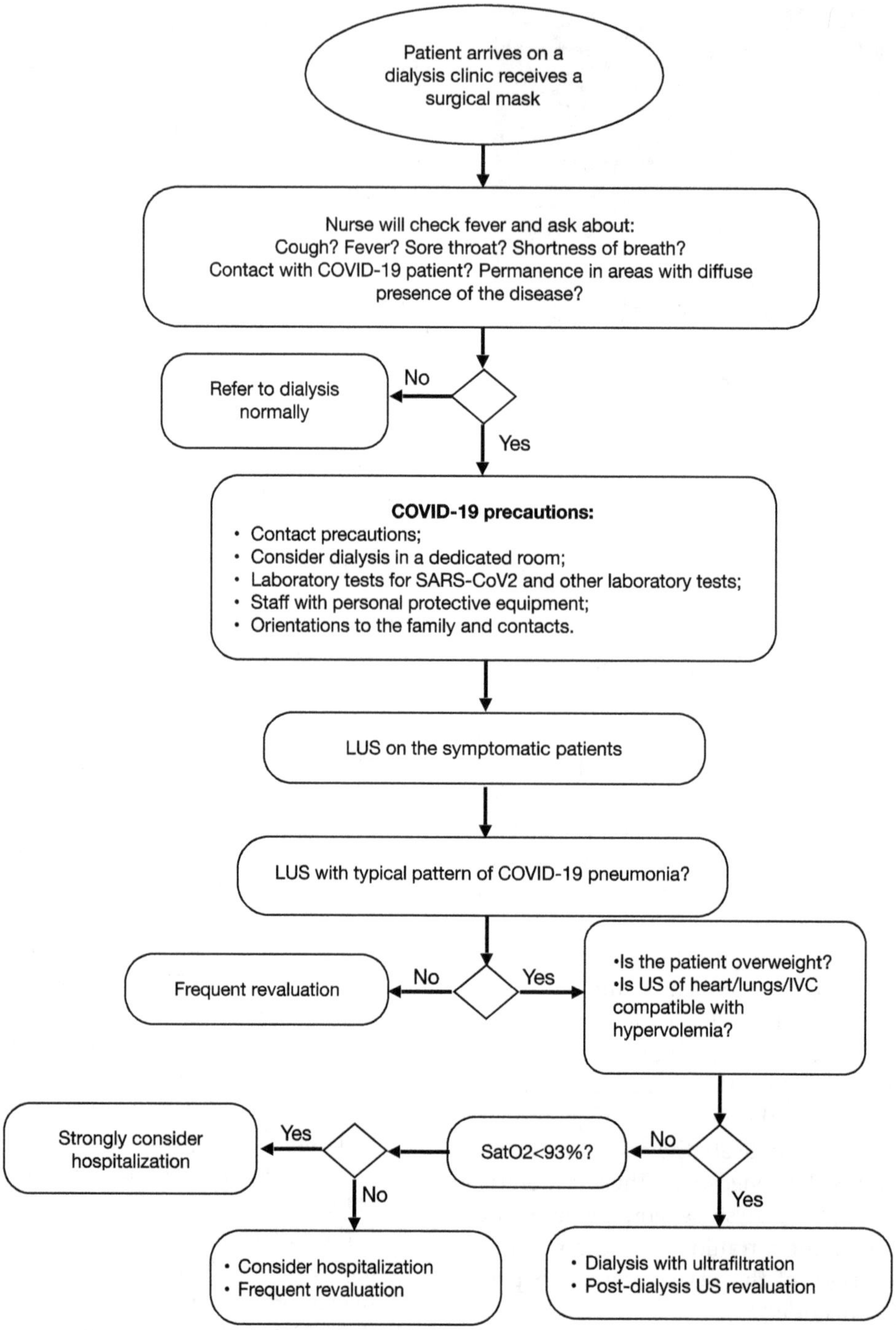

Fig. 9 Flowchart of our recommendations for management of dialysis patients in COVID-19 pandemic

for virus identification, and RT-PCR for SARS-CoV-2 can also be ordered, if available. Until the result of the test is obtained, all the family members should be alerted and the patient should maintain isolation for at least 14 days [29];

5. If the patient presents with signs and symptoms of the disease, all the previous measures should not only be adopted but the patient should also be studied by LUS at triage. The signs characteristic of the disease should be investigated, with a particular focus on the presence, characteristics and distribution of B-lines;
6. If the patient shows the typical LUS pattern of COVID-19 pneumonia without doubts about the alternative possibility of hydrostatic pulmonary edema, the next step is to assess the peripheral oxygen saturation. If saturation is below 93%, hospital

admission should be strongly considered. If saturation is above 93%, the cost–benefit ratio of hospitalization should be considered. Other factors, like adequate family support, comorbidities and socio-economic conditions, are important conditions that need to be investigated and considered. In the case a patient with positive signs of COVID-19 pneumonia is discharged to home, frequent clinical re-assessment should be programmed;

7. If the patient shows a pattern of B-lines not typical and hydrostatic edema remains a possible alternative, ideally, a more detailed ultrasound assessment should be performed, by extending the examination to the heart and IVC. If the ultrasound findings are compatible with hydrostatic edema, the patient should be submitted to dialysis with ultrafiltration and reassessed clinically and with ultrasound at the end of the procedure. If the clinical status and the LUS pattern improve significantly in terms of resolution of dyspnea and reduction in the number of B-lines, the possibility that the LUS pattern observed at triage was secondary to hypervolemia is reinforced. If there is no change in clinical and LUS parameters, the possibility of an infective origin of B-lines increases;
8. In the context of the pandemic that we are experiencing, it is essential to pay attention to measures of individual protection and the accurate cleaning and disinfection of the device and transducers after their use. The examiner must wear an apron, gloves (three pairs), glasses and N95 mask. The patient must wear a surgical mask during the examination [30]. To avoid contamination of the US device, it is recommended to cover the equipment keyboard with transparent plastic films to be changed after each use. It is also recommended to clean the device with gauze or similar material soaked in 70% alcohol and the transducers according to the manufacturer's guidelines (in general, compounds based on quaternary ammonia are recommended). The first pair of gloves should be removed after examining the patient, the second pair after disinfecting the equipment and the third pair together with the removal of the garment [31].

Conclusion

The world is witnessing a pandemic with disastrous effects due to the rapid spread of the SARS-CoV-2 virus and the huge demand for resources needed to contain COVID-19. In this context, LUS performed by the attending physician represents a safe, inexpensive, easily reproducible technique with a great potential in allowing to differentiate patients with signs of COVID-19 pneumonia. The screening performed by the LUS at the bedside allows defining the immediate management of dialysis patients, seen in dialysis units, where other propaedeutic resources are often not available. A strategy based on triaging suspected patients for COVID-19 pneumonia is potentially useful to prevent the dissemination of the virus and also to impact positively the prognosis of vulnerable dialytic patients.

Supplementary information

Additional file 1: Video 1. A-lines. Longitudinal scan on the anterior chest of a patient with aerated lung. The video demonstrates the A-lines.

Additional file 2: Video 2. Multiple B-lines. Oblique scan on the anterior chest of a hypervolemic patient with multiple (but not coalescent) B-lines.

Additional file 3: Video 3. Coalescent B-lines. Oblique scan on the lateral chest of a hypervolemic patient with coalescent B-lines.

Additional file 4: Video 4. Lung Consolidation and Pleural effusion. Scan of the right lung base of a patient with pneumonia. The video shows lung consolidation with dynamic air bronchogram and pleural effusion.

Additional file 5: Video 5. Pleural irregularity. Scan of a patient with COVID-19 performed by a hand-held device showing pleural irregularities.

Additional file 6: Video 6. "Light Beam" sign. Oblique scan of a patient with COVID-19 with "light beam" signs with on–off effect and separated by spared areas (A-lines).

Abbreviations

COVID-19: Corona Virus Disease-19; CT: Computed tomography; ESRD: End-stage renal disease; HD: Hemodialysis; IVC: Inferior vena cava; LUS: Lung ultrasound; RT-PCR: Reverse transcription polymerase chain reaction; SARS-CoV-2: Severe Acute Respiratory Syndrome Corona Virus; US: Ultrasound.

Acknowledgements

We sincerely thank Dr. Giovanni Volpicelli for image courtesy ("light beam" video) and for sharing his knowledge.

Authors' contributions

All the authors of the article are responsible for concept and writing. All authors read and approved the final manuscript.

Author details

[1] Department of Nephrology, Santa Casa de Misericórdia de Barbacena and University of Medicine of Barbacena Department of Point of Care Ultrasound, Minas Gerais, Brazil. [2] Department of Nephrology and Intensive Care Medicine, Santa Casa de Misericórdia de Barbacena and University of Medicine of Barbacena Department of Point of Care Ultrasound, Minas Gerais, Brazil. [3] Federal University of Juiz de Fora, Minas Gerais, Brazil. [4] Faculty at School of Medicine, UNIFAGOC and SUPREMA, Minas Gerais, Brazil.

References

1. Guan W, Ni Z, Hu Y et al (2020) Clinical characteristics of 2019 novel coronavirus infection in China. N Engl J Med 27:382
2. Deng Y, Liu W, Liu K et al (2020) Clinical characteristics of fatal and recovered cases of coronavirus disease 2019 (COVID-19) in Wuhan, China: a retrospective study. Chin Med J (Engl). https://doi.org/10.1097/cm9.0000000000000824
3. Peng Q, Wang X, Zhang L (2020) Findings of lung ultrasonography of novel corona virus pneumonia during the 2019–2020 epidemic. Intensive Care Med. https://doi.org/10.1007/s00134-020-05996-6
4. Fang Y, Zhang H, Xie J et al (2020) Sensitivity of chest CT for COVID-19: comparison to RT-PCR. Radiology. https://doi.org/10.1148/radiol.2020200432

5. Hope MD, Raptis CA, Henry TS (2020) Chest computed tomography for detection medicine. Ann Intern Med. https://doi.org/10.7326/m20-1382
6. Webster A, Nagler E, Morton R et al (2017) Chronic Kidney disease. Lancet 389(10075):1238–1252
7. Yiqiong M, Diao B, Xifeng L et al (2020) 2019 novel coronavirus disease in hemodialysis (HD) patients: report from one HD center in Wuhan, china. medRxiv. https://doi.org/10.1101/2020.02.24.20027201
8. Jody A. Charnow (2020) Dialysis Facilities Confront COVID-19. https://www.renalandurologynews.com/home/news/nephrology/hemodialysis/dialysis-facilities-brace-for-covid-19/. Accessed 12 Apr 2020
9. Lichtenstein D, Malbrain M (2017) Lung ultrasound in the critically ill (LUCI): a translational discipline. Anaesthesiol Intensive Ther 49:430–436
10. Huang Y, Wang S, Liu Y et al (2020) A Preliminary Study on the Ultrasonic Manifestations of Peripulmonary Lesions of Non-Critical Novel Coronavirus Pneumonia (COVID-19) https://ssrn.com/abstract=3544750 or http://dx.doi.org/10.2139/ssrn.3544750
11. Poggiali E et al (2020) Can lung US help critical care clinicians in the early diagnosis of novel coronavirus (COVID-19) pneumonia? Radiology. https://doi.org/10.1148/radiol.2020200847
12. Soldati G, Smargiassi A, Inchingolo R et al (2020) Is there a role for lung ultrasound during the COVID-19 pandemic? J Ultrasound Med. https://doi.org/10.1002/jum.15284
13. Volpicelli G, Gargani L (2020) Sonographic signs and patterns of COVID-19 pneumonia. Ultrasound J. https://doi.org/10.1186/s13089-020-00171-w
14. Volpicelli G, Lamorte A, Villen T (2020) What's new in lung ultrasound during the COVID-19 pandemic. Intensive Care Med. https://doi.org/10.1007/s00134-020-06048-9
15. BBC World News. https://www.youtube.com/watch?v=lq1kpx5LyQl&feature=youtu.be. Accessed 12 Apr 2020
16. Lichtenstein D, Axler O (1993) Intensive use of general ultrasound in the intensive care unit, a prospective study of 150 consecutive patients. Intensive Care Med 19:353–355
17. Arbelot C, Dexheimer Neto FL, Geo Y et al (2020) Lung ultrasound in emergency and critically ill patients: number of supervised exams to reach basic competence. Anesthesiology 132(4):899–907
18. Muniz Pazeli J et al (2014) Can nephrologists use ultrasound to evaluate the inferior vena cava? A cross-sectional study of the agreement between a nephrologist and a cardiologist. Nephron Extra. 4(1):82–88
19. Surekha M, Stephen M, Paul S et al (2018) Point-of-care ultrasound education to improve care of dialysis patients. Semin Dial 31(2):154–162
20. Lichtenstein DA (2010) Introduction to Lung Ultrasound. In: Lichtenstein DA (ed) Whole Body ultrasonography in the critically ill. Springer-Verlag, Heidelberg, pp 117–127
21. Gargani L, Volpicelli G (2014) How I do it: lung ultrasound. Cardiovasc Ultrasound 12:25
22. Lichtenstein D, Mezière G (2008) Relevance of lung ultrasound in the diagnosis of acute respiratory failure: the BLUE protocol. Chest 134:117–125
23. Demi M, Soldati G, Demi L (2018) On the artefactual information of ultrasound lung images: a lines and B lines. Proc Mtgs Acoust 35:020003
24. Volpicelli G et al (2012) International evidence-based recommendations for point-of-care lung ultrasound. Intensive Care Med 38:577–591
25. Mallamaci F, Benedetto F, Tripepi R et al (2010) Detection of pulmonary congestion by chest ultrasound in dialysis patients. JACC Cardiovasc Imag 3(6):586–594
26. Bucharles S, Varela A, Barberato S et al (2010) Assessment and management of cardiovascular disease in patients with chronic kidney disease. J Bras Nefrol 32(1):118–125
27. Noble V, Murray A, Capp R et al (2009) Ultrasound assessment for extravascular lung water in patients undergoing hemodialysis. Time course for resolution. Chest 135(6):1433–1439
28. Via G, Tavazzi G, Price S (2016) Ten situations where inferior vena cava ultrasound may fail to accurately predict fluid responsiveness: a physiologically based point of view. Intensive Care Med 42(7):1164–1167
29. Center for Disease Control and Prevention. Coronavirus Disease 2019 (COVID-19): Social Distancing, Quarantine, and Isolation. https://www.cdc.gov/coronavirus/2019-ncov/prevent-getting-sick/social-distancing.html. Accessed 12 Apr 2020
30. United States Department of Labor. https://www.osha.gov/SLTC/covid-19/controlprevention.html. Accessed 12 Apr 2020
31. ACEP Guideline on COVID-19: Ultrasound Machine and Transducer Cleaning. Approved March 31, 2020. https://www.acep.org/globalassets/new-pdfs/guideline-on-covid-19–ultrasound-machine-and-transducer-cleaning_policy_033120.pdf. Accessed 12 Apr 2020

11

Billing I-AIM: a novel framework for ultrasound billing

Daralee Hughes[1*], Michelle M. Corrado[2], Irene Mynatt[1], Michael Prats[1], Nelson A. Royall[3], Creagh Boulger[1] and David P. Bahner[1]

Abstract

Background: Point-of-care ultrasound (POCUS) has an ever-growing footprint in medicine. With this growth POCUS billing and reimbursement has become an area gaining quite a bit of attention as a means of funding and sustaining quality and education programs. Standardization across providers is needed to improve the financial viability of POCUS.

Results: We created an institutional collaborative which developed a framework to identify critical POCUS billing and reimbursement checkpoints. The framework, Billing I-AIM, provides a feasible structure to enhance provider-based reimbursement and perform quality improvement efforts across variable POCUS environments.

Conclusions: POCUS billing using the Billing I-AIM technique allows administrative oversight, quality assurance, and educational functions as well. A discussion of the framework and respective application is provided.

Keywords: Point-of-care ultrasound, Ultrasonography, Ultrasound billing, Ultrasound reimbursement, Emergency service, Bedside ultrasound

Background

Point-of-care ultrasound (POCUS) utilization in medicine is rapidly increasing in academic and community settings [1]. Numerous studies demonstrate that physician-performed POCUS improves patient care through increased diagnostic accuracy, decreased time to diagnosis and intervention, decreased procedural complications, decreased length of stay, and decreased patient care costs [1–10]. Although utilization of POCUS is increasing, standard procedures for ultrasound documentation and billing procedures have not been codified with standardized terminology in the published medical literature.

The American College of Emergency Physicians (ACEP), as well as organizations from other specialties, have defined the scope of practice for POCUS [10, 11]. These guidelines from 2016 establish four clinical categories for POCUS: resuscitative, diagnostic, symptom or sign-based procedure guidance, and therapeutic and monitoring [3]. Across all clinical categories, POCUS applications are accepted to be a separate billable procedure. To this point, unique codes exist for POCUS within Current Procedural Terminology (CPT) and International Classification of Disease Procedures Coding System (ICD-PCS). POCUS billing requires additional unique documentation and variable preservation of imaging based upon the clinical category and payer source, which differs from comprehensive radiology ultrasound exams. In POCUS, images and interpretations are completed by the same provider at the bedside, whereas comprehensive reports are completed by an ultrasonographer and then interpreted by a radiologist. Published information on billing and reimbursement for POCUS is limited, and many providers report a high rate of reimbursement denials related to this complex billing process unfamiliar to the average provider [1, 5].

*Correspondence: Daralee.hughes@osumc.edu

†Daralee Hughes and Michelle M. Corrado are co-principal investigators and co-first authors

[1] Department of Emergency Medicine, The Ohio State University College of Medicine, 750 Prior Hall, 376 W 10th Ave, Columbus, OH 43210, USA

Full list of author information is available at the end of the article

As providers are increasingly expected to learn the billing and reimbursement process, there is a need to streamline the billing for reimbursement. Given these challenges, The Ohio State University Wexner Medical Center created an institutional collaborative aimed at evaluating and enhancing the billing and reimbursement process for POCUS. Given the success of teaching mnemonics for acquisition of ultrasound, we proposed similar mnemonics would be beneficial for teaching the billing of POCUS [12]. The purpose of this article is to present concepts developed through the collaborative which facilitate reliable billing for POCUS. We aim to focus on the emergency department (ED) given our institutional experience, but these concepts apply to other hospital-based specialties as well [10].

Methods: the concept

Previously the concept of using a structured mnemonic to teach and perform POCUS has been published and is widely used. This concept, known as I-AIM, is the basis of the nomenclature in this paper used as a way to understand the requirements for POCUS billing and reimbursement [12]. It explains the components involved in the process of performing POCUS, documentation requirements, coding specifics, reasons for revenue loss, and the ways in which ultrasound scans can be classified based on the presence or absence of images and documentation.

The Billing I-AIM concept is (1) Indication, (2) Acquisition, (3) Interpretation, and (4) Money, and includes the components necessary for each of those steps to achieve revenue generation from performed POCUS (Fig. 1). A description of the Billing I-AIM concept is provided in Fig. 1 along with common barriers to reimbursement and nomenclature stratifying ultrasound exams on the presence of documentation and saved images. A discussion of this nomenclature is followed by more detailed information on the components of Billing I-AIM with examples to illustrate concepts.

Results

Ultrasound scan nomenclature

POCUS reimbursement relies upon Medicare standards for diagnostic imaging, which require documentation of the exam performed and images or video depicting the exam. A written interpretation of the indication and description of visualized structures and abnormalities, in addition to stored images within a database are

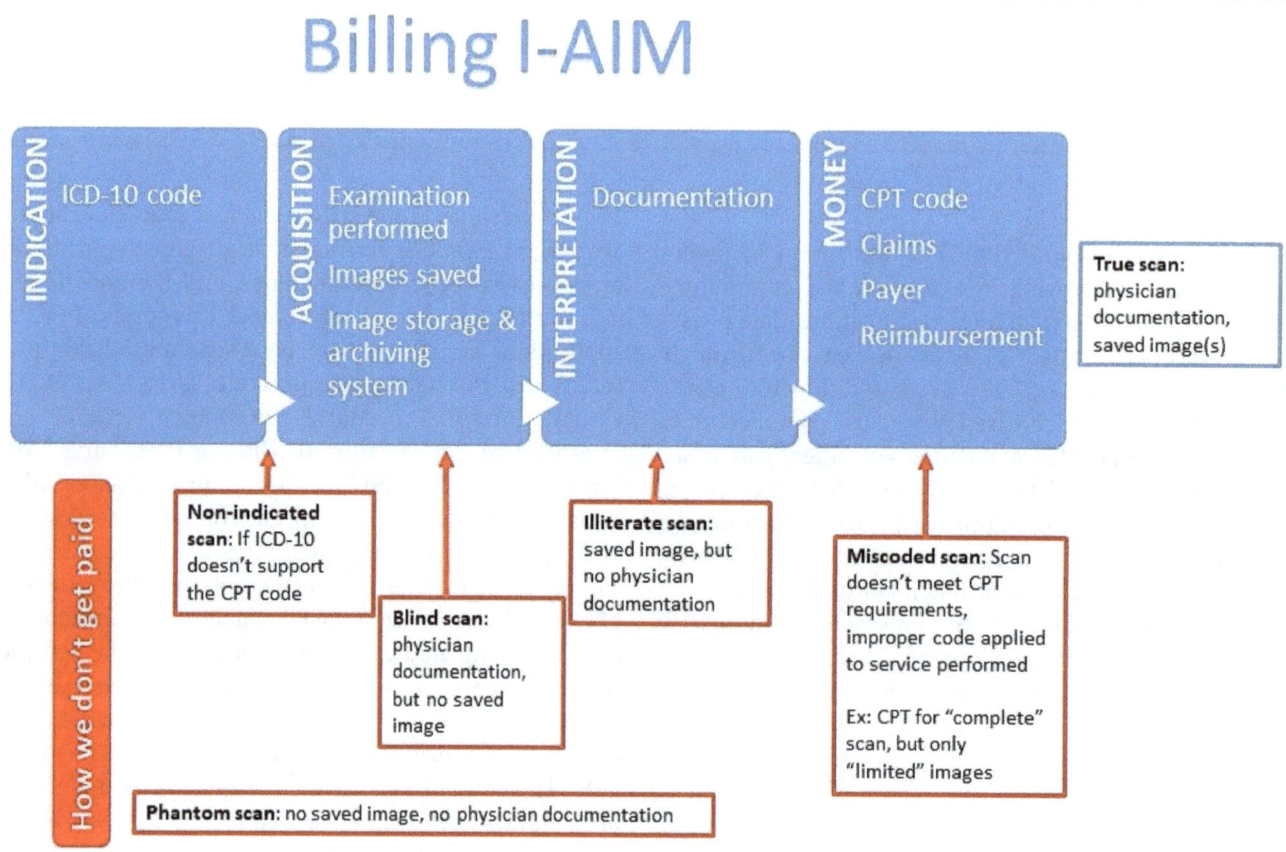

Fig. 1 Billing I-AIM is a simplified framework to enhance provider-based reimbursement and identify common errors

recommended by ACEP in order to fulfill Medicare and other payer requirements for ultrasound examinations [13]. The omission of either documentation or stored images potentially leads to lost revenue.

Given Medicare and ACEP criteria for POCUS examination reimbursement, the following nomenclature was developed to discriminate between properly and improperly completed examinations: phantom, blind, illiterate or true scans (Fig. 2).

Phantom scans are those with no saved images and no provider documentation. From a coding, billing, and medicolegal perspective, these scans never occurred. There is no way to bill for the services provided, and no opportunity for quality assurance.

Blind scans are those with no saved images, but with provider documentation of the scan and integration into the medical decision-making. Without images there can be no quality assurance or review by other providers. These scans are not able to be billed.

Illiterate scans are those with saved images, but without provider documentation. These scans have images that are available for quality assurance and patient care, but documentation is missing. Unlike blind scans, illiterate scans can be reviewed, rectified, and documented at a later time by the performing provider. Blind scans are unable to be retrospectively converted to true scans.

True scan is the final classification. These exams include an appropriate indication, saved images and provider documentation in the medical record. True scans can be coded and billed with the expectation of potential revenue generation.

There are additional permutations in the above-mentioned scans that impact the ability to generate revenue. If the patient's symptoms or diagnosis do not support the ultrasound examination performed, then the scan is not indicated and should not be coded or billed. Miscoded ultrasound exams can also limit revenue. This type of examination does not satisfy the requirements for billing or reimbursement based on the Current Procedural Terminology (CPT) code submitted, which is generally outside of the physician's ability to control. For example, if an ultrasound examination with images supporting only a limited CPT code is submitted under the complete CPT code, it may not be reimbursed. Details regarding limited versus complete scans and further information on CPT codes are discussed in subsequent sections.

Physician Documentation of Findings	Images or Video Recorded: Yes	Images or Video Recorded: No
Yes	True (+ +)	Blind (+ -)
No	Illiterate (- +)	Phantom (- -)

Fig. 2 For correct billing, both saved images and documentation of the scanning procedure are necessary

Billing for POCUS

There are specific reporting and documentation requirements for POCUS. The requirements are (1) test indication, (2) written report, and (3) interpretation [13]. The ultrasound exam must be medically necessary and the signs, symptoms or diagnoses prompting the ultrasound must be recorded in the EMR. There must be a written report signed by the performing physician for each procedure performed [13]. The ultrasound examination should be immediately interpreted and communicated to other providers via the patient's medical record. The documentation should describe the structures evaluated, the presence or absence of relevant anatomy or pathology, and the interpretation of findings [3, 13]. Incomplete or improper documentation prevents coding, billing, and physician compensation for patient care provided [5].

Indication

The indication for any ultrasound examination performed by the hospital-based physician is the complaint, exam finding, or other test result that demonstrates the medical necessity, which must be properly documented [13]. The protocol-driven use of ultrasound or a "screening examination" (such as for AAA in a patient with risk factors but without abnormal vital signs, classic symptoms or physical exam findings) may not be deemed medically necessary and may be denied payment as a non-indicated procedure performed [13].

Medical necessity is currently determined by the International Classification of Diseases (ICD), currently in the 10th edition. The ICD-10 is a code set published by the World Health Organization and is a cataloging tool developed for comparison of morbidity and mortality data [13]. Each code defines "the medical situation and conveys the necessity for subsequent medical services performed" [14]. The ICD-10 code is used by payers to determine why a procedure was performed. This differs from the CPT code which explains to the payer what procedure or service was performed [13]. The CPT codes are discussed further in the "Money" section.

If the patient's symptoms, test results, or diagnosis do not support the medical necessity of the performed procedure, or if the ICD-10 code is not covered by the payer, then the examination may be denied payment.

Acquisition

The acquisition of ultrasound images by the performing provider should be within the scope of practice as defined by their governing body. In order to perform an ultrasound at an institution, the provider should also be credentialed in this skill. Images and videos should clearly identify the relevant anatomy and any abnormal findings, if present. These ultrasound examinations should be linked to the patient's medical record. A unique accession number is created to link the ultrasound examination to the medical record. Saved images or recorded videos are then transmitted to an image archival system or database and permanently linked to the patient's medical record. Indefinite retention of images performed is preferred, but different areas of practice may have different requirements and this should be explored at the specific institution [15].

Ultrasound hardware with wireless connectivity, image archival systems, and integration with EMR allows images acquired to be accessible to other providers as well as coding specialists and payers, if requested [3]. This process is similar to how most radiology images and reports are linked to the patient's EMR. The use of an ultrasound management system allows administrative oversight, quality assurance, and educational functions as well [3].

The current guidelines specify that at least one image should be permanently retained; however, regulations do not specify the number of images required for reimbursement or the storage system utilized [13]. Improper image acquisition may result in reimbursement delay or denial.

For ultrasound-guided procedures, including vascular access, images must be saved before, during or after the procedure; real-time imaging is recommended but not required [16, 17]. A procedure note should document that ultrasound was used to obtain real-time visualization as well as a dedicated report for the ultrasound images (discussed in more detail below). The ultrasound examination and the procedure should both be billed. Procedures can also be ultrasound-assisted, in which ultrasound is utilized prior to the procedure but not during the procedure.

Interpretation

The ultrasound examination should ideally be immediately interpreted and entered into the patient's medical record. The documentation should describe the structures evaluated, the presence or absence of relevant anatomy or pathology, and the interpretation of findings [3, 13]. Incomplete or improper documentation prevents coding, billing, and provider compensation for patient care provided [5].

The scope of the study performed should be documented and include whether the examination was (1) limited versus complete, (2) a repeat examination by the same or subsequent physician with documentation on why it was repeated, and (3) if there is reduced level of service or any other relevant information regarding the scope of the study [13]. This additional information on the scope of the study performed is vital to proper coding and directly impacts the ability for reimbursement. Interpretation of the ultrasound examination should be completed prior to billing.

An example of proper documentation, modified from the previously published I-AIM method [12], and billing process is shown in Figs. 3 and 4.

Money

The Centers for Medicare and Medicaid Services (CMS) administers the Medicare and Medicaid programs which currently command the largest market share for healthcare payments [18]. Private payers tend to follow the CMS systems for reimbursement and payment, based on units of work performed (fee-for-service reimbursement system) [18].

A limited abdominal ultrasound examination was performed by the emergency department physician

Indication: right upper quadrant abdominal pain, nausea and vomiting

Acquisition: gallbladder was imaged in short and long axis

Interpretation: no evidence of gallstones, no anterior gallbladder wall thickening, no pericholecystic fluid, negative sonographic Murphy's sign

Medical Decision Making: No evidence of acute cholecystitis

Signed by the performing physician

Fig. 3 Example of proper documentation following the I-AIM method

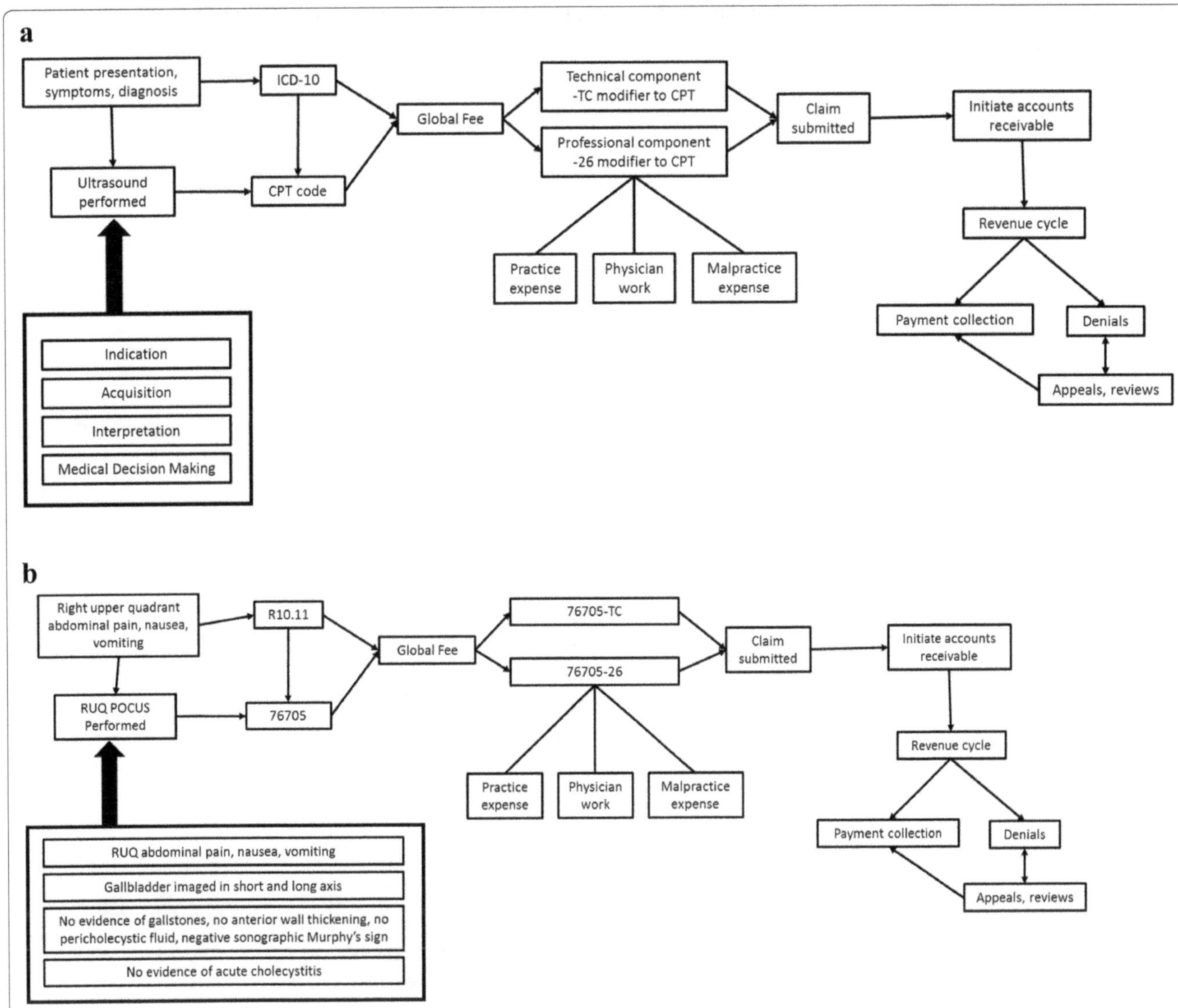

Fig. 4 Process flowchart illustrating the Billing I-AIM method in point-of-care ultrasound billing and coding

CPT codes are a system of descriptive terms to identify and report services that are performed [13]. This standardized code set is a communication tool between providers and payers to relay information about the medical care provided, and is used as a claims-processing tool by payers. Through an established formula, CPT codes attempt to quantify input costs of provider services and help payers determine the amount of reimbursement for services provided by being linked to relative value units (RVUs) to enable prediction of reimbursement [18]. Although the codes are standardized, the amount of reimbursement from the payer varies based on payer and local contracts [18, 19]. Multiple ultrasound CPT codes may be applied to the same patient during a single encounter if medically necessary [13]. See Table 1 for commonly used ultrasound CPT codes in the ED.

The revenue cycle, the full discussion of which is beyond the scope of this article, requires that the examination is completed, the report is signed, and the chart is properly coded (ICD-10 and CPT). Then a claim can be submitted initiating an accounts receivable (AR) that ultimately results in revenue collection [18].

Limited versus complete Ultrasound examinations are designated as either limited or complete. A complete examination attempts to visualize and evaluate all anatomic structures within a region and therefore is not routinely performed in POCUS. In contrast, a limited examination is focused on specific anatomic structures or a diagnostic question [19]. For example, a complete abdominal exam (CPT 76700) will evaluate and document the liver, gallbladder, common bile duct, pancreas, spleen, kidneys, upper abdominal aorta, and inferior vena cava,

Table 1 Common current procedural terminology (CPT) codes associated with point-of-care ultrasound

CPT code	Ultrasound study
93308	FAST (focused assessment of sonography in trauma): scan for hemopericardium and hemoperitoneum, may include lung ultrasound[a]
76705	For pneumothorax
76604	
76815	Pregnant transabdominal (TA)
76817	Pregnant transvaginal (TV)
76775	Retroperitoneal: aorta, renal
93308	Cardiac
76604	Thoracic (chest only)
76705	Biliary
76857	Bladder
93971	DVT—unilateral
93970	DVT—bilateral
Soft tissue ultrasound	
76536	Head/neck
76882	Axilla
76604	Chest wall
76641	Breast
76604	Upper back
76705	Lower back
76705	Abdominal wall
76857	Pelvic wall
76882	Extremity
76512	Ocular
76999	Miscellaneous ultrasound
Ultrasound-guided procedure codes[b]	
76930	Ultrasound-guided pericardiocentesis
76937	Ultrasound-guided vascular access placement
32555	Ultrasound-guided thoracentesis
49083	Ultrasound-guided paracentesis
76942	Miscellaneous ultrasound-guided procedure without catheter
76942	Ultrasound-guided abscess drainage
76942	Ultrasound-guided peritonsillar abscess drainage
76942	Ultrasound-guided lumbar puncture
76942	Ultrasound-guided suprapubic aspiration
76942	Ultrasound-guided fb removal
20604	Ultrasound-guided joint aspiration: small joint or bursa—finger, toe
20606	Ultrasound-guided joint aspiration: intermediate joint or bursa—elbow, wrist
20611	Ultrasound-guided joint aspiration: major joint or bursa—shoulder, hip, knee

[a] FAST: not a specific CPT code, FAST is a compilation of separate studies to evaluate areas potentially injured in trauma. Can bill for the specific components performed

[b] Can add the CPT code for the procedural component as well

tissue, vascular flow, and pathology. A limited abdominal exam (CPT 76705) could visualize and evaluate the right upper quadrant for signs of acute cholecystitis. If a limited and complete examination of the same anatomic region is performed on a patient during the same encounter, the limited portion is subsumed by the complete examination code [13].

Modifiers A CPT modifier is a two-digit code reported at the end of the five-digit CPT code to further classify the service provided [13]. Multiple modifiers can be reported for a patient if appropriate [13]. Table 2 lists a summary of common CPT modifiers applied for POCUS.

The most commonly applied CPT modifier in POCUS separates the billable expense into a professional and technical component (TC). Emergency physicians cannot bill the combined, professional plus technical, CPT for ultrasound performed in ED unless they directly own the ultrasound equipment [18–20]. In these settings, the physician reports using the -26 professional modifier and the facility reports using the -TC technical component modifier.

CPT codes ICD-10 codes applied to the patient encounter are used by payer sources to determine the medical necessity of reported CPT codes. National and Local Coverage Determinations (LCDs) are lists of pre-approved ICD-10 codes that support using a particular CPT code [13, 18]. If an ICD-10 is reported for an encounter which is listed on the LCD for a CPT code, then the probability of reimbursement is increased. The combination of ICD-10 codes on a particular LCD will vary based on regional Medicare Administrative Contractor (MAC) who developed the LCD for a state or region.

Submitted CPT codes for a particular patient encounter are compared with the ICD-10 diagnosis codes in a process termed Edits. Edits are policy-driven computer programs or manual reviews to check information on payment claim forms to determine coded services which have a high probability of being incorrect or medically unnecessary [13]. The charge is reimbursed through an appeal demonstrating medical necessity; termed a "diagnosis" or "payment" edit [13]. Other types of edits include procedure-to-procedure edits, frequency-to-time edits, and site of service edits. Procedure-to-procedure edits occur when the billed CPT code is compared to a second CPT code to ensure that the reporting of a group of procedures with related codes is given the most appropriate comprehensive code [13]. This occurs if the same physician attempts to bill a limited and complete exam of the same anatomic region during the same visit; the limited exam would be denied as it is subsumed by the complete exam which is the more appropriate and most comprehensive code. Frequency-to-time edits apply when multiple exams of the same anatomic region are performed during the same patient encounter and will be denied unless medical necessity for the repeated exam is documented. These subsequent exams would also require the modifiers as discussed above [13]. The classic example of this would be the blunt abdominal trauma patient who has a negative initial focused assessment with sonography in trauma (FAST) examination, but becomes hemodynamically unstable necessitating a repeat FAST examination to evaluate for intra-abdominal free fluid. Site of service edits are also performed in which the CPT code is compared to the site where the service is performed and if the global CPT code, without the -26 professional component modifier, is billed by a hospital-based emergency physician (EP), it would be rejected [13].

There are additional considerations for CPT codes submitted for standard POCUS examinations such as the FAST exam, soft tissue/musculoskeletal, pelvic ultrasound, and ultrasound-guided procedures. The FAST exam is not a single CPT code but actually two separately billed exams—limited abdomen (CPT 76705) and limited echocardiography (CPT 93308). If not all views of the FAST are performed, only the CPT code that accurately describes the anatomic regions evaluated should be used. Soft tissue and musculoskeletal ultrasound examinations are coded based on the location of the body examined and all are limited examinations, so the reduced service

Table 2 Common CPT modifier codes, to be added after the five-digit CPT code (see Table 1)

CPT modifier	Description of modifier	Example
26	Professional component of global fee	Physician component of global fee for professional services including interpretation of diagnostic tests with separate signed report
52	Partially reduced service provided	Transvaginal ultrasound in known pregnant patient (76817, no limited code exists), but POCUS does not include all anatomic structures in the region required for billing
59	Distinct procedural service—report procedures that are distinct but have the same CPT code[a]	Multiple soft tissue areas on different extremities examined for abscess vs cellulitis (76882)
76	Repeat procedure by the same physician[b]	Trauma patient requiring a repeat FAST examination by an emergency physician for a change in clinical stability such as hypotension
77	Repeat procedure by another physician[c]	Trauma patient requiring a repeat FAST examination by the trauma surgeon for a change in clinical stability such as hypotension

[a] *CPT* current procedural terminology

[b] Same physician—providers who are under the same group Medicare provider number on the same date of service or patient encounter

[c] Another physician—provider with a different group Medicare provider number on the same date of service or patient encounter

modifier (– 52) is not required [13] Pelvic ultrasound also has some special considerations in regard to CPT codes selected. The initial determination is whether the patient is known, prior to performance of the ultrasound, to be pregnant or not regardless of the final ultrasonographic findings. In general, pelvic ultrasound performed in the ED will be on a "known" pregnant patient to evaluate for intrauterine pregnancy and/or fetal cardiac activity. These CPT codes are 76815 for transabdominal pelvic ultrasound in a pregnant patient and 76817 for transvaginal pelvic ultrasound in a pregnant patient. If both transabdominal and transvaginal examinations are medically necessary, both can be performed, coded and billed. This may be necessary if, in an early first trimester pregnancy, the provider performed transabdominal ultrasound cannot rule-in intrauterine pregnancy and then the same provider performs a transvaginal ultrasound to rule-in intrauterine pregnancy (76817-26,-52). If the provider cannot rule-in intrauterine pregnancy via transabdominal or transvaginal ultrasound, a comprehensive radiology performed transvaginal ultrasound can be ordered to determine if an intrauterine or ectopic pregnancy is present. The provider can bill for both ultrasounds and radiology can bill for the comprehensive transvaginal ultrasound 76817-77 (CPT modifier -77 for repeat examination by second physician with a different group Medicare provider number) [13]. It is inappropriate to routinely perform a transabdominal and then a transvaginal ultrasound on all pregnant patients as each ultrasound performed must be medically necessary.

Ultrasound-guided procedures are another area of special consideration with regard to coding and billing. Diagnostic POCUS and related ultrasound-guided CPT codes can be reported only if the procedural code does not subsume the diagnostic code. For example, if a patient undergoes an ultrasound-guided pericardiocentesis after identifying a pericardial effusion with tamponade with POCUS, the physician should report a limited echocardiography (93308-26), ultrasound-guided pericardiocentesis (76930-26), and pericardiocentesis (33010) [13].

Discussion

POCUS has rapidly expanded as a standard component of emergency medicine practices. While emergency medicine programs have readily adopted POCUS programs and increasingly adopted quality improvement processes for image review, the development of fiscally sustainable models has been difficult due to the myriad of variables affecting image storage, documentation, coding, denials, and reimbursement. Many POCUS programs within emergency medicine practices currently are either operating without a formal billing process or lack a feasible reimbursement pattern [21, 22].

A lack of understanding regarding the intricacies of billing for POCUS can be an impediment to its use. A program that is able to show evidence of income is more readily supported by administrators concerned with return on investments. Conversely, without any reimbursement from POCUS, it is harder to justify the benefits to those who are not using this valuable modality clinically. It is apparent that POCUS can offer advantage to patients and health systems alike when decreasing costs for the same level of care. Studies have shown improved patient safety when using POCUS for procedures or eliminating the need for a procedure, increased patient satisfaction, improved department resource utilization, reduction in more costly or invasive procedures, and improved clinical decision-making [3, 13]. Unfortunately, many of these benefits will not be realized if there is no initial investment in POCUS programs. A well-organized and successful billing program can be an asset to both developing and established programs.

The Billing I-AIM model creates an understandable outline of the steps that need to take place for reimbursement. At each step there are potential pitfalls and barriers to success. The indication for each POCUS should be clear, including what focused questions are being asked. It is valuable to understand that what constitutes an appropriate indication will be determined based on the diagnosis in the form of ICD-10 codes. Documentation of the indication, and specifically the medical necessity, is especially important for repeat examinations that may necessitate further CPT modifiers. With regard to acquisition, it is necessary to save images in a permanent database. Ideally this will be linked to patients' medical record. Phantom scans without saved images or documentation are unacceptable and will result in no reimbursement. Having no images saved leads to a blind scan which is also not billable.

The interpretation of the POCUS exam should be well documented. Poor compliance with timely documentation of exams can be a disservice to the patient and other providers caring for them, as well as impeding the billing process. This deserves special attention, because it is a common barrier encountered that can significantly impact billing patterns. An exam without documentation is considered illiterate and non-billable. Reports that are not completed in a timely fashion may not allow coders sufficient documentation to support medical necessity of the exam or include the exam in the billable patient encounter [5]. Certain conditions may improve compliance. Web-based workflow and archival systems with a user-friendly interface can be valuable. It is additionally useful if offering remote access so providers can complete documentation from outside of the work place. Wirelessly transferring images to the system is efficient and advantageous compared to manually exporting and uploading ultrasound exams. Ongoing education and productivity reports distributed to faculty and trainees can increase compliance with workflow requirements. Reminder emails from administrators or ultrasound faculty can also improve completion of charting. Quality assurance is also an important component in ensuring the accuracy of interpretation. This can also be means of providing feedback for future improved quality of acquisition and interpretation. Efforts to improve compliance with documentation of POCUS exams can lead to rectification of these illiterate exams to true billable examinations.

Reimbursement for POCUS can increase the E&M code as well, and thus reimbursement for the ED encounter, by increasing the complexity of the medical decision-making [1]. Reimbursement rates affect the amount of income generated which is dependent on the payer mix of the region in which the ED is located and is also determined by the payers' concept of accepted professional medical standards, even though these may not always be based on the most current literature [1].

Although the nomenclature described in this article represents an initial attempt to differentiate causes for inadequately documented POCUS scans, there are several limitations. First, use of the nomenclature has not been externally validated to produce a significant difference in identifying quality improvement for POCUS scans within emergency ultrasound programs. A larger and prospective application of the nomenclature within multiple emergency ultrasound programs is required prior to its application for the purposes of quality improvement.

Conclusions

The Billing I-AIM model serves as both a mnemonic and a checklist for the process of billing a POCUS examination. By breaking down a potentially intimidating process into its core components of indication, acquisition, interpretation, and money, practitioners of POCUS can easily remember and understand the steps necessary for successful reimbursement. The proposed nomenclature allows differentiation of POCUS examinations performed for the purposes of quality improvement and improved reimbursement. Future studies can examine how incorporating this model into a POCUS billing system may increase revenue from POCUS examinations. As successful billing can solidify the longevity of a POCUS program, our hope is that improvement on this front will facilitate further use of this valuable modality.

Abbreviations

AAA: Abdominal aortic aneurysm; ACEP: American College of Emergency Physicians; CMS: Centers for Medicare and Medicaid Services; CPT: Current Procedural Terminology; E&M: Evaluation and management; EMR: Electronic medical record; IAIM: Indication, Acquisition, Interpretation, Money; ICD-PCS: International Classification of Disease Procedures Coding System; LCD: Local coverage determinations; POCUS: Point-of-care ultrasound; TC: Technical component; TVUS: Transvaginal ultrasound; US: Ultrasound; WHO: World Health Organization.

Acknowledgements

The authors would like to thank the billing and imaging informatics departments at The Ohio State University Wexner Medical Center, and the 2017 American Institute of Ultrasound in Medicine annual meeting for accepting this abstract for oral presentation.

Authors' contributions

DH developed the concept of the Billing I-AIM method and was major contributor to the writing and revision of the manuscript. MC developed the concept of the Billing I-AIM method and was a major contributor to the writing and revision of the manuscript. IM contributed to the development of the Billing I-AIM method and was a major contributor to the revision of the manuscript. MP contributed to the development of the Billing I-AIM method and was a major contributor to the revision of the manuscript. NR developed the concept of the quality improvement ultrasound nomenclature and was a major contributor in the revision of the manuscript. CB contributed to the development of the Billing I-AIM method and was a major contributor to the revision of the manuscript. DB developed the concept of the quality improvement ultrasound nomenclature and the Billing I-AIM method and was a major contributor in the revision of the manuscript. All authors read and approved the final manuscript.

Author details

[1] Department of Emergency Medicine, The Ohio State University College of Medicine, 750 Prior Hall, 376 W 10th Ave, Columbus, OH 43210, USA.
[2] Children's Hospital Colorado, The University of Colorado, Denver, CO, USA.
[3] Department of Surgery, The University of Oklahoma College of Medicine, Tulsa, OK, USA.

References

1. Adhikari S, Amini R, Stolz L et al (2014) Implementation of a novel point-of-care ultrasound billing and reimbursement program: fiscal impact. Am J Emerg Med 32(6):592–595. https://doi.org/10.1016/j.ajem.2014.02.051
2. Rosenkrantz AB, Bilal NH, Hughes DR, Duszak R (2014) National specialty trends in billable diagnostic ultrasound in the ED: analysis of Medicare claims data. Am J Emerg Med 32(12):1470–1475. https://doi.org/10.1016/j.ajem.2014.09.002
3. American College of Emergency Physicians. Ultrasound guidelines: emergency, point-of-care, and clinical ultrasound guidelines in medicine. 2016: Emergency Ultrasound Section. https://www.acep.org/Clinical—Practice-Management/Ultrasound/#sm.0001wi32c84dcew4yrs2erxapx6h1. Accessed June 2017
4. Moore CL, Copel JA (2011) Point-of-care ultrasonography. N Engl J Med 364(8):749–757. https://doi.org/10.1056/nejmra0909487
5. Lewiss RE, Cook J, Sauler A et al (2016) A workflow task force affects emergency physician compliance for point-of-care ultrasound documentation and billing. Crit Ultrasound J. https://doi.org/10.1186/s13089-016-0041-0
6. Melniker LA, Leiber E, McKenney MG, Lopez P, Briggs WM, Mancuso CA (2006) Randomized controlled clinical trial of point-of-care, limited ultrasonography for trauma in the emergency department: the first sonography outcomes assessment program trial. Ann Emerg Med 48(3):227–235
7. Blaivas M, Adhikari S, Lander L (2011) A prospective comparison of procedural sedation and ultrasound-guided interscalene nerve block for shoulder reduction in the emergency department. Acad Emerg Med 18(9):922–927
8. Jones BP, Tay ET, Elikashvili I et al (2016) Feasibility and safety of substituting lung ultrasonography for chest radiography when diagnosing pneumonia in children. Chest. 150(1):131–138
9. McCarthy ML, Shokoohi H, Boniface KS et al (2016) Ultrasonography versus landmark for peripheral intravenous cannulation: a randomized controlled trial. Ann Emerg Med 68(1):10–18
10. Koenig SJ, Lou BX, Moskowitz Y et al (2019) Ultrasound billing for intensivists. Chest 156(4):792–801

11. American College of Emergency Physicians (2001) American college of emergency physicians use of ultrasound imaging by emergency physicians. Ann Emerg Med 38:469–470
12. Bahner DP, Hughes D, Royall NA (2012) I-AIM: a novel model for teaching and performing focused sonography. J Ultrasound Med 31(2):295–300. https://doi.org/10.7863/jum.2012.31.2.295
13. Facep SH, Facep ED. Ultrasound coding and reimbursement document 2009 Table of Contents. 2009
14. WHO (2016) ICD-10 Version:2016. WHO, Berlin. https://doi.org/10.1177/1071100715600286
15. University of Florida Emergency Medicine Department. How to Send Ultrasounds to PACS 2013. http://emergency.med.ufl.edu/files/2013/02/How-to-Send-Ultrasounds-to-PACS.pdf. Accessed July 2017
16. Moore CL (2011) Credentialing and reimbursement in point-of-care ultrasound. Clin Pediatr Emerg Med. 12(1):73–77. https://doi.org/10.1016/j.cpem.2010.12.001
17. Flannigan MJ, Adhikari S (2017) Point-of-care ultrasound work flow innovation: impact on documentation and billing. J Ultrasound Med. 36(12):2467–2474
18. Lam DL, Medverd JR (2013) How radiologists get paid: resource-based relative value scale and the revenue cycle. Am J Roentgenol 201(5):947–958. https://doi.org/10.2214/ajr.12.9715
19. CPT® (Current Procedural Terminology) | American Medical Association. https://www.ama-assn.org/practice-management/cpt-current-procedural-terminology. Accessed 23 Jan 2018
20. Levin DC, Parker L, Rao VM (2017) The recent losses in medicare imaging revenues experienced by radiologists, cardiologists, and other physicians. J Am Coll Radiol. 14(8):1007–1012. https://doi.org/10.1016/j.jacr.2017.02.044
21. Soremekun OA, Noble VE, Liteplo AS, Brown DFM, Zane RD (2009) Financial impact of emergency department ultrasound. Acad Emerg Med 16(7):674–680. https://doi.org/10.1111/j.1553-2712.2009.00447.x
22. Moore CL, Gregg S, Lambert M (2004) Performance, training, quality assurance, and reimbursement of emergency physician-performed ultrasonography at academic medical centers. J Ultrasound Med 23(4):459–466. https://doi.org/10.7863/jum.2004.23.4.459

12

Stab wound of the superficial femoral artery early diagnosed by point-of-care Doppler ultrasound

Pablo Blanco[1,2*] and María Fernanda Menéndez[3]

Abstract

Background: Traumatic vascular injury of the limbs has the potential to cause substantial patient morbidity and mortality, and therefore, early recognition and treatment are crucial to improve outcomes. While patients with hard signs of arterial injury mandate for an immediate surgical intervention, patients presenting with soft signs of arterial injury need further diagnostic evaluation.

Case presentation: A 24-year-old male was admitted to the emergency department after suffering a stab wound in the anterolateral aspect of his left upper thigh. Entry wound measures approximately 3 cm × 0.7 cm; no exit wound was observed. On examination of the injured limb, the thigh was swollen and painful. Skin color was mildly pale and skin temperature was slightly diminished in his leg; leg numbness was also pointed out by the patient. Common femoral artery pulse was normal, while distal pulses were diminished. Point-of-care Doppler ultrasound (DUS) showed a subfascial hematoma in the thigh, which filled on color Doppler, corresponding to a pseudoaneurysm. On spectral Doppler, signs of distal low blood supply were noted. The patient was immediately transferred to the operating room where a 1-cm laceration was found in the anterior aspect of the superficial femoral artery. The involved artery was successfully repaired and distal flow was reestablished, as assessed by clinical examination, pulse palpation and DUS.

Conclusions: Based on its several advantages, DUS should be considered as the first-line diagnostic tool in the diagnostic workup of patients with soft signs of arterial injury.

Keywords: Point-of-care, Doppler ultrasound imaging, Trauma, Vascular injuries

Introduction

Vascular injuries represent less than 3% of all traumatic findings and have a potential to cause morbidity and mortality if they are not timely recognized and treated [1–4]. The majority of vascular injuries occur in the extremities and may result from penetrating trauma, blunt trauma, or both. Among them, gunshot injury is the leading cause, followed by stab wounds and blunt trauma [1]. Mortality is mainly related to hypovolemia after a major vessel is injured, while morbidity may result secondary to compartment syndrome, arteriovenous fistula, limb loss or wound infections [1–4].

Vascular injury can be arterial, venous or mixed [2]. Serious arterial injury may result from transection, laceration or dissection while venous injury is mainly related to vein rupture or thrombosis and rarely from venous wall dissection [2].

Among patients with arterial injury, those presenting with "hard signs" of arterial injury (e.g., pulsatile bleeding, expanding hematoma, absent distal pulses, cold/pale limb, palpable thrill or an audible bruit) mandate for an immediate surgery and vascular repair without the support of diagnostic imaging techniques. On the other hand, patients with "soft signs" of arterial injury such as diminished pulses, small and non-expanding hematoma

*Correspondence: ohtusabes@gmail.com; deihospitalferreyra@gmail.com
[1] Intensive Care Unit, Clínica Cruz Azul, 2651, 60 St, Necochea 7630, Argentina
Full list of author information is available at the end of the article

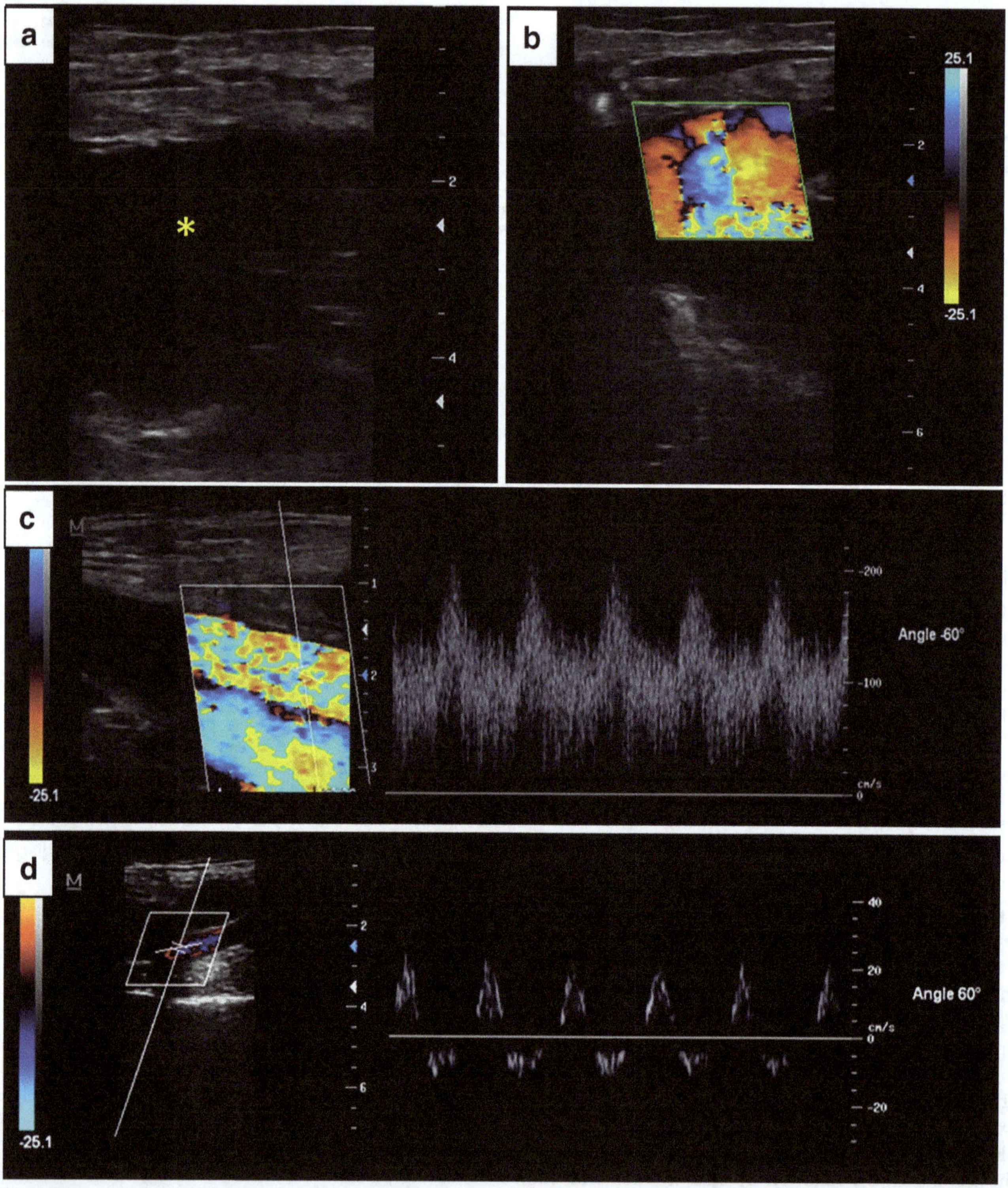

Fig. 1 Stab wound of the left-sided superficial femoral artery. **a** Subfascial fluid collection corresponding to a hematoma (asterisk); **b** Color Doppler demonstrating flow in the hematoma, corresponding to a pseudoaneurysm; **c** spectral Doppler of the superficial femoral artery proximal to the site of injury, showing high-velocity monophasic waveforms, indicating a reduction in the vascular resistance distal to the insonation site (arterial laceration) and compensatory flow; **d** spectral Doppler in arteries distal to the site of injury, showing low-velocity biphasic waveforms, indicating low blood supply

or proximity of wound to a major vessel require further diagnostic evaluation [1, 5], such as the ankle-brachial pressure index (ABPI), angiography, or Doppler ultrasound (DUS).

We present hereby the case of a patient with stab injury of the superficial femoral artery demonstrated by point-of-care DUS and how the use of this method impacted in decision-making.

Case report

A 24-year-old male was brought to the emergency department (ED) immediately after suffering a stab injury in his left thigh which he alleged to be produced during a neighborhood altercation. A kitchen knife entered from the anterolateral aspect of the upper third of his left thigh, leaving a 3 cm × 0.7 cm entry wound which penetrates into the deep tissues; no exit wound was found. On admission, tachycardia (120 beats/min) and mild arterial hypotension (80/50 mmHg) were observed. On the injured limb, physical examination showed a painful and swollen tight. He was able to move the entire limb; however, he noted numbness of his leg. Below the knee, skin color was mildly pale and temperature was slightly diminished. A prolonged capillary refill time was observed in his foot. Common femoral artery pulse was normal, while diminished pulses were palpated in popliteal, tibial anterior and tibial posterior arteries. A point-of-care DUS showed a large hypoechoic slightly pulsating hematoma in the subfascial compartment (Fig. 1a), which filled with a turbulent flow on color Doppler (Fig. 1b), consistent with a pseudoaneurysm. On spectral Doppler, common femoral artery and superficial femoral artery proximal to the hematoma showed a high velocity low-resistance profile (Fig. 1c), while popliteal, tibial posterior and tibial anterior arteries showed low-velocity biphasic waveforms (Fig. 1d), consistent with a proximal blood leak and reduced distal blood supply. Common femoral and femoral veins were patent and compressible.

Given that arterial injury sounded unequivocal based on clinical examination and DUS findings, the patient was immediately transferred to the operating room for surgical exploration. A 1-cm longitudinal laceration was found in the anterior aspect of the superficial femoral artery (Fig. 2); deep veins were not compromised. The injured vessel was successfully repaired and then the patient was transferred to the intensive care unit for postoperative care. On the next day, skin color and temperature of the affected limb were normal, the patient indicated disappearance of his leg numbness, and distal pulses were full. DUS showed normal velocity triphasic waveforms in the proximal and distal arteries (Fig. 3). Patient follow-up was uneventfully and he was discharged from the hospital on day 5.

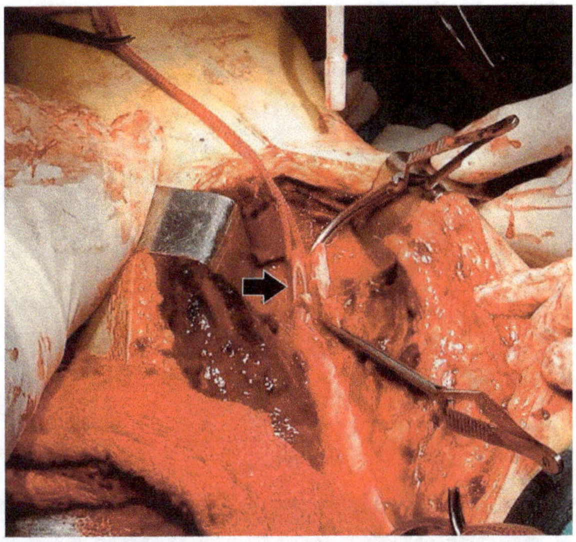

Fig. 2 Surgery demonstrating a 1-cm laceration in the anterior aspect of the superficial femoral artery (arrow)

Discussion

There are several methods varying in availability, complexity and costs for evaluating the patient with suspicion of arterial injury.

The ankle-brachial pressure index (ABPI), a simple, non-invasive, inexpensive and easy to perform vascular test, is considered by some authors as the first-line diagnostic tool for patients with "soft signs" of arterial injury of the lower limbs [5]. An ABPI > 1 practically excludes an arterial injury, while an ABPI < 1 warrants further investigation, such as DUS or angiography [5]. In the upper limbs, the wrist-brachial index can be used, with the same cutoff described for the ABPI. However, for practitioners working in emergency settings, the ABPI is poorly known, is not widely available and thus it is rarely used in this scenario.

Conventional angiography, which is considered the gold standard, or currently computed tomography angiography (CTA) or magnetic resonance angiography (MRA) aid in providing a definite diagnosis. However, these methods require transferring the patient to the Cath lab or the radiology department, use iodinated contrast media and ionizing radiation (CTA), or paramagnetic contrast media (MRA), and are expensive.

In contrast to the aforementioned techniques, DUS is nowadays widely available in the emergency department, is non-invasive, does not emit ionizing radiation and has demonstrated a good diagnostic accuracy for the diagnosis of vascular injury. Regarding the latter, the reported sensitivity of DUS is 95–97%, specificity of 95–98% and accuracy of 98% in assessment of peripheral vascular injuries [2]. A recent study showed a sensitivity

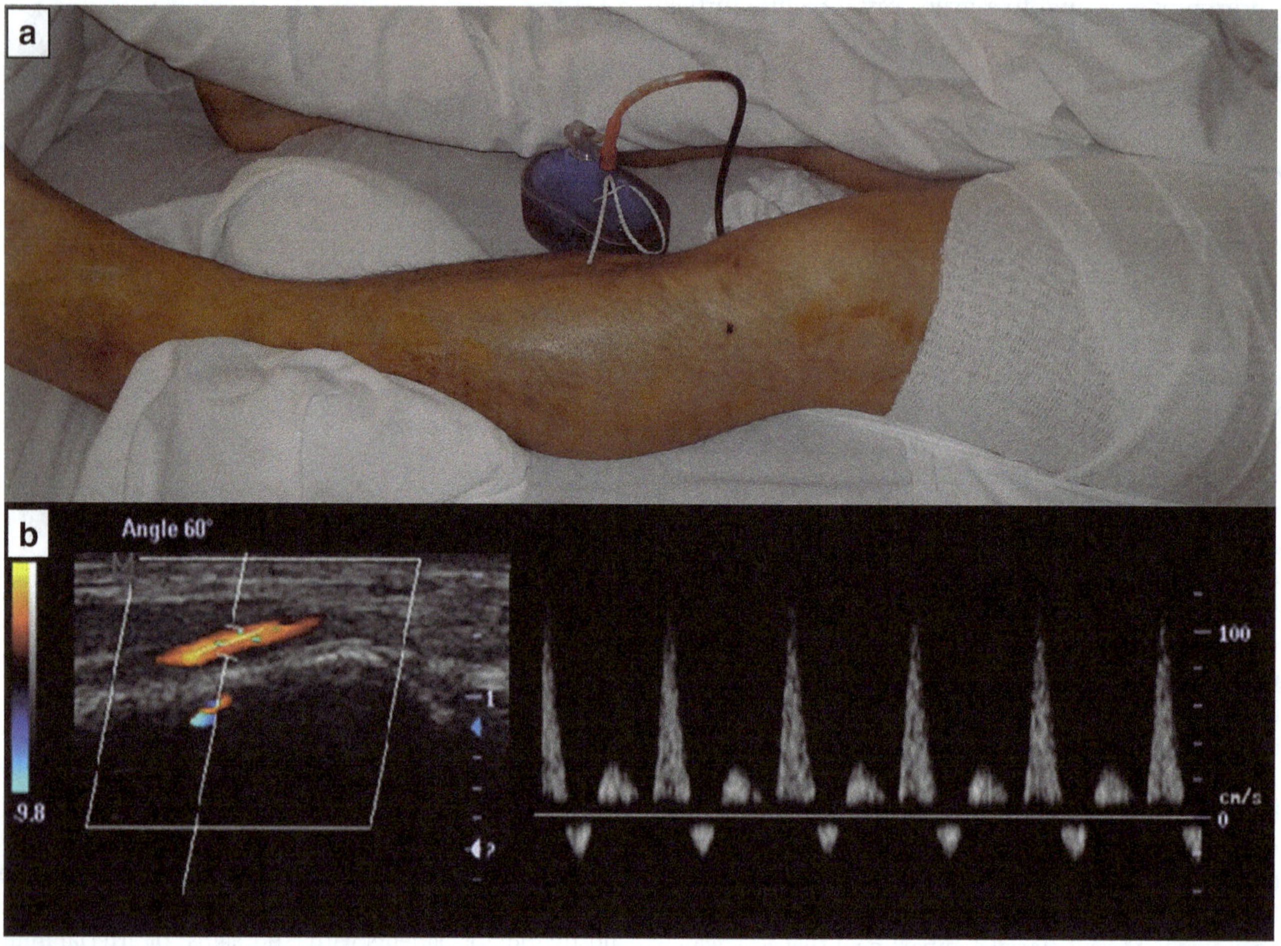

Fig. 3 Postoperative care. **a** The patient's left lower limb shows normal perfusion; **b** spectral Doppler shows normal-velocity triphasic waveforms in proximal and distal arteries (tibial posterior artery is only shown)

and specificity of 100% to rule out a severe arterial injury when a triphasic flow was present [6]; the detection of other patterns (e.g., biphasic, monophasic flows) points toward the need of further investigations (see below). Two-dimensional imaging may show signs of vascular injury, such as a pseudoaneurysm, as seen in our patient, an intimal flap in the case of arterial dissection, or a partial or complete arterial thrombus [2]. Color Doppler may demonstrate a diminished or even the absence of flow, flow in the true and false lumen (arterial dissection) or the filling of the pseudoaneurysm (as shown in our presented case) [2]. In addition to two-dimensional and color Doppler imaging, spectral Doppler findings are of paramount importance. Normal arterial waveforms of the resting limbs typically show a triphasic pattern: the first corresponds to the rapid antegrade flow reaching a peak during systole; the second to a transient reversal of flow during early diastole which is secondary to the high vascular resistance imposed by the resting muscles, and the third to a slow antegrade flow during late diastole, resulting from wall recoil [2, 6–8]. As mentioned above, as a normal triphasic flow is detected, a severe arterial injury may be ruled out [6]. While biphasic, monophasic or even an absent flow is expected in patients with a severe acute arterial injury, changes in the spectral waveforms may be observed in several other circumstances as well [2, 6–8]. For example, given that the arterial wall becomes more rigid with advancing years, the third component is often lost in old-aged people. Other conditions include non-resting limbs, chronic arterial stenosis/occlusion and collateral circulation or infections (e.g., cellulitis). For that reasons, specificity of DUS for detecting a severe arterial injury is not guaranteed and further investigations should be considered when a non-triphasic flow is observed. Other aspect that is often assessed with DUS is flow velocity. As a rule of thumb, normal arterial peak systolic velocities (PSV) are around 100 cm/s in proximal arterial segments (e.g., common femoral artery), while distal segments show velocities of about 50 cm/s (e.g., posterior tibial artery) [8]. Low flow velocities or even an absent flow is expected in severe arterial injury. Similar to spectral waveforms, several factors may impact velocities, such as technical factors (wrong angle between flow and ultrasound beam), arterial hypo/hypertension, non-resting limbs or chronic arterial stenosis/occlusion. Given that interpretation of low flow velocities may be cumbersome in practice, it seems more reliable to base the DUS diagnosis on spectral waveforms (triphasic vs non-triphasic flow/no flow).

While a full lower limb DUS scan is time consuming and is nowadays reserved to radiologists, a focused DUS examination is desirable in point-of-care settings, as is the FAST D protocol, where a two-point DUS is proposed (posterior tibial artery and dorsalis pedis artery) [6]. While promising, the feasibility and reliability of the FAST D protocol in the hands of emergency or critical care physicians should be assessed in further studies.

As was demonstrated in our presented case, an abnormal flow pattern was clearly demonstrated, indicating low blood supply distal to the site of injury. High-velocity monophasic waveforms proximal to the injury site, as observed in our patient, may be explained by the arterial tear which lowers the vascular resistance distal to the insonated artery, and compensatory flow.

Conclusions

DUS should be considered as the first-line method to detect a vascular injury of the limbs for the patient with soft signs of arterial injury in the emergency department. When there is suspicion of arterial injury, DUS aids in decision making, ruling out a severe arterial injury when triphasic waveforms are present; and pointing out to perform further investigations when non-triphasic waveforms/no flow is detected. Serial POCUS DUS examinations aid for the patient's follow-up as well.

Abbreviations

ABPI: Ankle-brachial pressure index; DUS: Doppler ultrasound; CTA: Computed tomography angiography; MRA: Magnetic resonance angiography; PSV: Peak systolic velocity.

Acknowledgements

None.

Authors' contributions

PB observed the case, performed the ultrasound examinations, collected the data and contributed significantly to the drafting and editing of the manuscript, performed the literature review and created the figures. MFM observed the case and contributed to the drafting and editing of the manuscript. Both authors read and approved the final manuscript.

Author details

[1] Intensive Care Unit, Clínica Cruz Azul, 2651, 60 St, Necochea 7630, Argentina. [2] Department of Teaching and Research, Hospital "Dr. Emilio Ferreyra", 4801, 59 St, Necochea 7630, Argentina. [3] Intensive Care Unit, Hospital "Dr. Emilio Ferreyra", 4801, 59 Ave, Necochea 7630, Argentina.

References

1. Topal AE, Eren MN, Celik Y (2010) Lower extremity arterial injuries over a six-year period: outcomes, risk factors, and management. Vasc Health Risk Manag 6:1103–1110
2. Montorfano MA, Pla F, Vera L, Cardillo O, Nigra SG, Montorfano LM (2017) Point-of-care ultrasound and Doppler ultrasound evaluation of vascular injuries in penetrating and blunt trauma. Crit Ultrasound J 9(1):5
3. Jacob AO, Boseto F, Ollapallil J (2017) Epidemic of stab injuries: an Alice Springs dilemma. ANZ J Surg 77(8):621–625
4. Hugar BS, Bhagavath P, Harish SH, Anitha S (2014) Atypical fatal entry wound to the thigh—a case report. Med Leg J 82(3):116–118
5. Kurtoğlu M, Dolay K, Karamustafaoğlu B, Yanar H, Kuzkaya M (2009) The role of the ankle brachial pressure index in the diagnosis of peripheral arterial injury. Ulus Travma Acil Cerrahi Derg 15(5):448–452
6. Montorfano MA, Montorfano LM, Perez Quirante F, Rodríguez F, Vera L, Neri L (2017) The FAST D protocol: a simple method to rule out traumatic vascular injuries of the lower extremities. Crit Ultrasound J 9(1):8
7. Gupta P, Lyons S, Hedgire S (2019) Ultrasound imaging of the arterial system. Cardiovasc Diagn Ther 9(Suppl 1):S2–S13
8. Sánchez L, Dellamea M, Sanjuan I, Sáez A, Togni F, Sosa M (2016) Monophasic distal flow: It does not always mean atherosclerosis. Revista Argentina de Diagnóstico por Imágenes 5(13): 6–12. http://webcir.org/revistavirtual/articulos/2016/3_agosto/argentina/fed_arg/monophasic_distal_flow.pdf

13

Point-of-care ultrasound for evaluating intra-abdominal calcification in the pediatric emergency department: case series and review of literature

Vigil James[1*], John Samuel[2], Chor Yek Kee[3] and Gene Yong-Kwang Ong[1]

Abstract

Background: The presence of intra-abdominal calcification in the pediatric population can be due to a wide range of conditions. Calcification in the abdomen can be seen in normal or abnormal anatomical structures. In some patients, abnormal calcification points towards the pathology; whereas in others, calcification itself is the pathology. After a thorough history and clinical examination, point-of-care ultrasound (POCUS) would complement the assessment of acute abdominal pain, based on the list of differentials generated as per the abdominal region. The main objective of this article is to review commonly encountered causes of intra-abdominal calcifications in the pediatric population and help in clinical decision-making in a Pediatric Emergency Department.

Case presentation: We describe a series of pediatric patients who presented to the Pediatric Emergency Department with acute abdominal pain, in whom point-of-care ultrasound helped expedite the diagnosis by identifying varying types of calcification and associated sonological findings. For children who present to the Pediatric Emergency Department with significant abdominal pain, a rapid distinction between emergencies and non-emergencies is vital to decrease morbidity and mortality.

Conclusions: In a child presenting to the Pediatric Emergency Department with abdominal pain, POCUS and the findings of calcifications can narrow or expand the differential diagnosis when integrated with history and physical exam, to a specific anatomic structure. Integrating these findings with additional sonological findings of an underlying pathology might raise sufficient concerns in the emergency physicians to warrant further investigations for the patient in the form of a formal radiological ultrasound and assist in the patient's early disposition. The use of POCUS might also help to categorize the type of calcification to one of the four main categories of intra-abdominal calcifications, namely concretions, conduit wall calcification, cyst wall calcification, and solid mass-type calcification. POCUS used thoughtfully can give a diagnosis and expand differential diagnosis, reduce cognitive bias, and reduce physician mental load. By integrating the use of POCUS with the history and clinical findings, it will be possible to expedite the management in children who present to the Pediatric Emergency Department with acute abdominal pain.

Keywords: Ultrasound, Intra-abdominal, Calcification, Pediatric emergency, Point-of-care ultrasound, POCUS

Background

The presence of intra-abdominal calcification in the pediatric population can be due to a wide range of conditions. Calcification in the abdomen can be seen in normal or abnormal anatomical structures. In some

*Correspondence: vigiljames@gmail.com
[1] Children's Emergency, C/O KK Women's and Children's Hospital PTE. LTD, 100 Bukit Timah Road, Singapore 229899, Singapore
Full list of author information is available at the end of the article

patients, abnormal calcification points towards the pathology; whereas in others, calcification itself is the pathology [1]. The presence of intra-abdominal calcification may be diagnostic in some patients, and in some patients, it might raise enough concerns to warrant further investigations in the patient.

Intraabdominal calcifications in children can occur due to a broad spectrum of conditions ranging from benign causes to adverse conditions like malignancy. These can be broadly divided into concretions, conduit calcifications, cystic calcifications, and solid mass calcifications [1]. Concretions are discrete precipitates in an organ or vessel like renal, ureteric, vesical, and gall bladder calculi. Conduit calcifications are calcifications seen in the walls of any fluid-filled hollow tubular structures like pancreatic duct calcifications and vascular wall calcifications [1]. The cystic calcifications arise in the wall of a cyst or pseudocyst. Solid mass calcification shows extensive, but variable calcification with a dense center and irregular margins like mesenteric lymph nodes, adrenals, and metastasis [1].

Intra-abdominal calcification is detected on the ultrasound by the presence of a hyperechoic area in the abdominal organs. Calcium obstructs ultrasound more than any natural substance and results in the formation of an area of sonological opacity (signal void) called the posterior acoustic shadowing [2]. Once the intra-abdominal calcification is detected on ultrasound, the addition of accessory sonographic features of specific pathologies will help confirm the suspected pathologies.

Point-of-care ultrasound (POCUS) of the abdomen performed by emergency physicians is increasingly being used to evaluate clinical manifestations and to facilitate accurate diagnoses in the emergency departments [3–6]. For children who present to the Pediatric Emergency Department (PED) with significant abdominal pain, a rapid distinction between emergencies and non-emergencies is vital to decrease morbidity and mortality. We describe a series of pediatric patients who presented to the PED with acute abdominal pain, in whom POCUS helped expedite the diagnosis by identifying varying types of intra-abdominal calcification and associated sonological findings. Using the case series for illustration, we hope to provide a general approach in the POCUS evaluation of intra-abdominal calcifications and their additional sonological findings in pediatric patients in the emergency department setting. For the narrative review of this article, we searched medical databases for studies of any design and in any setting that included pediatric patients describing POCUS, intra-abdominal calcification, and abdominal pain.

Case presentation

Case 1

A 10-year-old boy was brought to the PED with fever for four days with associated poor appetite and abdominal pain for three days. He had tenderness and guarding in the right iliac fossa. The patient was clinically suspected of having acute appendicitis.

A POCUS examination of the abdomen was performed using a curvilinear transducer (2–5 MHz), which showed a distended appendix (16 mm in diameter) with wall thickening (Fig. 1) and associated probe-induced tenderness. An appendicolith with its posterior acoustic shadowing was seen in the distal appendix lumen (Fig. 1). A formal radiology ultrasound confirmed the diagnosis of acute appendicitis, and the patient was admitted for further inpatient management.

Case 2

A 15-year-old adolescent girl was brought to the PED with fever for four days with progressively worsening right upper abdominal pain for three days. She had tenderness and guarding in the right hypochondria of the abdomen. She was clinically suspected of having acute cholecystitis.

A POCUS examination of the abdomen was performed using a curvilinear transducer (2-5 MHz) and showed hyperechoic areas in the gall bladder with well-defined posterior acoustic shadowing (Fig. 2) and associated probe-induced tenderness. The patient was admitted for further management, and the radiological ultrasound confirmed acute cholecystitis.

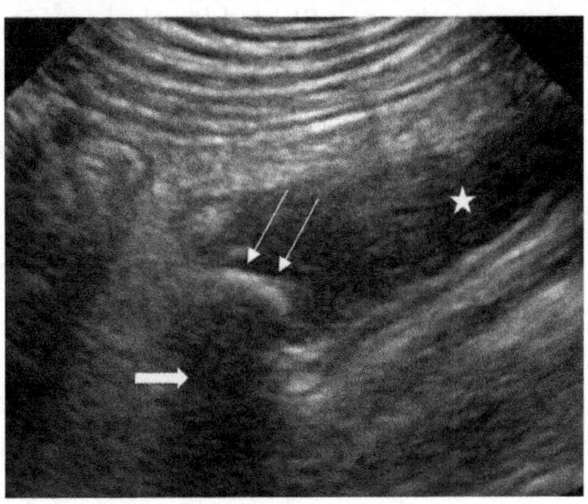

Fig. 1 Appendicolith: Ultrasound abdomen of the right lower quadrant showing an appendicolith (long thin arrows), which is the echogenic area within the appendix lumen (distal appendix) (star). There is a posterior acoustic shadowing seen behind the echogenic foci (thick arrow). The largest appendix diameter measured was 16 mm

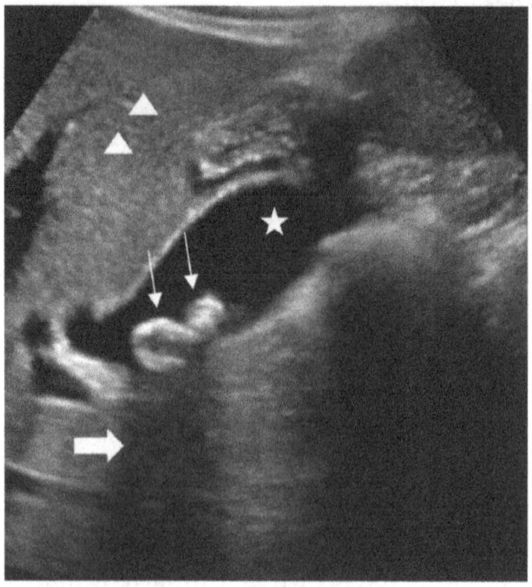

Fig. 2 Gall bladder calculi: Gall bladder calculi appears as a highly reflective echogenic focus (long thin arrows) within gallbladder lumen (star), with prominent posterior acoustic shadowing (thick arrows). The liver parenchyma (arrowheads) can be seen on the superior aspect of the acoustic window

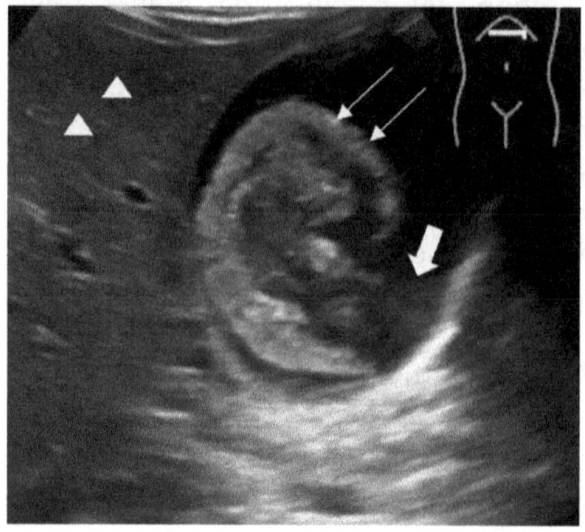

Fig. 3 Gall bladder sludge: Gall bladder sludge (long thin arrows), which appears as low-amplitude homogeneous echoes, layering (thick arrow) on the posterior wall of the gall bladder with posterior acoustic enhancement due to change in reflective surface. The liver parenchyma (arrowheads) can be seen on the superior aspect of the acoustic window

Case 3

A 13-year-old girl was brought to the PED with right upper abdominal pain for three days and fever for two days. She had similar abdominal pain in the past which resolved with oral analgesics. The examination of the abdomen revealed tenderness in the right hypochondria with guarding. She was clinically suspected of having acute cholecystitis.

A POCUS examination of the abdomen was performed using a curvilinear transducer (2–5 MHz), which showed hyperechoic areas in the gall bladder, which appeared as low-amplitude homogeneous echoes layering on the posterior wall of the gall bladder with no posterior acoustic shadowing suggestive of gall bladder sludge (Fig. 3) and associated probe-induced tenderness. The patient was admitted for further management, and formal radiological ultrasound confirmed the diagnosis of acute cholecystitis.

Case 4

A 16-year-old boy presented to the PED with severe abdominal pain for the past six hours, radiating from the left lower abdomen to the groin area. Examination of the abdomen revealed tenderness in the left lumbar area with no guarding.

A POCUS examination of the abdomen performed using a curvilinear transducer (2–5 MHz), showed a hyperechoic area in the renal pelvis with pelvicalyceal dilatation (Fig. 4). A comprehensive ultrasound by the radiologist was suggestive of left-sided renal calculi with mild hydronephrosis.

Case 5

A 2-year-old boy with underlying complex congenital cyanotic heart disease was brought into the PED with fever, abdominal pain, multiple episodes of non-bilious vomiting, and diarrhea for 3 days. His cardiac examination revealed a continuous murmur over the right upper sternal border. The room air oxygen saturation was 84%. The abdomen was distended and non-tender.

A POCUS examination of the abdomen was performed using a curvilinear probe (2–5 MHz) to evaluate the

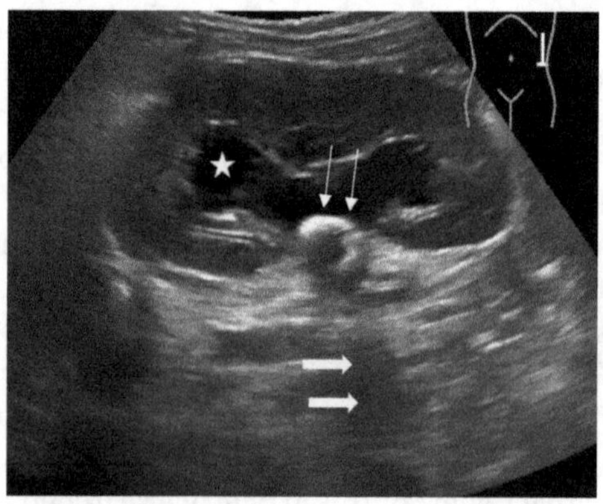

Fig. 4 Renal calculi: Renal calculi seen in the renal pelvis as an echogenic focus (long thin arrows). There is associated posterior acoustic shadowing seen behind the echogenic foci (thick arrows). Pelvicalyceal dilation is also seen secondary to obstructive uropathy (star)

abdominal distension and revealed no free fluid in the abdomen and no abnormally distended bowel loops. The renal POCUS showed calcification of the renal medulla in bilateral kidneys, appearing as hyperechoic areas in the renal pyramids with coarse echotexture, suggestive of suspected nephrocalcinosis (Fig. 5a, b). The patient was admitted for further workup, and the formal radiological ultrasound confirmed medullary nephrocalcinosis secondary to underlying medullary sponge kidney and current presentation due to viral gastroenteritis.

Case 6

A sixteen-year-old girl presented to the PED with pain in the upper abdomen for three days. There was also associated severe nausea and three episodes of non-bilious vomiting. She had one episode of similar abdominal pain 2 years back and was managed conservatively. Her abdominal examination revealed tenderness in the epigastric region with guarding.

An ultrasound examination of the abdomen was performed by an expert emergency physician trained in abdominal ultrasound, using a curvilinear probe (2–5 MHz), and showed a heterogenous pancreas with parenchymal calcification, cystic areas, and ductal calculus (Fig. 6a). Dense posterior shadowing from intraductal calculus was seen in the epigastric region (Fig. 6b). An initial impression of acute pancreatitis in the background of chronic calcific pancreatitis was considered. The patient was admitted for further workup, and formal radiology ultrasound confirmed the diagnosis of acute pancreatitis in chronic calcific pancreatitis.

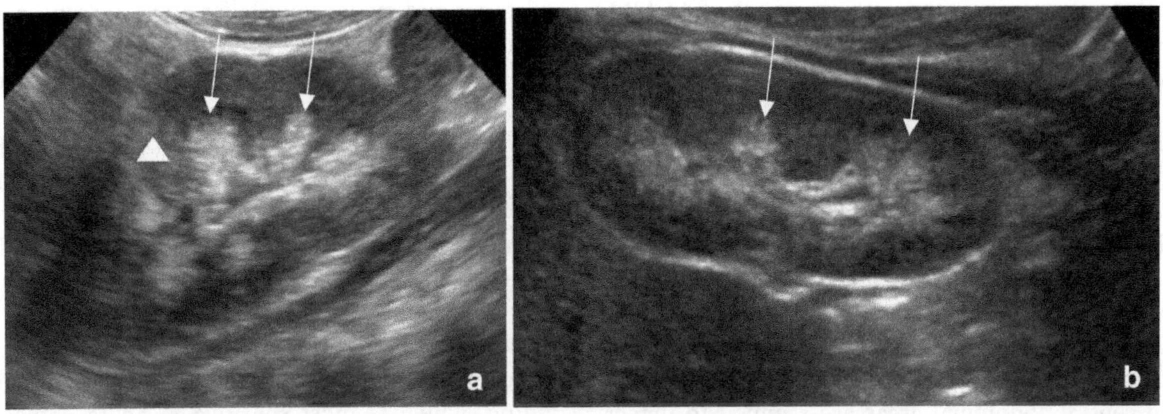

Fig. 5 Nephrocalcinosis: **a** Right kidney: Ultrasound of the right kidney showing hyper-echogenicity of the renal pyramids with coarse echotexture (long thin arrows). There is no associated posterior acoustic shadowing seen. Loss of cortico-medullary differentiation (arrowheads) can also be seen. **b** Left kidney: Ultrasound of the left kidney showing hyper-echogenicity of the renal pyramids with coarse echotexture (long thin arrows)

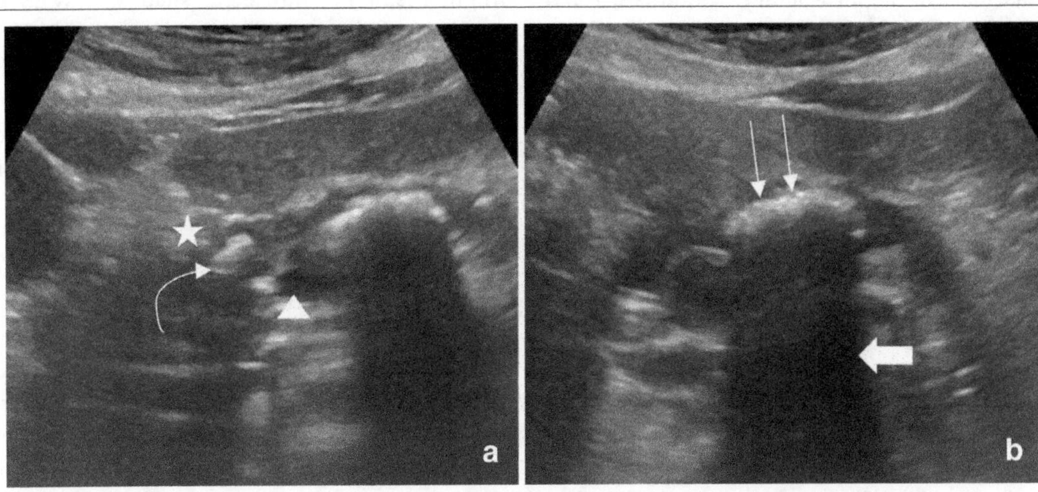

Fig. 6 Calcific pancreatitis: **a** Heterogenous pancreatic tissue (star) with parenchymal calcifications (curved arrow) and cystic areas (arrowhead) seen in the pancreas. **b** Dense posterior acoustic shadowing (thick arrows) from intraductal calculus (long thin arrows) is also seen

Discussion

POCUS examination of the abdomen performed by emergency physicians is increasingly being used to evaluate clinical manifestations and to facilitate accurate diagnoses in the emergency departments due to accessibility and portability of ultrasound machines [3–6]. The assessment of acute abdominal pain with POCUS must be done in conjunction with a thorough history and clinical examination generating a list of differentials as per the region of the abdomen. POCUS abdomen has been shown to aid and expedite the diagnosis in patients with abdominal trauma with hemoperitoneum, characterize systemic hypoperfusion and shock, detect gallstones, acute cholecystitis, and diagnose ureterolithiasis and assess for pyelonephritis [7–10]. It can be a useful adjunct for bedside diagnosis of digestive tract diseases such as intussusception, appendicitis, small bowel obstruction, and bowel perforation [3, 11–13]. POCUS can be a valuable imaging tool for assessing a pediatric patient with abdominal pain, in whom stringent adherence to the principle of ALARA is paramount [14]. A POCUS done by the emergency physician is shown to be associated with faster diagnosis time and expediting the disposition from the emergency department in a large variety of conditions [15, 16].

Abdominal POCUS is performed with the patient laying in the supine position. A low-frequency transducer is used to scan for focused findings (e.g., free fluid) [4]. A high-frequency linear probe can then be used to study the bowel, looking for abnormalities in the intramural areas and bowel wall thickening, as well as for the evaluation of the mesentery and surrounding lymph nodes [4]. The central abdominal areas are scanned to detect abnormal lymph nodes and abnormal dilatation of the small bowel [11]. After a thorough clinical history and physical examination, the differential diagnosis derived can guide further selective POCUS imaging of any of the following areas like the hepato-biliary structures, renal parenchyma, and bladder for hyperechoic lesions, calcifications, or abnormal dilation. The physician sonographer must bear in mind that these are not standard POCUS examinations. The presence of any abnormal sonological findings must be confirmed with a formal, comprehensive radiology ultrasound. This is especially important if the POCUS findings are out of the scope of Pediatric Emergency Medicine (PEM) POCUS, as currently described in the literature [4]. Additional scanning can be done in the subxiphoid window to evaluate for the presence of pericardial effusion and in bilateral upper quadrants for an anechoic area in the supradiaphragmatic area to detect the presence of pleural effusion [8].

POCUS is a valuable assessment tool for abdominal pain. The finding of different types of calcifications on POCUS can narrow down the differential diagnosis. When using POCUS to assess right lower quadrant pain, thoroughly interrogate for sonological features of acute appendicitis [4, 17]. The use of POCUS in these patients also demonstrated significantly decreased length of stay in the PED [4, 18]. The presence of a target sign with diameter >6 mm, non-compressibility of the appendix, free fluid surrounding the appendix, and increased echogenicity of local mesenteric fat will facilitate the diagnosis of acute appendicitis [18, 19]. An appendicolith is a calcified deposit within the appendix, which may be an incidental finding, but it may also cause appendicitis [20]. On the ultrasound, an appendicolith will appear as a hyperechoic area within the appendix lumen, casting a posterior acoustic shadow (Fig. 1). Lack of consistent visualization of the appendix is a limitation when assessing the right lower quadrant, with the visualization rates ranging from 22 to 98% [21]. The use of additional sonological findings in these patients might help in the diagnosis.

POCUS of the hepato-biliary system is done to detect gallstones and evidence of biliary obstruction or inflammation [4]. Ultrasound is considered the gold standard for detecting gallstones [22]. On the greyscale ultrasound, the gallbladder calculi appear as a highly reflective hyperechoic focus within gallbladder lumen, with prominent posterior acoustic shadowing (Fig. 2) [23]. Upon changing the position of the patient, a gravity-dependent movement is often seen, and this is called the "rolling stone sign." Gallbladder sludge appears as low-amplitude homogeneous echoes, layering on the posterior wall of the gall bladder (Fig. 3) [24]. The sludge does not cause posterior acoustic shadowing [25]. POCUS finding, which is most sensitive in acute cholecystitis, is the presence of cholelithiasis in combination with the sonographic Murphy sign, gallbladder wall thickening (>3 mm), and pericholecystic fluid [4, 26]. A single large stone or a collection of stones within the gall bladder might result in "wall echo shadow" (WES sign), which results in failure to identify the gall bladder [4]. Biliary POCUS could be technically difficult to perform due to the presence of overlying fat, bowel gas, and abdominal discomfort [4]. The presence of gallstones might be an incidental finding on POCUS, and the PED physician must be vigilant not to overlook other life-threatening emergencies in children [4].

POCUS can be a useful adjunct in the assessment of the kidneys and urinary tract for the presence of hydronephrosis, calculi, cysts, and abscesses [4]. Urolithiasis is the presence of calculi anywhere along the course of the urinary tracts [27]. Ultrasound features of renal calculi include a hyperechoic focus in the renal pelvis (Fig. 4) or along the ureter or bladder. There is associated posterior acoustic shadowing seen behind the hyperechoic foci (Fig. 4). Ultrasound might not be able to detect the calcified stones in the ureters unless they are close to the renal pelvis or in close proximity to the bladder at the vesico-ureteric junction because the ureters are often covered by the bowel gas in the retroperitoneum [4, 28]. However, symptomatic patients with new-onset hydronephrosis and correlating abnormal bladder jet (either absent or very high/low velocity) might suggest a blocked ureter [28]. This is especially concerning if there are symptoms suggesting of urinary tract infection. Also, other differential diagnoses that must be considered in this situation are posterior urethral valves and external mass effect from constipated stool or tumor, which are beyond the scope of POCUS.

Nephrocalcinosis, which is the calcification of renal parenchyma, is seen as secondary to hyperparathyroidism, renal tubular acidosis, and medullary sponge kidney [29]. Ultrasound features of medullary nephrocalcinosis include hyper-echogenicity in the periphery of the pyramids in the early phase of the disease, progressing to coarse calcification in the late phase (Fig. 5) [30]. The presence of nephrocalcinosis is not a real PEM POCUS finding. The nephrocalcinosis can be seen in the PEM POCUS, but this is not included in the PEM POCUS syllabus [4]. A formal, comprehensive radiological ultrasound assessment must always confirm the incidental presence of renal parenchymal calcification detected on the POCUS examination.

Bedside ultrasound for assessment of the pancreas, and its pathology is out of the scope of PEM POCUS as currently described in the literature [4]. However, suggestive history and clinical findings, along with gross calcifications that might be seen in the upper abdomen, should raise the possibility of pancreatitis. Pancreatic calcifications are generally seen with chronic pancreatitis, although it can be seen in rarer conditions like hyperparathyroidism and hemochromatosis [31]. Typically, the calcification appears speckled (Fig. 6a) as the calcium gets deposited on the network of pancreatic ducts. The presences of intraductal calcifications with small cysts, which appear as hyperechoic foci in the epigastric region (Fig. 6b), combined with history and clinical features of recurrent pancreatitis, are pathognomonic for chronic pancreatitis.

In addition to the above causes of intra-abdominal calcifications, neuroblastoma, calcified lymph nodes, an ovarian dermoid, peri-portal calcified lymph node, fecalith, and calcified granulomas in the spleen will appear as a hyperechoic area on the POCUS imaging of the abdomen [1]. By correlating the location of the calcification with the underlying anatomical structure and integrating the findings with history and clinical details, pediatric emergency physicians can derive a focused set of differential diagnoses (Table 1).

There could be numerous pitfalls while performing POCUS abdomen in PED. The presence of abdominal pain might make the child uncooperative for the abdominal POCUS examination. Similarly, intestinal gas and fecal matter might obscure the underlying structures [32]. Calcifications on ultrasound can be challenging to detect or differentiate from bowel gas to the novice and even expert eyes. The posterior acoustic shadowing or signal void seen behind the calcified structures, which is an accessory finding in calcifications, will be absent in biliary sludge and nephrocalcinosis [23, 24, 29]. Misidentification of the anatomy might lead to misdiagnosis. For example, small bowel might be confused for appendix, portal vein or inferior vena cave or hepatic cysts can be mistaken for gall bladder, and ovarian cysts might be mistaken for urinary bladder [4].

Table 1 Differential diagnosis for calcified echogenic structures on POCUS abdomen in various anatomical areas

Right hypochondriac region	Epigastric region	Left hypochondriac region
Gall stones Peri-portal calcified lymph node Calcified granuloma liver	Chronic calcific pancreatitis (body)	Chronic calcific pancreatitis (tail) Calcified granuloma spleen
Right lumbar region	**Umbilical region**	**Left lumbar region**
Renal calculi Nephrocalcinosis Neuroblastoma	Calcified lymph nodes Neuroblastoma	Renal calculi Nephrocalcinosis Neuroblastoma
Right iliac region	**Hypogastric region**	**Left iliac region**
Calcified lymph nodes Appendicolith Ovarian dermoid Urinary tract calculi	Bladder calculi Vesico-ureteric junction calculi	Fecalith Calcified lymph nodes Ovarian dermoid Urinary tract calculi

Conclusions

In a child presenting to the Pediatric Emergency Department with abdominal pain, POCUS and the findings of calcifications can narrow or expand the differential diagnosis when integrated with history and physical exam, to a specific anatomic structure. Integrating these findings with additional sonological findings of an underlying pathology might raise sufficient concerns in the emergency physicians to warrant further investigations for the patient in the form of a formal radiological ultrasound and assist in the patient's early disposition. The use of POCUS might also help to categorize the type of calcification to one of the four main categories of intra-abdominal calcifications, namely concretions, conduit wall calcification, cyst wall calcification, and solid mass-type calcification. POCUS used thoughtfully can give a diagnosis and expand differential diagnosis, reduce cognitive bias, and reduce physician mental load. By integrating the use of POCUS with the history and clinical findings, it will be possible to expedite the management in children who present to the Pediatric Emergency Department with acute abdominal pain.

Acknowledgements

We thank Dr. Lee Khai Pin, Senior Consultant and Head of Children's Emergency, KK Women's and Children's Hospital, Singapore, for advice and technical support.

Authors' contributions

VJ and JS contributed to concept and design of the study along with drafting the manuscript. CYK revised the manuscript critically for important intellectual content. GYKO contributed to the acquisition of data and interpretation of data, revising it critically for important intellectual content. All authors read and approved the final manuscript.

Author details

[1] Children's Emergency, C/O KK Women's and Children's Hospital PTE. LTD, 100 Bukit Timah Road, Singapore 229899, Singapore. [2] Department of Radiodiagnosis, Christian Fellowship Hospital, Oddanchatram, Tamilnadu 624619, India. [3] Paediatric Intensive Care Unit, Department of Pediatrics, Sarawak General Hospital, Kuching, Malaysia.

References

1. Bassano JM (2006) Abdominal calcifications and diagnostic imaging decision making: a topic review. J Chiropr Med 5:43–52
2. Baad M, Lu ZF, Reiser I et al (2017) Clinical Significance of US Artifacts. Radiogr Rev Publ Radiol Soc N Am Inc 37:1408–1423
3. Kameda T, Taniguchi N (2016) Overview of point-of-care abdominal ultrasound in emergency and critical care. J Intensive Care 4:53
4. Marin JR, Abo AM, Arroyo AC et al (2016) Pediatric emergency medicine point-of-care ultrasound: summary of the evidence. Crit Ultrasound J. https://doi.org/10.1186/s13089-016-0049-5. (**Epub ahead of print 3 November 2016**)
5. Moore CL, Copel JA (2011) Point-of-care ultrasonography. N Engl J Med 364:749–757
6. Becker DM, Tafoya CA, Becker SL et al (2016) The use of portable ultrasound devices in low- and middle-income countries: a systematic review of the literature. Trop Med Int Health TM IH 21:294–311
7. Alpert EA (2019) The ABCDs of ResUS—resuscitation ultrasound. Cureus. https://doi.org/10.7759/cureus.4616
8. Seif D, Perera P, Mailhot T et al (2012) Bedside ultrasound in resuscitation and the rapid ultrasound in shock protocol. Crit Care Res Pract. https://doi.org/10.1155/2012/503254. (**Epub ahead of print 2012**)
9. Tzou DT, Usawachintachit M, Taguchi K et al (2017) Ultrasound use in urinary stones: adapting old technology for a modern-day disease. J Endourol 31:S89–S94
10. Hilsden R, Leeper R, Koichopolos J et al (2018) Point-of-care biliary ultrasound in the emergency department (BUSED): implications for surgical referral and emergency department wait times. Trauma Surg Acute Care Open. https://doi.org/10.1136/tsaco-2018-000164. (**Epub ahead of print 30 July 2018**)
11. James V, Alsani FS, Fregonas C et al (2016) Point-of-care ultrasound in pediatric small bowel obstruction: an ED case series. Am J Emerg Med 34:2464.e1-2464.e2
12. James V, Warier A, Lee KP et al (2017) Point-of-care ultrasound identification of pneumatosis intestinalis in pediatric abdominal pain: a case report. Crit Ultrasound J 9:2
13. Benabbas R, Hanna M, Shah J et al (2017) Diagnostic accuracy of history, physical examination, laboratory tests, and point-of-care ultrasound for pediatric acute appendicitis in the emergency department: a systematic review and meta-analysis. Acad Emerg Med Off J Soc Acad Emerg Med 24:523–551
14. Strauss KJ, Kaste SC (2006) The ALARA (as low as reasonably achievable) concept in pediatric interventional and fluoroscopic imaging: striving to keep radiation doses as low as possible during fluoroscopy of pediatric patients—a white paper executive summary. Pediatr Radiol 36:110–112
15. Stanley A, Wajanga BMK, Jaka H et al (2017) The impact of systematic point-of-care ultrasound on management of patients in a resource-limited setting. Am J Trop Med Hyg 96:488–492
16. Harel-Sterling M, Diallo M, Santhirakumaran S et al (2019) Emergency department resource use in pediatric pneumonia: point-of-care lung ultrasonography versus chest radiography. J Ultrasound Med 38:407–414
17. Sivitz AB, Cohen SG, Tejani C (2014) Evaluation of acute appendicitis by pediatric emergency physician sonography. Ann Emerg Med 64(358–364):e4
18. Elikashvili I, Tay ET, Tsung JW (2014) The effect of point-of-care ultrasonography on emergency department length of stay and computed tomography utilization in children with suspected appendicitis. Acad Emerg Med Off J Soc Acad Emerg Med 21:163–170
19. Mostbeck G, Adam EJ, Nielsen MB et al (2016) How to diagnose acute appendicitis: ultrasound first. Insights Imaging 7:255–263
20. Kaya B, Eris C (2011) Different clinical presentation of appendicolithiasis. The Report of three cases and review of the literature. Clin Med Insights Pathol 4:1–4
21. Taylor GA (2004) Suspected appendicitis in children: in search of the single best diagnostic test. Radiology 231:293–295
22. Kothari SN, Obinwanne KM, Baker MT et al (2013) A prospective, blinded comparison of laparoscopic ultrasound with transabdominal ultrasound for the detection of gallbladder pathology in morbidly obese patients. J Am Coll Surg 216:1057–1062
23. Brink JA, Simeone JF, Mueller PR et al (1989) Routine sonographic techniques fail to quantify gallstone size and number: a retrospective study of 111 surgically proved cases. AJR Am J Roentgenol 153:503–506
24. Shaffer EA (2001) Gallbladder sludge: what is its clinical significance? Curr Gastroenterol Rep 3:166–173
25. Wilkinson LS, Levine TS, Smith D et al (1996) Biliary sludge: can ultrasound reliably detect the presence of crystals in bile? Eur J Gastroenterol Hepatol 8:999–1001
26. Hwang H, Marsh I, Doyle J (2014) Does ultrasonography accurately diagnose acute cholecystitis? Improving diagnostic accuracy based on a review at a regional hospital. Can J Surg 57:162–168
27. Brisbane W, Bailey MR, Sorensen MD (2016) An overview of kidney stone imaging techniques. Nat Rev Urol 13:654–662
28. Wong C, Teitge B, Ross M et al (2018) The accuracy and prognostic value of point-of-care ultrasound for nephrolithiasis in the emergency department: a systematic review and meta-analysis. Acad Emerg Med Off J Soc Acad Emerg Med 25:684–698
29. Shavit L, Jaeger P, Unwin RJ (2015) What is nephrocalcinosis? Kidney Int 88:35–43

30. Boyce AM, Shawker TH, Hill SC et al (2013) Ultrasound is superior to computed tomography for assessment of medullary nephrocalcinosis in hypoparathyroidism. J Clin Endocrinol Metab 98:989–994
31. Lesniak RJ, Hohenwalter MD, Taylor AJ (2002) Spectrum of causes of pancreatic calcifications. AJR Am J Roentgenol 178:79–86
32. Blanco P, Volpicelli G (2016) Common pitfalls in point-of-care ultrasound: a practical guide for emergency and critical care physicians. Crit Ultrasound J. https://doi.org/10.1186/s13089-016-0052-x. (**Epub ahead of print 26 October 2016**)

14

Are seminal vesicles a potential pitfall during pelvic exploration using point-of-care ultrasound (POCUS)?

Antoine Fasseaux[1*], Philippe Pès[2], Françoise Steenebruggen[3] and Florence Dupriez[3]

Abstract

Background: Trauma is a major cause of death among the working population. Many countries have now adopted a structured approach to trauma management in which ultrasound is used as a primary evaluation tool. While its use has direct therapeutic benefits, many artifacts and pitfalls are inherent to the technique. Knowledge of the most frequently encountered pitfalls in practice could thus help reduce the risk of error and lead to more accurate trauma assessments.

Objective: This study evaluates a potential pitfall caused by seminal vesicles during focused assessment with sonography for trauma examinations of the male pelvis performed by an emergency physician with experience in point-of-care ultrasound.

Methods: We took five static and five dynamic (3-s loops) transverse ultrasound images of the pelvis in five healthy males. The images and videos were then incorporated into an online survey and emailed through the World Interactive Network Focused On Critical UltraSound (WINFOCUS) in France and the Ultrasound and Emergency Medicine (UEM) Organization in Belgium. A questionnaire asked anonymous participants to assess the presence of free fluid in the static and dynamic images and to share information about their training and experience in point-of-care ultrasound. To validate the static and dynamic images, the survey was sent to three external radiologists for independent verification.

Results: A total of 191 individuals responded fully or partially to the survey, 114 of whom completed it. Among the 114 participants who completed the survey, the misinterpretation rate was 0.55 (95CI 0.51–0.60) for all static and dynamic ultrasound transverse pelvic views. The misinterpretation rate was 0.61 (95CI 0.55–0.66) and 0.50 (95CI 0.45–0.55) for static and dynamic ultrasound transverse pelvic views, respectively. The three external radiologists answered the questionnaire correctly without misinterpreting the survey ultrasound views.

Conclusions: Seminal vesicles are a potential pitfall when interpreting transverse ultrasound images of the male pelvis in the context of point-of-care ultrasound.

Keywords: Focused assessment with sonography for trauma (FAST), Pitfall, Emergency physician, Seminal vesicle, Point-of-care ultrasound, Ultrasound, Bedside ultrasound, Emergency ultrasound, Clinical ultrasound

Background

Injuries are the leading cause of death for people aged between 1 and 44 years [1]. A structured approached to trauma management is followed in many countries using the Advanced Trauma Life Support (ATLS) protocol for the initial assessment of patients. The ATLS, Western Trauma Association, and Eastern Association for the

*Correspondence: afasseaux@gmail.com
[1] Department of Emergency Medicine, CHR Jolimont, 7100 La Louvière, Belgium
Full list of author information is available at the end of the article

Surgery of Trauma guidelines all support the use of ultrasound during the assessment of severe trauma [2–4]. As a result, clinical ultrasound use in emergency departments has increased considerably since its introduction more than 30 years ago [5]. Without interrupting management, bedside ultrasounds allow the rapid evaluation of patients to determine the presence of free fluid in the peritoneum or pericardium. Focused assessment with sonography for trauma (FAST) is a point-of-care ultrasound (POCUS) examination of four sites: Morrison's pouch between the liver and right kidney, the splenorenal recess, the pelvic area, and the pericardial space [6].

Extended focused assessment with sonography for trauma (E-FAST) incorporates four additional areas: the two pulmonary apex and the two pulmonary bases. The exploration of these areas aims to identify the presence of free fluid in the pleura or clinically significant pneumothorax [7]. In unstable patients, E-FAST identifies the pericardial, peritoneal, or pleural location of the bleeding for faster surgical management [8]. FAST ultrasound examinations are now an integral part of emergency physician training [9]. Yet despite the large number of courses available around the world, ultrasound curricula suffer from a lack of standardization. Consequently, skill acquisition is less systematic, depending particularly on the types of cases encountered and the number of examinations carried out before clinical POCUS use [10].

Like other clinical ultrasound examinations, FAST can be prone to pitfalls and artifacts, leading to the misinterpretation of the acquired images. A recent meta-analysis involving 8635 patients showed a sensitivity of 0.74 (95CI 0.65–0.81) and a specificity of 0.96 (95CI 0.94–0.98) when E-FAST is performed by an emergency physician [11].

In some ultrasound curricula, seminal vesicles are reported as a source of misinterpretation when assessing the male pelvis [12]. Located behind the bladder, seminal vesicles have a hypoechoic appearance that can be mistaken for free fluid. Misinterpretation of a FAST could have a direct therapeutic impact. A literature search did not reveal any evidence of seminal vesicles as a source of pitfall during FAST. The main goal of this study is therefore to verify whether seminal vesicles may be a source of false-positive POCUS results performed by an emergency physician trained in POCUS.

Methods

Five healthy male volunteers were scanned using a Philips Sparq® and a C6 2–6 MHz convex probe. The abdomen preset of the ultrasound machine was chosen for the ultrasound examination and image registration. Each volunteer was scanned to obtain static and dynamic ultrasound transverse views of the pelvis. The dynamic image was a 3-s loop showing transverse ultrasound images of the pelvis from the pubic symphysis toward the apex of the bladder, obtained by fanning the probe. The seminal vesicles were visible on each ultrasound image. The static and dynamic images were incorporated into an online survey via SurveyMonkey® using a high image resolution in JPEG format. After validation, the survey was sent by email to the networks of the World Interactive Network Focused On Critical UltraSound (WINFOCUS) in France and the Ultrasound and Emergency Medicine (UEM) Organization in Belgium. Only the anonymous participants who described themselves as familiar with FAST ultrasound were given the opportunity to complete the survey in French or in Dutch. (available at https://fr.surveymonkey.com/r/MQ297W2) After recording the demographic and professional (Table 1) profile and clinical ultrasound background of the participating emergency physicians, they were asked whether they saw free fluid on the recorded static and dynamic images. For the analysis of the ultrasound images, apart from the gender of the volunteers and the ultrasound view setting (i.e., male transverse pelvic view), no other clinical information was given to participants. Only the results of fully completed questionnaires were included in the study. The

Table 1 Profile of participants

Profile	Total ($n=114$)
Experience in emergency medicine	
< 5 years	38 (33%)
5–10 years	34 (29.83%)
10–20 years	30 (26.32%)
20–30 years	10 (8.77%)
> 30 years	2 (1.75%)
Total	114 (100%)
Ultrasound training	
None	1 (0.88%)
Short course	61 (53.51%)
Validated short course	6 (5.26%)
Long course	29 (25.44%)
Multiple training courses (2 or more)	17 (14.91%)
Total	114 (100%)
Ultrasound frequency of use	
Daily	71 (62.28%)
Weekly	37 (32.46%)
Monthly	4 (3.51%)
Rarely	2 (1.75%)
Total	114 (100%)
Ultrasound availability at work	
Yes	111 (97.37%)
No	3 (2.63%)
Total	114 (100%)

participants were not given the opportunity to repeat the survey or review the images and change their responses after seeing the next question. To independently validate the selected static and dynamic ultrasound images, the survey was taken by three external radiologists.

For the statistical analysis, the calculations were performed using the software Excel® (Microsoft, Redmond (Washington), United States). A paired data t-test was used to compare the results of the static and dynamic sections.

Results

Between February 1 and March 31, 2020, 191 people responded to the survey. Overall, 77 people were excluded from the study because they did not complete the questionnaire, while 114 completed it entirely. Table 1 reports the profile of participants.

The misinterpretation rate was 0,55 (95CI 0.51–0.60) for all static and dynamic ultrasound transverse pelvic views. The misinterpretation rate was 0.61 (95CI 0.55–0.66) and 0.50 (95CI 0.45–0.55) for static and dynamic ultrasound transverse pelvic views, respectively. The difference in misinterpretation rate for static and dynamic images was 0.53 (p-value 0.0001).

Given the large heterogeneity in the number of participants in the different subgroups, no statistically significant correlation was found in terms of professional experience, frequency of ultrasound use, or training background. The misinterpretation rates according to the different subgroups are described in Table 2. The three external radiologists all correctly answered the questionnaire and did not mistake the seminal vesicles for free fluid.

Discussion

Many emergency departments use ultrasound on a daily basis to assess patients. The FAST protocol and its variant e-FAST allow the rapid assessment of severe trauma patients. However, there is a lack of standardization in the different training programs and especially in the teaching of the FAST protocol [10].

Located in the retroperitoneum, the seminal vesicles contain fluid that can have a hypoechoic appearance in the ultrasound images of the male pelvis (Fig. 1, Additional file 1: video S1). Although poorly studied, this hypoechoic structure may be misinterpreted as free fluid. In male patients, free fluid is located in the Douglas pouch, never next to or directly above the prostate, but rather more cranially at the level of the bladder. Figure 2 shows a transverse ultrasound view of the male pelvis above the seminal vesicles, whereas Fig. 3 and Additional file 2: video S2 show a pathological ultrasound view of the male pelvis with free fluid. Our study suggests that the seminal vesicles are a potential

Table 2 Mean misinterpretation rate in participant subgroups

	Total ($n=10$)	Static views ($n=5$)	Dynamic views ($n=5$)
All categories combined	5.54 ± 0.46	3.04 ± 0.28	2.51 ± 0.24
Experience in emergency medicine			
< 5 years	5.55 ± 0.78	3.06 ± 0.48	2.49 ± 0.42
5–10 years	5.58 ± 0.83	3.06 ± 0.51	2.52 ± 0.45
10–20 years	5.58 ± 0.90	3.06 ± 0.55	2.53 ± 0.49
20–30 years	5.59 ± 1.75	3.05 ± 1.08	2.50 ± 0.93
> 30 years	5.86 ± 17.44	3.14 ± 12.41	2.72 ± 9.57
Ultrasound training			
None (1 response)	9	5	4
Short course	5.56 ± 0.62	3.05 ± 0.38	2.51 ± 0.33
Validated short course	5.65 ± 2.56	3.06 ± 1.57	2.59 ± 1.33
Long course	5.65 ± 0.91	3.10 ± 0.56	2.55 ± 0.49
Multiple training courses (2 or more)	5.18 ± 1.35	2.88 ± 0.80	2.29 ± 0.65
Ultrasound frequency of use			
Daily	5.59 ± 0.56	3.07 ± 0.34	2.51 ± 0.31
Weekly	5.54 ± 0.81	3.04 ± 0.50	2.50 ± 0.43
Monthly	5.71 ± 3.79	3.05 ± 2.31	2.66 ± 2.04
Rarely	6.00 ± 21.18	3.30 ± 10.42	2.70 ± 12.02
Ultrasound available at work			
Yes	5.54 ± 0.46	3.04 ± 0.28	2.51 ± 0.25
No	5.72 ± 5.78	3.12 ± 3.55	2.61 ± 3.17

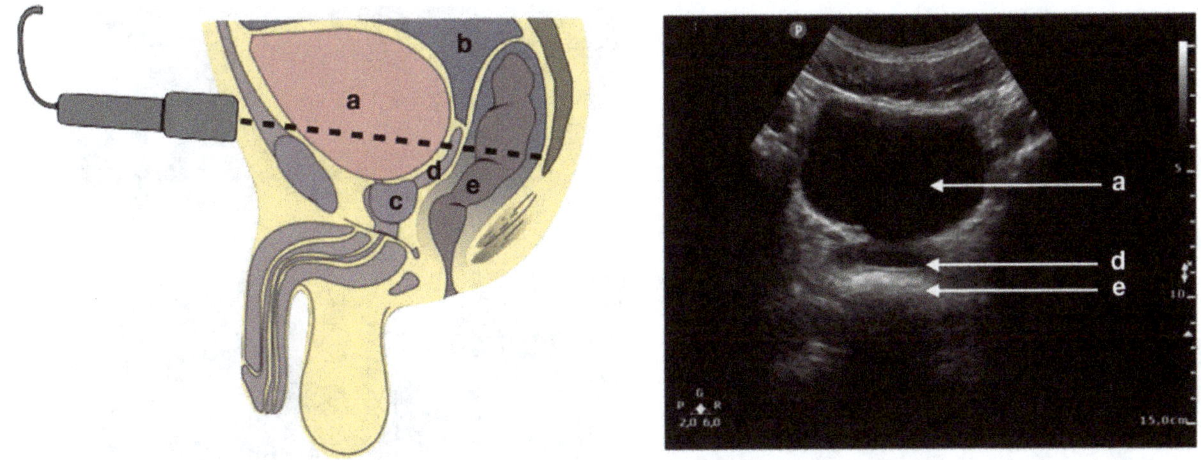

a: bladder, b peritoneal space, c prostate, d seminal vesicles, e rectum, f free fluid

Fig. 1 Transverse ultrasound view of the male pelvis—probe oriented towards the seminal vesicles

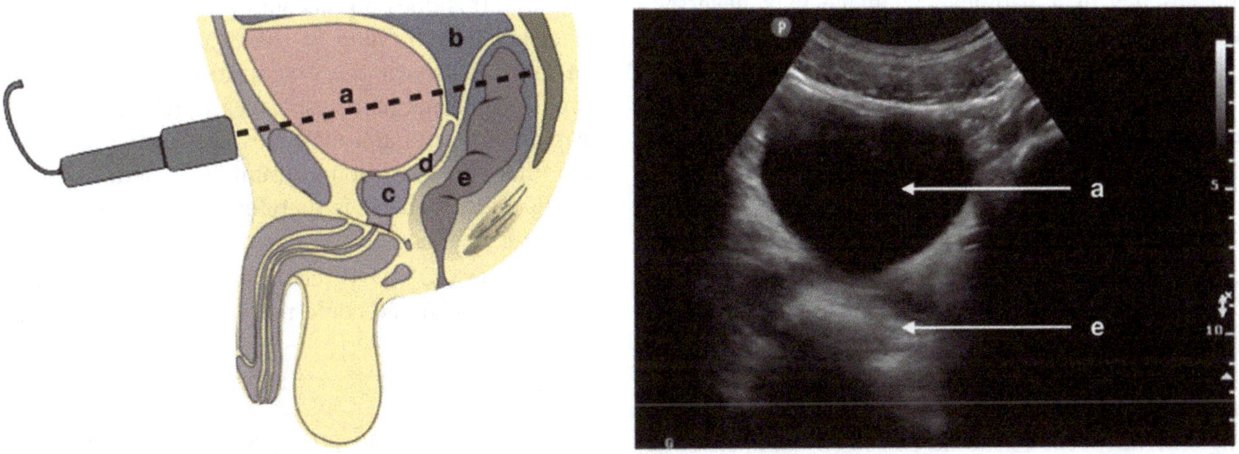

a: bladder, b peritoneal space, c prostate, d seminal vesicles, e rectum, f free fluid

Fig. 2 Transverse ultrasound view of the male pelvis—probe oriented towards the peritoneal space

POCUS pitfall when assessing the presence of free fluid in the male pelvis. Among the ultrasound images included in the survey, only the seminal vesicles could be the source of misinterpretation for free fluid. The completion of the survey by three external radiologists to confirm the quality of the chosen ultrasound transverse pelvic views gives methodological strength to this study.

Although participants were given information about the view and location of the ultrasound images as well as the gender of the volunteers, seminal vesicles were not specially mentioned in order to avoid influencing responses. All included participants described themselves as familiar with the FAST protocol, and only one participant had not received clinical ultrasound training. Participants' knowledge may thus be considered representative of ultrasound training courses, as they had a heterogeneous background in ultrasound imaging. This study also significantly demonstrates that dynamic examinations of the pelvic region reduce the number of misinterpretations compared to static images. This enlightens the importance of using dynamic, rather than static, assessment of ultrasound images during a FAST examination. This dynamic assessment should cover the region. As the participants were not given the opportunity to repeat the survey or return to a previous question, their initial responses could not be changed after the subsequent viewing of static or dynamic images. Since this study only aims to highlight the false-positive rate, no pathological image was included in the survey.

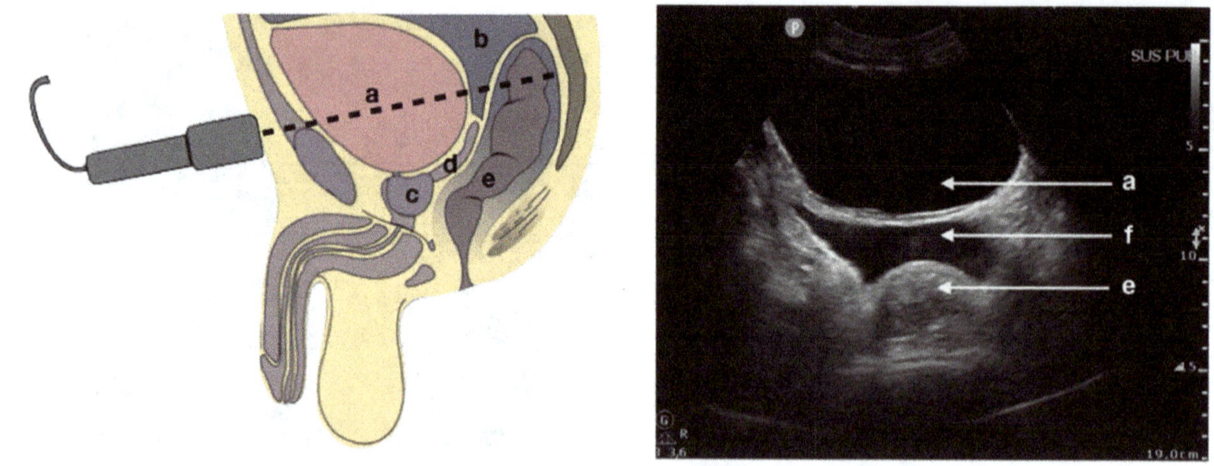

a: bladder, b peritoneal space, c prostate, d seminal vesicles, e rectum, f free fluid

Fig. 3 Transverse ultrasound view of the male pelvis with free fluid—probe oriented towards the peritoneal space

The absence of a pathological image may nevertheless have influenced the certainty index of participants' responses, as they may have interpreted images according to the following yes–no question: is free fluid visible in this transverse ultrasound image of the male pelvis? However, the survey used carefully chosen sentences to avoid influencing participants about the possible absence or presence of free fluid.

The exclusive use of a transverse section view without a longitudinal view may be cited as a limitation of this study. Indeed, the e-FAST protocol strictly recommends the use of a transverse view along with a longitudinal view to assess the presence of free fluid in the pelvis [13]. Complementary studies should therefore clarify whether the additional use of a longitudinal ultrasound view decreases the number of misinterpretations.

Another limitation of this study relates to its setting. Indeed, a questionnaire is far removed from the clinical setting. However, responses provided without the stress of a pathological setting could be considered even more accurate than answers given in the stress of a severe trauma assessment. Complementary studies are nevertheless required to avoid this bias. FAST and, more broadly, POCUS aim to clinically interpret the images obtained as part of a comprehensive approach to patient care. In addition, ultrasound is an operator-dependent examination, which gives the questionnaire setting of this study another substantial bias. This bias can be partially attenuated given that the quality of the images was independently and successfully validated by three radiologists.

Another limitation of this work is the selection bias due to the inclusion of physicians registered in the database of two ultrasound training providers in France and Belgium. This does not account for the fact that participants received training in these organizations. Indeed, the mailing lists of the organizations included participants with other courses' background, although their proportion could not be assessed. Both organizations only offer short ultrasound training programs. The background heterogeneity is therefore substantial in the different subgroups.

Given the COVID-19 crisis, the follow-up email that was initially planned could not be returned by these two organizations.

Conclusion

The FAST ultrasound protocol is now standard in the management of trauma patients in many countries. Seminal vesicles can nevertheless be a source of misinterpretation when evaluating transverse ultrasound images of the male pelvis. However, this is significantly diminished by the interpretation of dynamic views. This potential pitfall should be addressed in the various teaching methods and available curricula. Ultrasound instructors should also stress the importance of the dynamic assessment of the pelvis using a fanning movement. Further studies are required to determine whether the addition of a longitudinal view helps decrease the incidence of this newly studied pitfall. We believe that ultrasound curricula available around the world should introduce seminal vesicles as a potential pitfall when using POCUS.

Supplementary Information

Additional file 1: Video S1. Normal transverse ultrasound view of the male pelvis.

Additional file 2: Video S2. Pathological transverse ultrasound view of the male pelvis—free fluid.

Abbreviations
POCUS: Point-of-care ultrasound; WINFOCUS: World Interactive Network Focused On Critical UltraSound (WINFOCUS) UEM: Ultrasound and Emergency Medicine; FAST: Focused assessment with sonography for trauma; ATLS: Advanced Trauma Life Support; E-FAST: Extended focused assessment with sonography for trauma; COVID-19: Coronavirus disease 2019.

Acknowledgements
Not applicable.

Authors' contributions
AF: elaboration of the survey, interpretation of data, drafting of the manuscript; PP: critical revision of the manuscript; FS: translation of the survey; FD: critical revision of the methodology and the manuscript. All authors read and approved the final manuscript.

Author details
[1] Department of Emergency Medicine, CHR Jolimont, 7100 La Louvière, Belgium. [2] Department of Emergency Medicine, CHU Nantes, Nantes Univer sity Hospital, 44000 Nantes, France. [3] Department of Emergency Medicine, Cliniques Universitaires Saint Luc, 1200 Brussels, Belgium.

References
1. Centers for Disease Control and Prevention (2018) National center for injury prevention and control. https://www.cdc.gov/injury/images/lc-charts/leading_causes_of_death_by_age_group_2018_1100w850h.jpg. Accessed 6 May 2020.
2. American College of Surgeons. Advanced trauma life support. 10th edition. Chicago: American College of Surgeons, Committee on Trauma; 2018.
3. Kozar RA et al (2009) Western Trauma Association critical decisions in trauma: nonoperative management of adult blunt hepatic trauma. J Trauma 67(6):1144–1148 (**discussion 1148–1149**)
4. Hoff WS et al (2002) Practice management guidelines for the evaluation of blunt abdominal trauma: the East practice management guidelines work group. J Trauma 53(3):602–615
5. Kimura A, Otsuka T (1991) Emergency center ultrasonography in the evaluation of hemoperitoneum: a prospective study. J Trauma 31(1):20–23
6. Scalea TM, Rodriguez A, Chiu WC, Brenneman FD, Fallon WF Jr, Kato K, McKenney MG, Nerlich ML, Ochsner MG, Yoshii H (1999) Focused Assessment with Sonography for Trauma (FAST): results from an international consensus conference. J Trauma 46(3):466–472
7. Montoya J, Stawicki SP, Evans DC, Bahner DP, Sparks S, Sharpe RP, Cipolla J (2016) From FAST to E-FAST: an overview of the evolution of ultrasound-based traumatic injury assessment. Eur J Trauma EmergSurg 42(2):119–126
8. Melniker LA, Leibner E, McKenney MG, Lopez P, Briggs WM, Mancuso CA (2006) Randomized controlled clinical trial of point-of-care, limited ultrasonography for trauma in the emergency department: the first sonography outcomes assessment program trial. Ann Emerg Med 48(3):227–235
9. Lewiss RE, Pearl M, Nomura JT, Baty G, Bengiamin R, Duprey K, Stone M, Theodoro D, Akhtar S (2013) CORD-AEUS: consensus document for the emergency ultrasound milestone project. AcadEmerg Med 20(7):740–745
10. Russell L, Østergaard ML, Nielsen MB, Konge L, Nielsen KR (2018) Standardised assessment of competence in Focused Assessment with Sonography for Trauma. Acta AnaesthesiolScand. https://doi.org/10.1111/aas.13141
11. Stengel D, Leisterer J, Ferrada P, Ekkernkamp A, Mutze S, Hoenning A (2018) Point-of-care ultrasonography for diagnosing thoracoabdominal injuries in patients with blunt trauma. Cochrane Database Syst Rev 12(12):Cd012669
12. Ducros L. Echographie en situation d'urgence, JRUR; 2009
13. Bloom BA, Gibbons RC (2020) Focused Assessment with Sonography for Trauma (FAST). StatPearls. StatPearls Publishing, Treasure Island

15

POCUS and POCDUS: essential tools for the evaluation and management of carotid artery pseudoaneurysms after a gunshot wound

Lisandro Montorfano[1], Marianna Sarkissyan[2], Matthew Wolfers[1], Federico Rodríguez[2], Fernando Pla[2] and Miguel Montorfano[2*]

Abstract

Background: Evaluation of asymptomatic penetrating vascular injuries can be done with Point-of-care ultrasound (POCUS) and Point-of-care Doppler ultrasound (POCDUS).

Case presentation: A 21-year-old woman was admitted to the Emergency Department with a small wound and pain on the left side of her neck. The patient stated she was standing outside her home and suddenly felt acute pain in the neck. She denied trauma or being assaulted and reported no significant past medical or surgical history. On physical exam the only positive finding was a small gunshot entry wound on the left side of her neck without hard signs of vascular injury. Bedside POCUS demonstrated soft tissue swelling and a hematoma next to the left carotid artery. A round in shape bullet was visualized in contact with the posterior left common carotid artery wall and two small saccular pseudoaneurysms were seen at left common carotid artery wall. POCDUS showed a patent left carotid artery and turbulent flow in the two saccular aneurysms. A computed tomography angiogram (CTA) was performed confirming the findings and a stent in left carotid artery was placed. The patient tolerated the procedure well and was discharged 4 days after the procedure. At the sixth month follow-up, Doppler ultrasound showed patent stent and resolution of the muscular hematoma.

Conclusions: Penetrating trauma-related vascular injuries are complex cases to handle within an acute setting. POCUS and POCDUS are increasingly being used for the workup and decision-making process of gunshot-related vascular injuries to the neck and are a fundamental part of the follow-up after definitive therapy.

Keywords: Point-of-care ultrasound, Point-of-care Doppler ultrasound, Doppler ultrasound, Penetrating trauma, Vascular injury, Carotid injury, Pseudoaneurysm, POCUS, POCDUS

Background

Violence and crime in Latin America have been considered "the social pandemic of the 20th century" [1]. Traumatic vascular injuries represent approximately 3% of all traumatic injuries. The majority of these lesions are caused by gunshot wounds, stab wounds, and blast injuries or from penetrating debris [2]. Mortality from high-velocity traumatic injuries, such as gunshot wounds, specifically to the neck, is estimated to be as high as 5%. Hence, expedited diagnosis and treatment are essential to reduce disabilities and to prevent death [2–7]. When patients present with hard signs of vascular injury (such as external bleeding, expanding hematoma, absent distal pulses, palpable thrill, and audible bruit) surgical exploration is mandatory. When soft signs or no clear signs of vascular injury are present and the patient is hemodynamically stable, vascular injuries present a challenge.

*Correspondence: miguel.montorfano@winfocus.org
[2] Department of Ultrasound and Vascular Doppler, Hospital de Emergencias "Dr. Clemente Alvarez", Av. Pellegrini 3205, Rosario, Santa Fe, Argentina
Full list of author information is available at the end of the article

Traditionally, the approach to treatment of penetrating vascular injuries to the neck has been guided by damage to the anatomic zone [8, 9]. In brief, Zone III spans the neck from base of skull to the angle of mandible, Zone II from the angle of mandible to cricoid cartilage, and Zone I from cricoid cartilage to the thoracic inlet. Injury to Zone II is most common, and injury to Zone I is more life-threatening and traditionally most likely to require immediate surgical exploration. Penetrating neck injuries can involve laryngotracheal anatomy resulting in respiratory distress and symptoms, pharyngoesophageal injuries that can affect the aerodigestive functions, or involve the nervous system injuries, which can impact autonomic and even spinal functions. Vascular injuries are the most common cause of immediate mortality due to exsanguination, with the highest rate related to carotid artery injury [9].

Imaging can be useful in the diagnosis, management, and follow-up of vascular injuries [3, 10, 11]. Angiographic evaluation of these injuries continues to be the gold standard; however, noninvasive modalities such as CTA, magnetic resonance angiography, and Doppler ultrasound represent valid alternatives [11–17].

Point-of-care ultrasound (POCUS) and Point-of-care Doppler ultrasound (POCDUS) are cheaper, noninvasive and faster alternatives to diagnose vascular injuries [14, 15]. Bergstein et al. found that, using arteriography as the gold standard, Color Flow Doppler (CFD) had a specificity of 99%, sensitivity of 50%, and Fry et al. described 100% sensitivity and specificity of Doppler ultrasound compared with the conventional arteriography and operative exploration [12, 13]. In our previous study using a FAST Doppler examination (FAST D protocol), we found 100% sensitivity and specificity to rule out vascular injury in penetrating gunshot wounds of the lower limbs [15]. In many facilities, POCUS and POCDUS are the first diagnostic modality available, and are used for a whole body examination, from head to toe, allowing for an integrated management of the trauma patient [14–16]. Moreover, in some rural or remote places, those are the only diagnostic resource available. The aim of this study is to describe POCUS and POCDUS characteristics of an asymptomatic penetrating vascular injury to the neck after a gunshot wound.

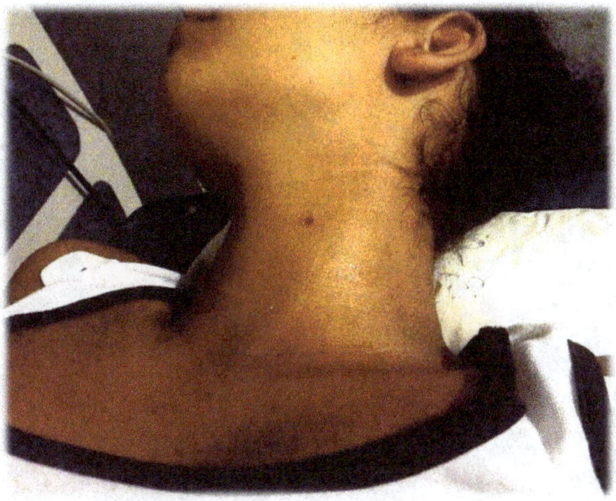

Fig. 1 Gunshot wound to the neck

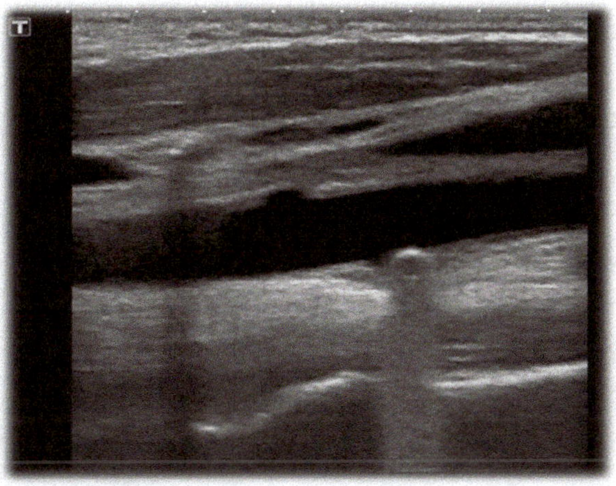

Fig. 2 Ultrasound view of left common carotid artery demonstrating two saccular pseudoaneurysms and bullet

Case report

A 21-year-old woman was admitted to the Emergency Department with neck pain and a small wound on the left side of her neck (Fig. 1). The patient stated she was standing outside her home and suddenly felt acute pain in the left side of the neck. She denied trauma or being assaulted at the time of the occurrence and reported no significant past medical or surgical history. On physical exam, the patient was in no acute distress, and vital signs were stable and within normal limits. The only positive physical exam finding was a small gunshot entry wound on the left side of her neck without hard signs of vascular injury.

Bedside POCUS was performed and demonstrated soft tissue swelling and a hematoma next to the left carotid artery. A round in shape bullet, with metallic like reverberation artifact, was visualized in contact with the posterior left common carotid artery wall. Two small saccular pseudoaneurysms were seen at left common carotid artery wall (Fig. 2). POCDUS showed a patent left carotid artery and turbulent flow in the two saccular aneurysms (Fig. 3). The studies were performed with a broadband linear array transducer with a frequency range of 5–12 MHz (Toshiba Xario;

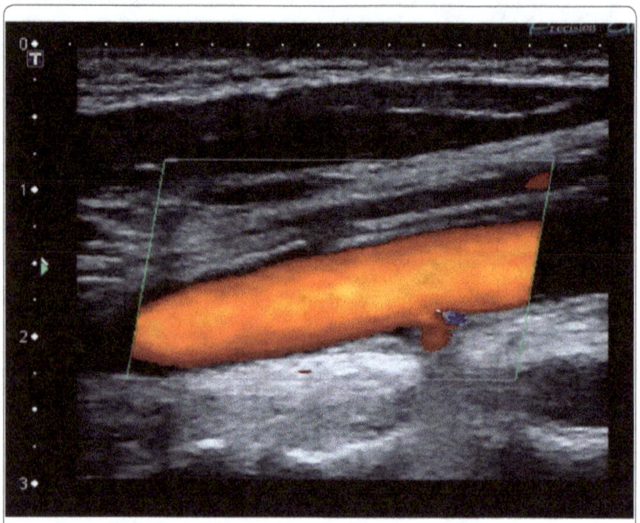

Fig. 3 Color Doppler Imaging of carotid demonstrating turbulent flow in the posterior wall pseudoaneyrysm

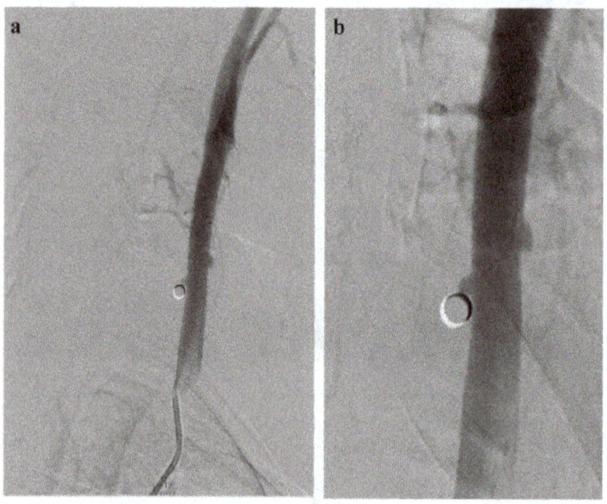

Fig. 4 **a**, **b** Views of angiography of the left carotid artery showing the two pseudoaneurysms and bullet

Tokyo, Japan). Patient was scanned in a supine position. Transverse and longitudinal scans of the vessel were performed. Due to the findings on ultrasound and color Doppler, a computer tomography angiogram was performed. The CTA confirmed these findings (Figs. 4a, b) and the decision was made to consult interventional radiology. Interventional radiology placed a left carotid stent (Figs. 5, 6, 7) and anti-platelet aggregators were given. The patient tolerated the procedure well and was discharged 4 days after the procedure. At the sixth month follow-up, Doppler ultrasound showed patent stent and resolution of the muscular hematoma next to the left carotid artery.

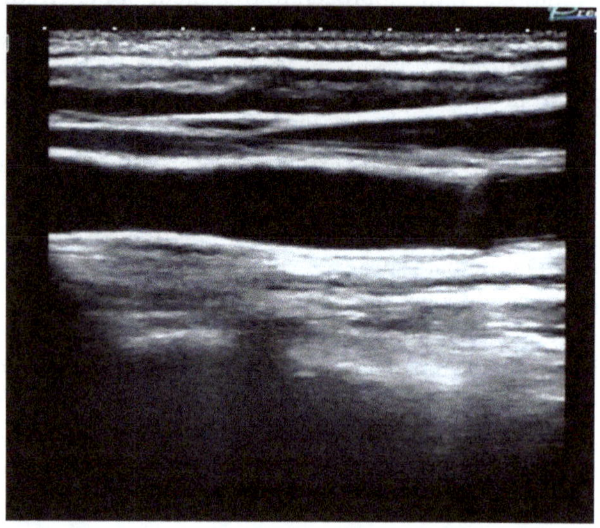

Fig. 5 Ultrasound of carotid after stenting: Longitudinal view

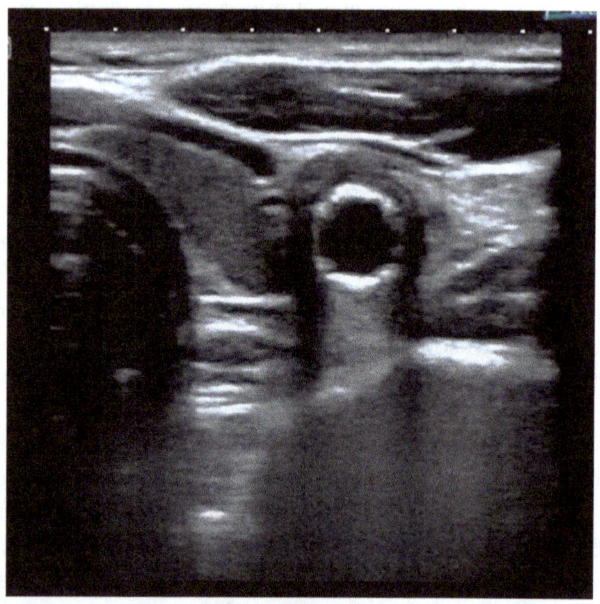

Fig. 6 Ultrasound of carotid after stenting: Transverse view

Discussion

Penetrating trauma-related vascular injuries are challenging. When patients present with hard signs of vascular injury such as hemorrhage or expanding hematomas, surgical exploration is mandatory [9]. When soft signs or no clear signs of vascular injury are present and the patient is hemodynamically stable, imaging methods could be useful tools in the diagnosis and management of these patients. CTA continues to be the gold standard for the diagnosis of these injuries. However, POCUS and POCDUS are a cheaper,

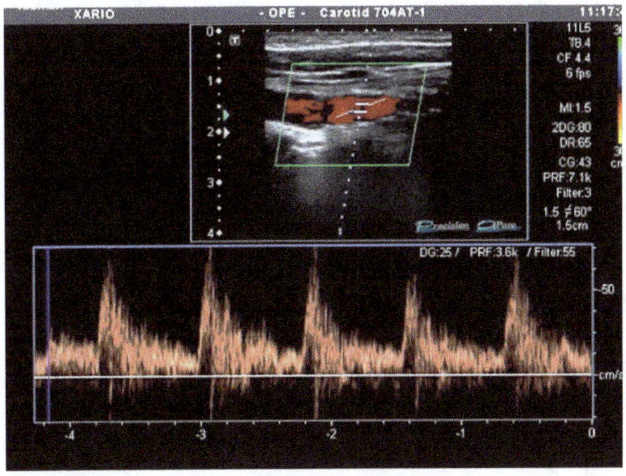

Fig. 7 Color and pulsed Doppler demonstrating restored normal flow in common carotid artery at the site of the stent

noninvasive and faster alternative to diagnose these injuries. As described in this manuscript, these tools can provide valuable information at the bedside and guide the decision-making process and follow-up of these patients.

High-frequency linear probes are the probes of choice because higher resolution and lower penetration are needed to assess this kind of injuries. When evaluating a penetrating vascular injury, it is important to scan the region of the trauma in a transverse and longitudinal fashion with B-mode. Flows should be investigated with Color and Duplex Doppler ultrasound. For comparative purposes, it is advised to evaluate both sides of the neck—affected and unaffected sides. Veins in the neck are oval in shape and are compressible. The Duplex Doppler evaluation shows a continuous flow pattern with respiratory variations. Arteries are round in shape and non-compressible. Doppler ultrasound is a useful tool for the assessment of anatomy and flow dynamics of the carotid arteries. The Duplex Doppler evaluation shows a pulsatile flow pattern with low resistance in the common and internal carotid artery and high resistance in external carotid artery.

Large hematomas, subcutaneous air, morbid obesity or large open wounds can represent a challenge, yet several studies have shown that POCUS and Doppler ultrasound remain useful tools to rule in or rule out trauma-related vascular injuries [11, 12, 14, 15]. As described in a previous paper, in patients with clinical suspicion of a vascular injury, POCUS and POCDUS are used to answer 2 basic questions [15]:

1. Does the patient have a vascular lesion? Yes or no?
2. If the answer is yes: What kind of lesion?

Two pseudoaneurysms of the left common carotid artery were found in this patient. A pseudoaneurysm is the result of a partial rupture of an artery wall, which causes accumulation of periarterial blood. The accumulated blood is surrounded and contained by the adventitia or adjacent hematomas or soft tissues. Traumatic carotid injuries are divided into grades, which can assist in guiding management [18]. Grade I injuries are mild intimal injuries which do no cause significant hemodynamic injury, grade II involve dissections and hematomas which do impact vascular hemodynamics, grade III are pseudoaneurysms (such as in this case), and grade IV and V are occlusions and transection with extravasation, respectively [18]. In this case report, the small pseudoaneurysms could have been caused by direct hit or by the heat the bullet generated next to the artery. Pseudoaneurysms always communicate with the arterial lumen by the pseudoaneurysm neck. While penetrating trauma is a common cause [19, 20], the most common cause is iatrogenic pseudoaneurysm [11, 21].

Evaluation of pseudoaneurysms with Doppler ultrasound on B-mode will demonstrate an anechoic or hypoechoic image containing moving echoes. It may increase in size during systole. The presence of a partially filled lumen by echogenic structures may represent a thrombus. The color flow evaluation will demonstrate the typical swirling motion known as the Yin–Yang sign, which is caused by the circular motion of the blood inside the pseudoaneurysm. During systole, the flow goes toward the pseudoaneurysm and during diastole the blood moves back to the arterial lumen [20, 21]. Spectral analysis will demonstrate turbulent flow. The pulse Doppler with the sample volume placed at the level of the neck of the pseudoaneurysm will show a flow pattern known as "to-and-fro", a bidirectional flow caused by the continuous entry and exit of blood from the artery to the pseudoaneurysm and vice versa.

The management of traumatic carotid injuries are guided by grade and appropriate and timely interventions are warranted to prevent sequelae, such as stroke and occlusions, causing permanent central nervous system-related morbidity and mortality [18, 22–24]. Traditionally, grade I and II have been successfully managed with anticoagulants or anti-platelet equivalents (if there are no contraindications precluding its use). Among patients being managed with anti-coagulant therapy, PT/INR ratio should be maintained between 2 and 3, for 3–6 months [18, 22–24]. Unlike grade I–II injuries, however, grade III–V injuries require invasive therapies, either endovascular or surgical.

Grade III blunt carotid injuries have a stroke rate as high as 33% and mortality up to 11% [18, 24] with grade IV and V having even higher risks. Hence, timely and effective treatment often combining anticoagulation with procedural intervention is advisable. Endovascular interventions such as stenting present reasonable alternatives to open surgical techniques. A review by Morr et al. evaluated various stenting interventions to traditional open surgery methods such as endarterectomy [25]. Many factors of the stent characteristics themselves, including bare-metal vs. covered, tapered vs. untampered, and drug eluting vs. cutting/balloon based are pertinent to the discussion. Overall, stenting is a safe alternative to traditional surgical techniques such as carotid endarterectomies in some situations. Complications from endovascular procedures around stenting have been limited to few cases of carotid artery spasm, which can be medically managed with nitrates or calcium channel blockers.

A meta-analysis by Pham et al. evaluated the utility of endovascular stenting in carotid pathologies and included 31 studies with over 140 patients. The review showed that 98.4% of pseudoaneurysm cases were either successfully stented or occluded when appropriate [26]. Endovascular stenting is a safe and appropriate alternative to surgical intervention but randomized clinical trials are still needed. Maras et al. also reviewed the safety and short-term efficacy of covered stents for traumatic extracranial carotid artery pseudoaneurysms [27]. The review included 20 patients with carotid pseudoaneurysms secondary to traumatic injury and demonstrates that endovascular approaches can spare the morbidity and risk of surgical repair while providing similar efficacy in maintaining patency. Notably, endovascular approaches are less likely to result in cranial nerve injuries which are associated with open surgical approaches. While together these reviews and studies suggest a strong role for stenting in grade III blunt carotid injuries, longer follow-up on more patients is needed to further examine this promising treatment in addition to randomized clinical trials.

Conclusions

POCUS and POCDUS are widely available, noninvasive, sensible and specific techniques that are increasingly used for the diagnosis and decision-making process of penetrating vascular injuries to the neck and are a fundamental part of the follow-up after definitive therapy.

Acknowledgements
Not applicable.

Authors' contributions
LM, MS, MW: Manuscript writing and edition. FR: Point-of-care ultrasound, Follow-up ultrasound, Consent for case report and IRB approval. FP: Point-of-care ultrasound, Doppler ultrasound, Follow-up ultrasound. MM: Consent for case report and IRB approval, Point-of-care ultrasound, Doppler ultrasound, Follow-up ultrasound, Manuscript writing and edition. All authors read and approved the final manuscript.

Author details
[1] Department of General Surgery, Cleveland Clinic Florida, Weston, FL, USA.
[2] Department of Ultrasound and Vascular Doppler, Hospital de Emergencias "Dr. Clemente Alvarez", Av. Pellegrini 3205, Rosario, Santa Fe, Argentina.

References

1. Chelala C (1997) Violence in the Americas: the social pandemic of the 20th century. Pan American Health Organization, Washington, DC
2. Martín Trenor A (2005) Traumatismos vasculares periféricos. Rev Med Univ Navarra 49(2):24–31
3. Rozycki GS et al (2003) Blunt vascular trauma in extremities: diagnosis, management and outcome. J Trauma 55:814–824
4. Soto GS et al (2004) Trauma vascular periférico. Cuad Cir 18:91–97. https://doi.org/10.4206/cuad.cir.2004.v18n1-15
5. Torres Carranza SA (2006) Trauma vascular de las extremidades y un poco de su historia. Trauma 9(3):83–86
6. Suárez CA et al (2007) Heridas por armas de fuego y traumas vasculares: una ventana a la violencia civil en Caracas. Gac Méd Caracas 115(4):304–312
7. Sonneborn R et al (2002) Vascular trauma in Latin America. A regional survey. Surg Clin North Am 82:189–194
8. Thal ER, Meyer DM (1992) Penetrating neck trauma. Curr Prob Surg 29:5–56. https://doi.org/10.1016/0011-3840(92)90031-w
9. McConnell DB, Trunkey DD (1994) Management of penetrating trauma to the neck. Adv Surg 27:97–127
10. Frykberg ER (1995) Advances in the diagnosis and treatment of extremity vascular trauma. Surg Clin North Am 75:207–223. https://doi.org/10.1016/S0039-6109(16)46584-9
11. Gaitini D et al (2008) Sonographic evaluation of vascular injuries. J Ultrasound Med 27:95–107
12. Bergstein JM, Blair JF, Edwards J et al (1992) Pitfalls in the use of color-flow duplex ultrasound for screening of suspected arterial injuries in penetrated extremities. J Trauma 33:395–402. https://doi.org/10.1097/00005373-199209000-00010
13. Fry WR, Smith RS, Sayers DV, Henderson VJ, Morabito DJ, Tsoi EK et al (1993) The success of duplex ultrasonographic scanning in diagnosis of extremity vascular proximity trauma. Arch Surg 128(12):1368–1372
14. Montorfano MA, Montorfano LM, Perez Quirante F, Rodríguez F, Vera L, Neri L (2017) The FAST D protocol: a simple method to rule out traumatic vascular injuries of the lower extremities. Crit Ultrasound J. 9(1):8. https://doi.org/10.1186/s13089-017-0063-2
15. Montorfano MA, Pla F, Vera L, Cardillo O, Nigra SG, Montorfano LM (2017) Point-of-care ultrasound and Doppler ultrasound evaluation of vascular injuries in penetrating and blunt trauma. Crit Ultrasound J. 9(1):5. https://doi.org/10.1186/s13089-017-0060-5
16. Neri L, Storti E, Lichtenstein D (2007) Towards an ultrasound curriculum. Crit Care Med 35(5):S290–S304. https://doi.org/10.1097/01.CCM.0000260680.16213.26
17. Schoder M, Prokof M, Lammer J (2002) Traumatic injuries: imaging and intervention of large arterial trauma. Eur Radiol 12:1617–1631. https://doi.org/10.1007/s00330-002-1487-y
18. Biffl WL, Moore EE, Offner PJ et al (1999) Blunt carotid arterial injuries: implications of a new grading scale. J Trauma Inj Infect Crit Care 47:845. https://doi.org/10.1097/00005373-199911000-00004
19. Olinde AJ (1989) Traumatic subclavian axillary artery aneurysm. J Vasc Surg 11:848–849. https://doi.org/10.1016/0741-5214(90)90085-O
20. Yetkin U, Gurbuz A (2003) Post-traumatic pseudoaneurysm of the brachial artery and its surgical treatment. Tex Heart Inst J 30:293–297
21. Mitchell DG, Needleman L, Bezzi M, Goldberg BB et al (1987) Femoral artery pseudoaneurysm: diagnosis with conventional duplex and Color Doppler US. Radiology 165:687–690. https://doi.org/10.1148/radiology.165.3.3317501
22. Bromberg WJ, Collier BC, Diebel LN et al (2010) Blunt Cerebrovascular Injury Practice Management Guidelines & colon; The Eastern Association

for the Surgery of Trauma. J Trauma Inj Infect Crit Care 68:471–477. https://doi.org/10.1097/ta.0b013e3181cb43da
23. Biffl WL, Cothren CC, Moore EE et al (2009) Western Trauma Association Critical Decisions in trauma & colon; screening for and treatment of blunt cerebrovascular injuries. J Trauma Inj Infect Crit Care 67:1150–1153. https://doi.org/10.1097/ta.0b013e3181c1c1d6
24. Lee TS, Ducic Y, Gordin E, Stroman D (2014) Management of carotid artery trauma. Craniomaxillofac Trauma Reconstr 7:175–189. https://doi.org/10.1055/s-0034-1372521
25. Morr S, Lin N, Siddiqui AH (2014) Carotid artery stenting: current and emerging options. Med Devices Auckl N Z 7:343–355. https://doi.org/10.2147/mder.s46044
26. Pham MH, Rahme RJ, Arnaout O et al (2007) Endovascular stenting of extracranial carotid and vertebral artery dissections a systematic review of the literature. Neurosurgery 68:856–866. https://doi.org/10.1227/neu.0b013e318209ce03
27. Maras D, Lioupis C, Magoufis G et al (2006) Covered stent-graft treatment of traumatic internal carotid artery pseudoaneurysms: a review. Cardiovasc Intervent Radiol 29:958–968. https://doi.org/10.1007/s00270-005-0367-7

16

A point-of-care thoracic ultrasound protocol for hospital medical emergency teams (METUS) improves diagnostic accuracy

M. J Blans[1*], E Bousie[1], J. G van der Hoeven[2] and F. H Bosch[3]

Abstract

Background: Point-of-care ultrasound (POCUS) has proven itself in many clinical situations. Few data on the use of POCUS during Medical Emergency Team (MET) calls exist. In this study, we hypothesized that the use of POCUS would increase the number of correct diagnosis made by the MET and increase MET's certainty.

Methods: Single-center prospective observational study on adult patients in need for MET assistance. Patients were included in blocks (weeks). During even weeks, the MET physician performed a clinical assessment and registered an initial diagnosis. Subsequently, the POCUS protocol was performed and a second diagnosis was registered (US+). During uneven weeks, no POCUS was performed (US−). A blinded expert reviewed the charts for a final diagnosis. The number of correct diagnoses was compared to the final diagnosis between both groups. Physician's certainty, mortality and possible differences in first treatment were also evaluated.

Results: We included 100 patients: 52 in the US+ and 48 in the US− group. There were significantly more correct diagnoses in the US+ group compared to the US− group: 78 vs 51% ($P = 0.006$). Certainty improved significantly with POCUS ($P < 0.001$). No differences in 28-day mortality and first treatment were found.

Conclusions: The use of thoracic POCUS during MET calls leads to better diagnosis and increases certainty.

Background

Medical Emergency Teams (METs) are called to the bedside when patients on hospital wards deteriorate. [1, 2] METs use various algorithms to assess the patient's condition, most frequently the ABCDE method. The MET physician will use a combination of history, physical examination and point-of-care laboratory tests to assess the patient. The addition of point-of-care ultrasound (POCUS) could potentially improve diagnostic accuracy. [3] METs are associated with a reduction in patient mortality [4], but few data exist on differences in operation procedures by METs. The role of POCUS for instance during MET calls has not been investigated extensively yet, even though its role in the emergency room (ER) and intensive care unit (ICU) is well established [5–13]. Recently, Zieleskiewicz et al. published the first prospective observational study on the effect of the use of a multi-organ POCUS protocol during MET calls [14]. In this study, the use of a multi-organ POCUS protocol improved diagnostic accuracy of the MET significantly. We also designed a prospective trial hypothesizing that multi-organ POCUS would increase MET diagnostic ability and postulated that the use of POCUS would also increase the diagnostic certainty of the MET physician. Influence on certainty by the use of POCUS

*Correspondence: mblans@rijnstate.nl
[1] Department of Intensive Care, Rijnstate Hospital, PO box 9555, 6800 TA Arnhem, The Netherlands
Full list of author information is available at the end of the article

has been found in a study on ER patients [5] and improving certainty might also be important to attending MET physicians.

Because most MET calls are requested for respiratory and or hemodynamic deterioration [15], we designed a POCUS protocol consisting of cardiac and lung (thoracic) ultrasound.

Methods

Study design and setting

Design

This is a prospective observational study examining the use of thoracic POCUS in adult patients on the general ward treated by the MET. The Modified Early Warning Score (MEWS) was used to assess the need for MET assistance (figure of MEWS score in Additional file 1).

The study (METUS NL61884.091.17) was approved by the local ethical committee and conducted in a Dutch 750 bed teaching hospital (Rijnstate Hospital, Arnhem) from January 18, 2019 until February 1, 2020. The study was registered at ClinicalTrials.gov. (NCT03214809).

Characteristics of participants

All patients 18 years and older in all regular hospital wards in need of a MET call were included.

Exclusion criteria were:

- Pregnancy
- Acute illness requiring direct lifesaving intervention (e.g., intubation, cardiopulmonary resuscitation).
- Glasgow Coma Score < 9 or a decline of the Glasgow Coma Score ≥ 2 as the primary reason for MET attendance.

Patients consent was obtained directly after the MET call; in case of an incapacitated patient, the next of kin was contacted. Deferred consent was also permitted.

MET team staffing

The ICU of Rijnstate Hospital runs a MET since 1996. The MET is staffed by 2 intensive care nurses and 1 ICU resident physician. Board certified intensivists are available within 15 min. The ICU of Rijnstate Hospital uses POCUS since 2009. ICU residents are trained in basic POCUS shortly before ICU rotation. The training program consists of 4 training days in basic cardiac, lung and abdominal ultrasound, POCUS is part of daily care [16].

POCUS protocol

Our cardiac POCUS protocol consists of 5 straightforward questions combined with a simple qualitative interpretation. Standard transthoracic windows using only 2D-ultrasound were used [17].

The following questions were answered:

1. Is the left ventricle dilated?—yes/no/don't know. Is the left ventricle function hyperdynamic/normal/moderately decreased/severely decreased/don't know?
2. Is the right ventricle dilated?—yes/no/don't know
3. Is the right ventricle function normal/abnormal/don't know?
4. Is pericardial effusion present?—yes/no/don't know
5. Is pericardial tamponade present?—yes/no/don't know

From the subcostal view the inferior vena cava (IVC) was identified. The IVC was measured and categorized:

- Collapsed: < 1.5 cm.
- Normal: 1.5–2.5 cm.
- Dilated: > 2.5 cm.
- Not visualized.

Lung ultrasound was used according to the Blue protocol by Lichtenstein [18] with the following diagnostic profiles:

- A-profile: normal lung.
- A/A'-profile (one sided): suspect pneumothorax, atelectasis, pleurodesis, pneumonectomy.
- B-profile: (both sides) suspect pulmonary edema, acute respiratory distress syndrome (ARDS).
- A/B-profile (one sided B-lines): suspect pneumonia.
- C-profile (consolidation): suspect pneumonia, atelectasis or compression.

The MET physicians started with cardiac POCUS in case of primary hemodynamic problems and with the Blue protocol of the lungs in case of primary pulmonary problems.

We used a hand held ultrasound device (Philips Lumify® S4-1) connected to an Android tablet attached to the MET cart. The Lumify^R S4-1 is a phased array transducer with software for cardiac and lung ultrasound exams.

Data collection

Eligible patients were included consecutively: in even weeks the POCUS protocol was used (US+), in odd weeks standard care without the use of POCUS (US−) was deployed.

After the initial assessment, a diagnosis was registered by the MET physician.

In the US+ weeks, a second diagnosis was registered after subsequent use of the POCUS protocol. The attending MET physician could decide to use POCUS in the US- weeks after an initial diagnosis was made. This deviation of protocol was registered and, in these cases, also a second diagnosis (after the use of POCUS) was noted.

All diagnoses were recorded in a case research form (CRF).

An experienced intensive care consultant and member of the hospital mortality committee (independent expert) conducted a full chart review (electronical medical record, HIX®) on all enrolled patients to determine a definite diagnosis 2 weeks after inclusion. The independent expert was unaware of the ultrasound findings (recorded in a separate CRF), the initial diagnosis made by the attending MET physician and he had no other role in the study. After evaluation by the independent expert, the MET diagnosis was rated as completely correct or completely incorrect. In case of multiple definite diagnosis made by the independent expert (for instance, acute heart failure and COPD), the MET diagnosis could also be rated partially correct if not all elements of the definite diagnosis were recorded in the CRF.

Diagnostic certainty was scored on a visual analogue scale of 0 (no clue) to 10 (absolute certain). The 10 point VAS scale was used because all other clinical scoring in our hospital is done with the 10 points VAS score (for instance pain). Other scales like the 5-point Likert scale would be novel for our physicians to use thereby possibly clouding the results. Ten point VAS scores have been used in other studies before in certainty assessment [19]. In the US+ weeks the MET physician rated certainty before and after the use of POCUS. In the US− weeks certainty was scored without the use of POCUS and in case of protocol deviation also after the use of POCUS.

We also registered the reason the MET was called, baseline demographics (age, gender, previous medical history, weight and height), clinical and laboratory parameters (heart rate, blood pressure, temperature, serum lactate and white blood cell count) and 28-day mortality.

The MET physicians were asked to rate the quality of the POCUS studies (good, moderate, bad) and were encouraged to capture the POCUS studies for review. Two investigators (FHB and MJB) checked the stored studies.

Outcome measures

The primary outcome measure was the percentage of correct diagnoses made by the MET physician in the US+ and US− weeks. The second diagnosis after the use of POCUS in the US+ weeks and the initial diagnosis in the US− weeks without the use of POCUS were compared to the final diagnosis made by the independent expert.

Secondary outcome measures were a change in diagnosis after the use of POCUS in the US+ group and (after protocol deviation) in the US− group, percentage of correct diagnosis in the US− group after the use of POCUS, the change in diagnostic certainty before and after the use of POCUS and 28-day mortality. The MET physician also noted first treatment (intravenous fluids, diuretics, vasopressors/inotropes, anti-coagulants, anti-arrhythmic drugs, vasodilators, morphine/sedatives, intubation or non-invasive ventilation, O_2 supply, or other treatments and the need for supervisor attendance).

Statistical analysis

Descriptive statistics are presented as mean with standard deviation for normally distributed continuous data, median and inter-quartile range (IQR) for skewed continuous variables and as numbers and percentages for dichotomous and categorical variables. Differences between groups (US+ group and US− group) were tested using the Pearson Chi-square test, Fisher exact and Students' T test. In case of not normally distributed variables, differences between groups were tested using the Mann–Whitney U test. Changes within groups were tested using the Wilcoxon signed rank test and the McNemar–Bowker test. Statistical analysis was done using SPSS® software (version 25). Sample size was estimated to detect an increase in the number of correct diagnosis of 30% ($\alpha = 0.05$ and $\beta = 0.20$). Based on Jones et al. [13] we estimated that a total of 76 patients should be enrolled (38 patients per group). Because few data exist on the use of POCUS during MET calls we decided to include 100 patients in total.

Results

We included a total of 100 patients, 52 patients in the US+ group and 48 patients in the US− group. In 5 patients the independent expert could not determine a reliable definite diagnosis (2 in the US+ and 3 in the US− group). These patients were excluded from the comparison of initial/second diagnosis with the definite diagnosis, but were included in other analysis. In total, there were 310 MET calls during the study period.

Flowchart of study enrollment and exclusion reasons are in listed in Fig. 1.

Patients characteristics are described in Table 1.

Primary outcome

Percentage of correct diagnosis US+ versus US− group

In the US+ group 39 (78%) of the diagnoses after the use of POCUS was completely correct versus 23 (51.1%) of the diagnosis without the use of POCUS in the US− group (Pearson Chi Square Test: $P = 0.006$) (Table 2.)

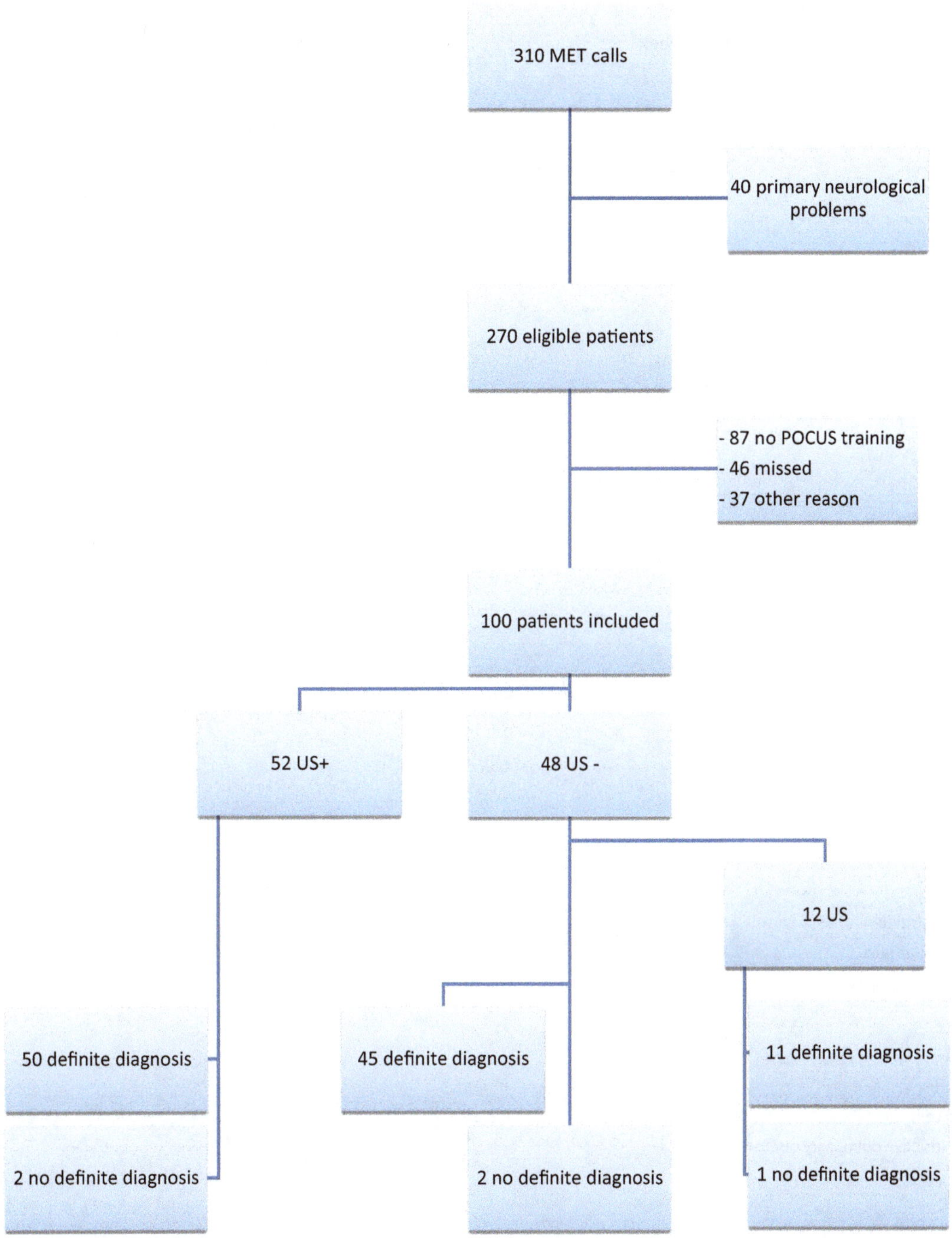

Fig. 1 Flowchart of patient study enrollment

Secondary outcomes

Change in diagnosis

In the US+ group, the initial diagnosis improved to partly correct in 3 (6%) and to completely correct in 10 (20%) of the patients (McNemar–Bowker test P = 0.004). In 3 (6%) patients an incorrect diagnosis was not improved with the use of POCUS and in 3 (6%) patients the diagnosis after ultrasound worsened from completely correct to partially correct. In no case the diagnosis changed from completely correct before to completely incorrect after the use of POCUS (Table 3).

Percentage of correct diagnosis in the US- group after the use of POCUS

In 12 (25%) patients in the US- group there was a protocol deviation. In 11 of these patients, a final diagnosis could be established. POCUS increased the agreement with the final diagnosis from 27.3% to 63.6%, but this

Table 1 Baseline characteristics

	Even week		Uneven week		*P* value
	N=52		N=48		
	Mean (SD)	N (%)	Mean (SD)	N (%)	
Age (years)	72.2 (15.0)		69.7 (12.1)		0.354
Gender, male		28 (53.8)		27 (56.3)	0.803
BMI[a] (kg/m^2)	26.5 (5.9)		28.2 (5.8)		0.175
Systolic BP (mmHg)	134 (36.5)		127 (42.9)		0.408
Diastolic BP (mmHg)	78 (22.0)		76 (26.2)		0.544
Heart rate (bpm)	110 (33.4)		111 (32.9)		0.870
Temperature (°C)	37.5 (1.6)		37.5 (1.2)		0.859
WBC[b] (× 10^9/L)	10.4 (5.2)		11.5 (7.6)		0.491
Plasma lactate (mmol/L)	3.1 (2.6)		3.3 (2.6)		0.731
Reason for call					
Anaphylaxis		0 (0.0)		1 (2.1)	0.296
Gastro-intestinal bleeding		2 (3.8)		0 (0.0)	0.175
Hypotension		16 (30.6)		18 (37.5)	0.469
Respiratory insufficiency		34 (65.4)		27 (56.2)	0.349
Tachycardia		0 (0.0)		2 (4.2)	0.137
Pre-existing condition					
Heart failure		14 (26.9)		5 (10.4)	0.037*
Myocardial infarction		12 (23.1)		4 (8.3)	0.045*
Peripheral vascular		9 (17.3)		5 (10.4)	0.323
COPD[c]		14 (26.9)		13 (27.1)	0.982
Renal insufficiency		16 (30.8)		7 (14.6)	0.056
Dialysis		1 (1.9)		1 (2.1)	0.943
Diabetes mellitus		8 (15.4)		8 (16.7)	0.860
Metastatic malignancy		4 (7.8)		7 (14.6)	0.281
Immunological insufficiency		1 (1.9)		2 (4.2)	0.503
Gastro-intestinal bleeding		2 (3.8)		0 (0.0)	0.175
Haematological malignancy		0 (0.0)		2 (4.2)	0.137

*$P < 0.05$

[a] BMI body mass index

[b] WBC white blood cells

[c] COPD chronic obstructive pulmonary disease

Table 2 Initial diagnosis versus final diagnosis US + and US

Initial diagnosis compared to final diagnosis	US+ weeks Number (%)	US− weeks Number (%)	Total Number (%)
Completely correct	39 (78.0)	23 (51.1)	62 (65.3)
Partly correct	8 (16.0)	9 (20.0)	17 (17.9)
Completely incorrect	3 (6.0)	13 (28.9)	16 (16.8)
Total	50 (100)	45 (100)	95 (100)

difference was not statistically significant, due to the small sample size.

The actual diagnoses before and after POCUS are listed in Table 4.

Certainty

Diagnostic certainty before the use of POCUS was the same in the US + and US− groups. In both groups the median certainty was 8 with comparable ranges. Certainty improved in the US+ group after the use of POCUS (Wilcoxon signed rank test $P < 0.001$) (Fig. 2).

Table 3 Initial versus diagnosis after POCUS in the US + group

Initial diagnosis before POCUS				
	Completely correct Number (%)	Partly correct Number (%)	Completely incorrect Number (%)	Total Number (%)
Diagnosis after POCUS				
Completely correct	26 (52)	3 (6.0)	10 (20.0)	39 (78.0)
Partially correct	1 (2.0)	7 (14.0)	0 (0.0)	8 (16.0)
Completely incorrect	0 (0.0)	0 (0.0)	3 (6.0)	3 (6.0)
Total	26 (53.1)	10 (20.0)	13 (26.0)	50 (100)

Table 4 List of diagnosis before and after ultrasound in the US+ and US− group

US+	
Diagnosis before ultrasound (completely incorrect)	**Diagnosis after ultrasound (completely correct)**
No diagnosis	Hypoventilation
No diagnosis	Respiratory problems due to abdominal disease
No diagnosis	Acute heart failure
Pneumonia	Acute heart failure + pneumonia
Acute heart failure	Pneumonia + septic shock
Acute pulmonary embolism	Hypoventilation
Acute heart failure	Underfilling
Acute exacerbation COPD	Pulmonary Fibrosis
Acute heart failure	Pneumonia
Acute exacerbation COPD	Acute heart failure
Diagnosis before ultrasound (partially correct)	**Diagnosis after ultrasound (completely correct)**
Pneumonia + atelectasis	Atelectasis
Acute exacerbation COPD	Acute heart failure + exacerbation COPD
Retention bladder	Septic shock + retention bladder
US−	
Diagnosis before ultrasound (completely incorrect)	**Diagnosis after ultrasound (completely correct)**
Pneumonia + exacerbation ILD	Acute heart failure
Tension pneumothorax	Haemothorax
Tension pneumothorax	Atelectasis
Diagnosis before ultrasound (partially correct)	**Diagnosis after ultrasound (completely correct)**
Septic shock	ARDS

COPD chronic obstructive pulmonary disease, *ILD* interstitial lung disease, *ARDS* acute respiratory distress syndrome

This was also found in the 12 patients from the US-group in which ultrasound was used (Fig. 2) Wilcoxon signed rank test $P=0.001$. In the minority of cases, the use of POCUS did not increase certainty.

Mortality

28-Day mortality rates were not statistically different: US+ weeks 14 (26.9%) and the US− weeks 13 (27.1%).

Initial treatment and need for immediate supervisor attendance

No statistically significant differences were found between the US+ and US− groups in first treatment (intravenous fluids, diuretics, vasopressors/inotropes, anti-coagulants, anti-arrhythmic drugs, vasodilators, morphine/sedatives, intubation or non-invasive ventilation, O_2 supply, or other treatments) nor in the number of times supervisor attendance was needed.

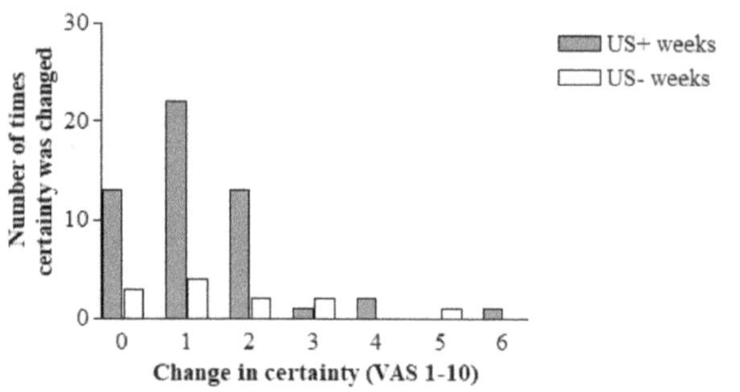

Fig. 2 Difference in certainty before and after US in US− weeks after the use of POCUS

Quality of POCUS exams

The MET physicians rated the quality of ultrasound exams as good in 25 (39%), moderate 27 (42%) and poor in 12 (19%). One in five studies were evaluated by two experts (FHB and MJB), in one case the quality was adjusted from good to moderate, in all other cases the experts agreed on the rating of POCUS study quality done by the MET physician.

Discussion

In this single-center prospective observational study the use of a thoracic POCUS protocol improved the number of correct diagnosis significantly. We also found that the number of correct diagnosis increased in the US+ group after the use of POCUS and that POCUS increased MET physician's certainty significantly. We did not find differences in mortality, first MET treatments or supervisor attendance.

There are multiple studies evaluating the use of POCUS in the ICU and ER department, until now only two studies focused on the use of POCUS during MET calls. Zieleskiewicz et al. published a paper [14] in which they evaluated the effect on diagnostic adequacy of thoracic POCUS during MET calls. As in our study, they found a significant increase in the number of correct diagnosis when POCUS was used (80% versus 94%). Furthermore, the time to first treatment was significantly lower in the POCUS group and there was an association with outcome parameters such as mortality, but the latter was not confirmed in the propensity score. Although this study has many similarities with ours, there are also some important differences. Both studies are single centered and prospective observational studies. The inclusion criteria are comparable as is the inclusion rate over time and the number of inclusions out of the total MET calls (34% Zieleskiewicz et al. versus 32% Blans et al.). In both studies, the protocol consisted of cardiac and lung POCUS, Zieleskiewicz et al. also used vascular POCUS to rule out lower extremity thrombosis, but the latter was used infrequently. Both studies found that the use of POCUS during MET calls improved the number of correct diagnosis made by the MET physician (primary endpoint). In both studies, chart review was used to establish a definite diagnosis, but there are some differences in the exact way in which this process was carried out. In contrast to the Zieleskiewicz et al. study, we used the term "partly" correct diagnosis if not all elements of the definite diagnosis made by the external expert were scored by the MET physician. If we add the partly correct to the completely correct numbers, our results would increasingly be comparable to the Zieleskiewicz results (US+ group 94% correct and US− group 69% correct).

Another important methodological difference with our study is the fact that Zieleskiewicz et al. used two MET teams, one which used POCUS and one did not. The two MET's alternated every other day. Both MET deployments (POCUS and not using POCUS) were considered standard therapy and therefore no consent was deemed necessary. We, however, choose to use the same MET but asked to use POCUS only during even weeks and discouraged the use of POCUS during odd weeks. Because Zieleskiewicz et al. used two separate METs, theoretically the difference in the number of correct diagnosis was not only the result of the use of POCUS, but also due to differences between the achievements of the two separate teams although a large number of seniors and juniors randomly composed each MET. In our study, the MET physician was the same during both weeks (US+ and US−).

Furthermore, it is unclear in the Zielskiewicz et al. study who exactly performed the POCUS protocol, their METs are staffed by junior and senior physicians (with minimally a level 2 in thoracic ultrasound). We also found a significant impact on diagnostic accuracy, but in our study POCUS was done by residents only, this aspect is worth emphasizing; POCUS can be of an extra value to the less experienced physician during MET calls. We found that without POCUS the number of correct diagnosis was relatively low (51.1%). Although this has been found before in studies in which POCUS was done by more experienced staff [11, 20], we think that this low percentage can also be partially explained by the fact that in our study less experienced physicians (residents) included the patients.

Several studies show that training programs for residents in multi-organ POCUS have satisfactory results in terms of acquiring adequate ultrasound skills and increasing diagnostic abilities. [21–28]. Our study supports the evidence that residents may obtain clinically relevant POCUS skills in a relatively short period of time, including making the right diagnosis during a MET call.

Our findings are of interest for other hospitals in which the MET is also staffed by residents; POCUS training will improve their diagnostic ability and certainty also during acute situations like MET deployments. Also important to stress is the fact that the use of the POCUS protocol never resulted in a change towards a completely incorrect diagnosis.

Because we asked the MET physician to note to a diagnosis before the use of POCUS and one after the use of POCUS, we could measure more precisely the effect of the use of POCUS and this was significant in the US+ group and also positive though not significant due to small numbers in the US− group. This also supports the fact that POCUS was the reason for more diagnostic accuracy.

The other study on the use of ultrasound by MET's was published by Sen et al. [29]. In this small study of 50 patients on the effect on diagnosis of a combined lung and lower extremity vascular POCUS protocol was evaluated. They showed that lung POCUS was feasible, but due to the small number of patients there was no statistically significant effect on the number of correct diagnosis. They therefore concluded that the use of lung ultrasound was non-inferior to MET clinical assessment. It could well be that by the addition of cardiac POCUS and the inclusion of more patients Zieleskiewicz et al. and we were able to prove a beneficial effect of POCUS on diagnosis during MET calls.

We also evaluated the effect of POCUS on physician's certainty. We showed that in the US+ and US− groups baseline certainty was quite high (eight on a 10 point VAS scale), but certainty increased significantly in the US+ group after the use of POCUS indicating that POCUS did not only improve certainty because certainty levels were low to begin with. There is one other study on the impact of POCUS on diagnostic certainty [5]. Shokoohi et al. looked at 118 ER patients and found that the use of a multi-organ POCUS protocol lowered uncertainty for a diagnosis. We are aware of the relatively small increase in certainty that was found in our study, but this finding could be psychologically important for residents during stressful clinical encounters such as MET calls. Junior physicians are less certain in the diagnostic process compared to more experienced colleagues [30].

We could not find differences in other outcome parameters (28-day mortality, initial treatment or supervisor attendance) possibly due to the small number of included patients. It will be difficult to design a study on the use of POCUS during MET calls large enough to detect differences in outcome parameters such as mortality. Preferably, a multicenter trial could help in including large enough numbers of patients. On the other hand, one could argue that the existing evidence is sufficient to support the incorporation of POCUS in MET protocols.

Our study has several limitations. This study was conducted in a single center and focused on ward patients with respiratory and or hemodynamic deterioration. Therefore, the presented results may not necessarily apply to other clinical settings. There were some differences in baseline characteristics between the US+ and US− groups. Significantly more patients in the US+ group had a history of myocardial infarction and heart failure. We have no reason to believe that these baseline differences had a significant impact on the study results. Our study design is prone to selection bias, but also has several advantages as discussed above. We decided to exclude the MET physicians without sufficient POCUS training from the trial. This resulted in a substantial number of non-included patients (87).

Our POCUS protocol consisted out of a combination of 5 basic cardiac questions and for the lung the Blue protocol was used which is consistent with current international POCUS practice. No further prespecified POCUS flow chart was used which makes our findings perhaps difficult to validate by others.

The diagnoses of the MET physicians were compared to the final diagnosis made by one blinded experienced intensive care consultant 2 weeks afterwards (independent expert) on the basis of a thorough chart review. This method remains challenging although often used in POCUS studies [12, 13]. In our study, only one independent expert reviewed the charts and was blinded to the ultrasound findings and diagnosis made by the attending MET physician. He had absolutely no other role in the study and because he is a member of the hospital mortality committee he is experienced in extracting official diagnoses from chart review.

Conclusion

We found that the use of a thoracic (cardiac and lung) POCUS protocol during MET calls due to respiratory and or hemodynamic deterioration has significant positive impact on establishing the correct diagnosis and a small but significant impact on MET physician's diagnostic certainty.

Abbreviations

POCUS: Point-of-care ultrasound; MET: Medical emergency team; US: Ultrasound; ER: Emergency room; ICU: Intensive care unit; MEWS: Modified Early Warning Score; IVC: Inferior vena cava; ARDS: Acute respiratory distress syndrome; AHF: Acute heart failure; AECOPD: Acute exacerbation of chronic obstructive pulmonary disease; CRF: Case research form; CPR: Cardiopulmonary resuscitation; N: Number; GI: Gastro-intestinal; AAD: Acute admission department; BMI: Body mass index; BP: Blood pressure; SD: Standard deviation; WBC: White blood cell count; COPD: Chronic obstructive pulmonary disease; ILD: Interstitial lung disease; VAS: Visual analogue scale.

Supplementary Information

Additional file 1. Figure of Modified Early Warning Score (MEWS).

Acknowledgements

Mrs L. Roovers, PhD helped with the statistical analysis

H.J. van Leeuwen, MD, PhD, reviewed the medical records and determined the final diagnosis

Authors' contributions

MJB, FHB and JGvdH designed the study; MJB and EB included the patients and MJB, EB, JGvdH and FHB contributed to the article. All authors have read and approved the final manuscript.

Author details

[1]Department of Intensive Care, Rijnstate Hospital, PO box 9555, 6800 TA Arnhem, The Netherlands. [2]Department of Intensive Care, Radboud University Medical Center, PO box 9101, 6500 HB Nijmegen, The Netherlands. [3]Department of Internal Medicine, Rijnstate Hospital, PO box 9555, 6800 TA Arnhem, The Netherlands.

References

1. Hillman KM, Chen J, Jones D (2014) Rapid response systems. Med J Aust 201(9):519–521
2. Ludikhuize J, Brunsveld-Reinders AH, Dijkgraaf MG, Smorenburg SM, de Rooij SE, Adams R et al (2015) Outcomes associated with the nationwide introduction of rapid response systems in The Netherlands. Crit Care Med 43(12):2544–2551
3. Narula J, Chandrashekhar Y, Braunwald E (2018) Time to add a fifth pillar to bedside physical examination: inspection, palpation, percussion, auscultation, and insonation. JAMA Cardiol 3(4):346–350
4. Maharaj R, Raffaele I, Wendon J (2015) Rapid response systems: a systematic review and meta-analysis. Crit Care 19:254
5. Shokoohi H, Boniface KS, Pourmand A, Liu YT, Davison DL, Hawkins KD et al (2015) Bedside ultrasound reduces diagnostic uncertainty and guides resuscitation in patients with undifferentiated hypotension. Crit Care Med 43(12):2562–2569
6. Sekiguchi H, Schenck LA, Horie R, Suzuki J, Lee EH, McMenomy BP et al (2015) Critical care ultrasonography differentiates ARDS, pulmonary edema, and other causes in the early course of acute hypoxemic respiratory failure. Chest 148(4):912–918
7. Bataille B, Riu B, Ferre F, Moussot PE, Mari A, Brunel E et al (2014) Integrated use of bedside lung ultrasound and echocardiography in acute respiratory failure: a prospective observational study in ICU. Chest 146(6):1586–1593
8. Pontet J, Yic C, Diaz-Gomez JL, Rodriguez P, Sviridenko I, Mendez D et al (2019) Impact of an ultrasound-driven diagnostic protocol at early intensive-care stay: a randomized-controlled trial. Ultrasound J 11(1):24
9. Laursen CB, Sloth E, Lassen AT, Christensen R, Lambrechtsen J, Madsen PH et al (2014) Point-of-care ultrasonography in patients admitted with respiratory symptoms: a single-blind, randomised controlled trial. Lancet Respir Med 2(8):638–646
10. Silva S, Biendel C, Ruiz J, Olivier M, Bataille B, Geeraerts T et al (2013) Usefulness of cardiothoracic chest ultrasound in the management of acute respiratory failure in critical care practice. Chest 144(3):859–865
11. Pirozzi C, Numis FG, Pagano A, Melillo P, Copetti R, Schiraldi F (2014) Immediate versus delayed integrated point-of-care-ultrasonography to manage acute dyspnea in the emergency department. Crit Ultrasound J 6(1):5
12. Volpicelli G, Lamorte A, Tullio M, Cardinale L, Giraudo M, Stefanone V et al (2013) Point-of-care multiorgan ultrasonography for the evaluation of undifferentiated hypotension in the emergency department. Intensive Care Med 39(7):1290–1298
13. Jones AE, Tayal VS, Sullivan DM, Kline JA (2004) Randomized, controlled trial of immediate versus delayed goal-directed ultrasound to identify the cause of nontraumatic hypotension in emergency department patients. Crit Care Med 32(8):1703–1708
14. Zieleskiewicz L, Lopez A, Hraiech S, Baumstarck K, Pastene B, Di Bisceglie M et al (2021) Bedside POCUS during ward emergencies is associated with improved diagnosis and outcome: an observational, prospective, controlled study. Crit Care 25(1):34
15. Mullins CF, Psirides A (2016) Activities of a Medical Emergency Team: a prospective observational study of 795 calls. Anaesth Intensive Care 44(1):34–43
16. Blans MJ, Pijl MEJ, van de Water JM, Poppe HJ, Bosch FH (2020) The implementation of POCUS and POCUS training for residents: the Rijnstate approach. Neth J Med 78(3):116–124
17. Blans MJ, Bosch FH, van der Hoeven JG (2019) A practical approach to critical care ultrasound. J Crit Care 51:156–164
18. Lichtenstein DA, Meziere GA (2008) Relevance of lung ultrasound in the diagnosis of acute respiratory failure: the BLUE protocol. Chest 134(1):117–125
19. Hobby JL, Tom BD, Todd C, Bearcroft PW, Dixon AK (2000) Communication of doubt and certainty in radiological reports. Br J Radiol 73(873):999–1001
20. Mantuani D, Frazee BW, Fahimi J, Nagdev A (2016) Point-of-Care Multi-Organ Ultrasound Improves Diagnostic Accuracy in Adults Presenting to the Emergency Department with Acute Dyspnea. West J Emerg Med 17(1):46–53
21. Jones AE, Tayal VS, Kline JA (2003) Focused training of emergency medicine residents in goal-directed echocardiography: a prospective study. Acad Emerg Med 10(10):1054–1058
22. Clay RD, Lee EC, Kurtzman MF, Dversdal RK (2016) Teaching the internist to see: effectiveness of a 1-day workshop in bedside ultrasound for internal medicine residents. Crit Ultrasound J 8(1):11
23. Mjolstad OC, Andersen GN, Dalen H, Graven T, Skjetne K, Kleinau JO et al (2013) Feasibility and reliability of point-of-care pocket-size echocardiography performed by medical residents. Eur Heart J Cardiovasc Imaging 14(12):1195–1202
24. Kimura BJ, Amundson SA, Phan JN, Agan DL, Shaw DJ (2012) Observations during development of an internal medicine residency training program in cardiovascular limited ultrasound examination. J Hosp Med 7(7):537–542
25. Croft LB, Duvall WL, Goldman ME (2006) A pilot study of the clinical impact of hand-carried cardiac ultrasound in the medical clinic. Echocardiography 23(6):439–446
26. Vignon P, Dugard A, Abraham J, Belcour D, Gondran G, Pepino F et al (2007) Focused training for goal-oriented hand-held echocardiography performed by noncardiologist residents in the intensive care unit. Intensive Care Med 33(10):1795–1799
27. Vignon P, Mucke F, Bellec F, Marin B, Croce J, Brouqui T et al (2011) Basic critical care echocardiography: validation of a curriculum dedicated to noncardiologist residents. Crit Care Med 39(4):636–642
28. Yamada T, Minami T, Soni NJ, Hiraoka E, Takahashi H, Okubo T et al (2018) Skills acquisition for novice learners after a point-of-care ultrasound course: does clinical rank matter? BMC Med Educ 18(1):202
29. Sen S, Acash G, Sarwar A, Lei Y, Dargin JM (2017) Utility and diagnostic accuracy of bedside lung ultrasonography during medical emergency team (MET) activations for respiratory deterioration. J Crit Care 40:58–62
30. Sklar DP, Hauswald M, Johnson DR (1991) Medical problem solving and uncertainty in the emergency department. Ann Emerg Med 20(9):987–991

17

Point-of-care ultrasound in cardiorespiratory arrest (POCUS-CA): narrative review article

Diana Ávila-Reyes[1*], Andrés O. Acevedo-Cardona[2,3], José F. Gómez-González[4,5], David R. Echeverry-Piedrahita[6], Mateo Aguirre-Flórez[7] and Adrian Giraldo-Diaconeasa[7]

Abstract

The POCUS-CA (Point-of-care ultrasound in cardiac arrest) is a diagnostic tool in the Intensive Care Unit and Emergency Department setting. The literature indicates that in the patient in a cardiorespiratory arrest it can provide information of the etiology of the arrest in patients with non-defibrillable rhythms, assess the quality of compressions during cardiopulmonary resuscitation (CPR), and define prognosis of survival according to specific findings and, thus, assist the clinician in decision-making during resuscitation. This narrative review of the literature aims to expose the usefulness of ultrasound in the setting of cardiorespiratory arrest as a tool that allows making a rapid diagnosis and making decisions about reversible causes of this entity. More studies are needed to support the evidence to make ultrasound part of the resuscitation algorithms. Teamwork during cardiopulmonary resuscitation and the inclusion of ultrasound in a multidisciplinary approach is important to achieve a favorable clinical outcome.

Keywords: Ultrasound, POCUS-point-of-care ultrasound, Cardiac arrest, Cardiopulmonary resuscitation, Echocardiography, Critical Care

Background

Cardiac arrest is the cessation of mechanical cardiac activity, as confirmed by the absence of circulation, and sudden cardiac arrest is an unexpected cardiac arrest that could result in attempts to restore circulation. If the attempts are unsuccessful, it is known as sudden cardiac death [1]. It is estimated that more than 356,000 out-of-hospital cardiac arrests occur annually in the United States of America. According to the American Heart Society's recent Heart and Stroke Statistics report, 90% of them are fatal [1]. After cardiac arrest, the survival at hospital discharge is approximately 10.4%, and survival with good functional status is 8.4% [2]. Around 209,000 in-hospital cardiac arrests occur in adults each year in the United States, with an average survival of 24.8% [3] and survival to discharge from hospital of 11.4% [3].

The mechanisms of cardiorespiratory a16 jrrest differ between out and in-hospital since in-hospital cardiac arrest is frequently the result of clinical deterioration, which typically occurs gradually for hours or days in the context of a critically ill patient. Cardiac arrest is frequently the result of noncardiac disorders of respiratory, hemodynamic, or neurological origin that cause a critical decrease in myocardial oxygenation, causing a reduction in contractility that culminates in pulseless electrical activity and ultimately asystole [4].

The basis for cardiac resuscitation includes the immediate provision of high-quality cardiopulmonary resuscitation combined with early defibrillation for defibrillable rhythms to impact the outcomes positively. These therapy bases lay the foundation for other possible interventions, such as medications, advanced airways, extracorporeal cardiopulmonary resuscitation, and post-cardiac arrest care, including targeted temperature control, cardiorespiratory support, and percutaneous coronary intervention [5]. Ultrasound is a diagnostic tool at the bedside of the patient that has been studied in the context of the patient

*Correspondence: diana.avila@utp.edu.co
[1] Department of Critical Care Medicine, Universidad Tecnológica de Pereira, Grupo de Investigación Medicina Crítica Y Cuidados Intensivos (GIMCCI), Pereira, Colombia
Full list of author information is available at the end of the article

in out and in-hospital arrest, and its importance has been suggested to be included in Advanced Cardiac Life Support (ACLS) algorithms [6–8].

The point of care ultrasound in cardiac arrest (POCUS-CA) conducted by a trained clinician allows the evaluation of the quality of the compressions, the quick diagnosis of reversible causes of arrest with non-defibrillable rhythms, the monitoring interventions, and its response to treatment. It also provides prognostic information regarding the possibility of a return to spontaneous circulation (ROSC) and survival [9].

During cardiopulmonary resuscitation (CPR), the POCUS-CA in the in-hospital setting, prioritizing the emergency department and the ICU, is a protocol to consider in the diagnosis of reversible causes of cardiac arrest in patients with non-defibrillable rhythms (pulseless electrical activity and asystole), such as cardiac tamponade, pulmonary embolism, tension pneumothorax, and hypovolemia [9], as well as to distinguish true asystole from fine ventricular fibrillation, conditions that have opposed therapeutic approaches. Current CPR guidelines recommend performing POCUS-CA when a reversible cause is suspected, although the impact on clinical outcomes is not yet clear [8, 10]. The literature mentions the importance of ultrasound in monitoring responses to interventions performed during resuscitation, real-time evaluation of the quality of compressions, and even as a guide to procedures such as decompression of tension pneumothorax and pericardiocentesis optimizing the safety and efficacy of the intervention [9, 11]. The most expert clinician must perform the POCUS-CA since the interpretation of images during compressions can be a challenge, and it entails the decisions to be taken in this context.

It is suggested that the POCUS-CA should be performed in the best possible window, ideally subxiphoid, and should not take more than 10 s, to minimize resuscitation interruptions [12, 13]. Given the importance that ultrasound has taken in this setting and its usefulness as a predictive tool, the importance of strengthening the available evidence through high-quality studies such as controlled clinical trials that allow integrating POCUS-CA into universal ACLS is highlighted.

Ultrasound in cardiac arrest

Ultrasound has become a safe and accurate diagnostic tool for critically ill patients in different settings. Greater accessibility and portability have made ultrasound at the point of care an available tool for the clinician [14]. Initially, ultrasound opened a field in the intensive care unit to insert the vascular catheter guided by ultrasound [15–17]. Wider applications have now been established to improve critical care practice [18]. During brain-cardio-pulmonary resuscitation (CPR) the POCUS-CA, is a protocol to consider in the diagnosis of reversible causes of cardiac arrest in patients with non-defibrillable rhythms (Pulseless electrical activity and asystole), using a rational "holistic" approach, always starting with cardiac imaging (subxiphoid window and inferior vena cava, and if not sufficient, advance to the visualization of the parasternal long axis or apical four-chamber window) and then explore the next area, if necessary, based on cardiac imaging, with the clinical correlation [9]. In general, the cardiac ultrasound in arrest should be performed by the most expert ultrasound clinician to interpret the findings correctly, and its evaluation should not interfere with the development of resuscitation. The ultrasound provider must make a visualization of the subxiphoid window during compressions, since it is the window that offers a more affordable visualization, in addition to avoiding interruptions of cardiac compressions, and during the 10 s defined by the American Heart Association (AHA) algorithm in which pulse and rhythm are verified [5]. The other available windows should be evaluated to achieve timely diagnoses.

Two studies have concluded that the use of ultrasound in patients with cardiac arrest delays the restart of compressions and generates an increase in interruptions during resuscitation [19, 20]. In this sense, medical specialists must be intervened in ultrasound training to minimize the required time to obtain and interpret images in stressful situations [12]. To achieve this, for example, the implementation of checklists could be carried out to allow rapid image acquisition and control of interruptions [21].

Technical aspects of the POCUS

POCUS-CA should ideally be performed with a probe appropriate to the expected objective. Lung evaluation requires a linear transducer with a 7–15 MHz frequency, which allows good resolution and low penetration. Cardiac evaluation requires a sectorial, low frequency (3.5–5 MHZ) transducer with high penetration for targeted assessment of structures. The convex transducer is preferred for the abdominal evaluation, which allows the assessment of deep tissues due to the high penetration, although with a lower resolution (frequency 2–5 MHz) [9]. POCUS-CA can be performed both transthoracic (TTE) and transesophageal (TEE). Using TTE, the clinician can assess the potentially reversible causes of cardiac arrest. By inserting the TEE probe into intubated patients, any reversible cause of arrest can be better elucidated, and the quality of chest compressions assessed, all while minimizing interruption of the compressions themselves. More studies are justified that evaluate echocardiography as a tool in cardiac arrest; however, TEE requires more training and level of expertise and presents certain limitations and risks [12].

POCUS-CA objectives

Cardiac activity

The objective is the visualization of cardiac activity, defined as any visible movement of the myocardium, excluding the movement of blood within the cardiac chambers or the movement of the isolated valve (Additional file 2: Video S1, Additional file 3: Video S3). The POCUS-CA allows the differential diagnosis between asystole and fine ventricular fibrillation (VF).

When POCUS-CA is used, studies have shown that 10 to 35% of patients with asystole have a demonstrable cardiac contraction. The demonstration of cardiac contraction on initial ultrasound is of vital prognostic importance since it would indicate the possibility of returning to spontaneous circulation. It helps decision-making in terms of continuity of effort during CPR regardless of the time of resuscitation. It means chances of survival at discharge [9]. In a multicenter study published in the "Resuscitation Journal" in the United States in 2016 [11] "REASON STUDY" included 793 patients with out-of-hospital cardiac arrest who presented non-defibrillable rhythms, cardiac activity was present in 33% of the patients. It was associated with ROSC (OR 2.8, 1.9–4.2), survival at hospital admission (OR 3.6, 2.2–5.9), and survival at hospital discharge (OR 5.7, 1.5–21.9). In contrast, patients who lacked detectable cardiac activity had a poor ROSC and a lower overall survival rate. In general, the ROSC rate was greater than 50% if the cardiac activity was detected with ultrasound. It should be noted that the detection of ROSC is dependent on other variables and diagnostic tools. A meta-analysis that included eight studies, with a total of 568 patients with arrest, also showed a low probability of ROSC and survival when no cardiac activity was detected on ultrasound, but a modest increase in these results if cardiac contraction was present. In a study with 49 patients in the intensive care unit, it was concluded that 34.7% were in asystole and 65.3% in pulseless electrical activity (PEA); the ROSC rates were lower in those with electromechanical dissociation. Ultrasound performed during cardiopulmonary resuscitation in intensive care unit (ICU) patients can be performed without interfering with care protocols and can contribute to the differential diagnosis of arrest and the identification of a subgroup of patients with a better prognosis [22]. Although the ROSC and the overall survival rate are low when the cardiac contraction was not observed there is no conclusive evidence to define a standard criterion for decision-making about not starting or stopping resuscitation efforts; since there are still a low number of patients who can come out of the arrest; especially those with witnessed arrest, early CPR, short downtime, or a potentially reversible cause [23, 24].

Efficacy of cardiac compressions

Another objective is to evaluate the effectiveness of compressions by providing direct, real-time observation of compression and relaxation of the cardiac chambers during the cardiac massage. Adequate or high-quality compressions are associated with ROSC and survival. Literature reports improper hand position during resuscitation may lead to compression of the ascending aorta, aortic root, or outflow tract of the left ventricle, but not the left ventricle [25, 26]. By using the POCUS-CA, you can help adjust the applied forces and the location of the hands to optimize compressions [9].

The method for the proper evaluation of the quality of the compressions is transesophageal echocardiography (TEE). This technique requires advanced training to achieve adequate images that allow for timely interpretation, but it has the advantage that it does not interfere with resuscitation and therefore does not generate interruptions [12]. Constant visualization of the heart during compressions allows an objective assessment of resuscitation quality, determining the proper location of the hands of the provider of CPR to avoid obstruction of the left ventricular outflow tract and allowing adequate ventricular relaxation, which guarantees an adequate preload and cardiac output [27]. The real-time evaluation of cardiac contractility during TEE allows determining prognostic factors and the response to procedures such as cardioversion [28], in addition to providing better visualization of pericardial effusion, signs of tamponade, cardiac rupture, pulmonary embolism, valve disease, thrombi, cardiac masses, and the differentiation between true asystole and fine ventricular fibrillation (which have opposed therapeutic measures) [29].

Practical approach use of the POCUS

Cardiorespiratory arrest corresponds to a stressful situation for medical personnel, and all interventions must be carried out in an organized manner, including the use of ultrasound. The practical approach of the POCUS-CA in the in-hospital setting, prioritizing the emergency department and the ICU, is described in the flowchart (Fig. 1). Initially, it is necessary to make the gain and depth adjustments, evaluate the transducers available for evaluation, and start the engraving process according to the characteristics of the ultrasound scanner, since some devices may have a delay in starting the recording function and must be considered the memory available for the process.

Once the patient is in arrest, the first cycle of CPR should be allowed to be performed, and the rhythm to

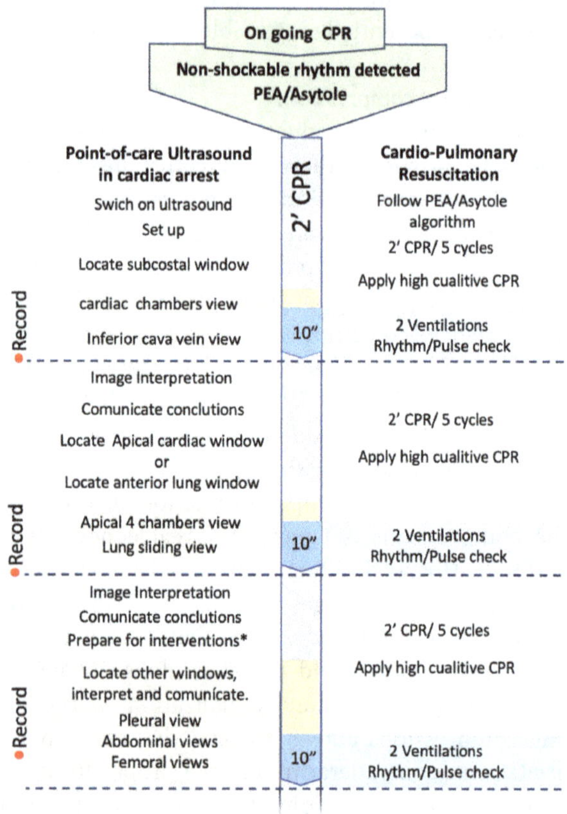

Fig. 1 POCUS-CA Flowchart. *Echo-guided pericardiocentesis or thoracostomy.CPR: cardiopulmonary resuscitation, PEA: pulseless electrical activity

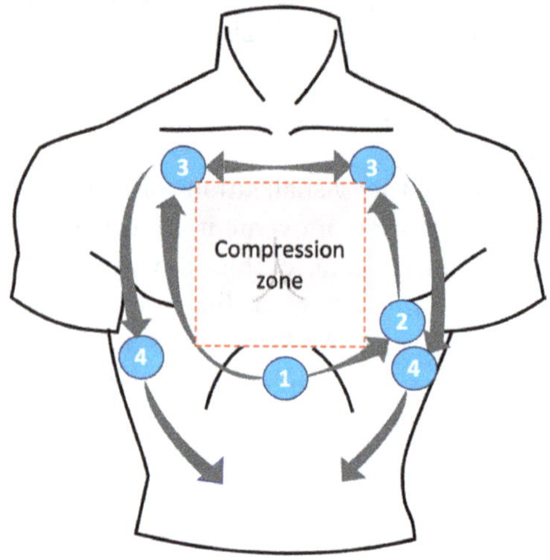

Fig. 2 POCUS-CA Windows

be defibrillable or non-defibrillable should be determined. During this cycle, the clinician in charge of performing the POCUS-CA prepares the equipment. Once the rhythm is described as non-defibrillable, it is recommended to start the POCUS-CA evaluation with the visualization of the subxiphoid window (subcostal 4 chambers) and obtain the image's recording. The evaluation of the images is not carried out during direct visualization, since this may delay the restart of the compressions, that means that the recording will be carried out for 10 s as indicated in the international resuscitation guidelines, and when the compressions are restarted, the clinician will evaluate the recording obtained to determine diagnostic findings, the findings are communicated and joint decision-making with the CPR team is carried out. The window used for assessing the patient with arrest during resuscitation is the subxiphoid window as the first option and the apical four chambers as the second option since they do not intervene with compressions (Fig. 2). During the pause for pulse taking and rhythm evaluation, the other windows available for diagnosis can be visualized, for a limit of 10 s, which are the pulmonary window in the assessment of pleural glide, the 4-chamber apical cardiac window, parasternal short axis, and as the last option the parasternal long axis. Windows can be used to evaluate pleural effusion, hemothorax, and free intra-abdominal fluid, described in the Extended Focused Assessment with Sonography in Trauma (FAST-E) protocol [30], which does not require synchronization with the CPR, and allow obtaining additional information on the patient's diagnosis. The POCUS-CA allows the determination of potentially reversible causes of arrest and should be integrated to the "5H's and 5 T's" checklist of cardiac arrest management (The **H's and T's** of ACLS; hypovolemia, cardiac tamponade, pneumothorax, and pulmonary embolism (Table 1) [8, 9, 12].

Diagnosis of reversible causes of cardiac arrest

The diagnosis of reversible causes allows early decision-making and could have a considerable impact on survival [12]. There are several echocardiography protocols in a patient with cardiac arrest. The Focus-Assessed transthoracic echocardiography (FATE) protocol, published by Jensen et al., was performed on 210 patients in 20 intensive care units and evaluated the subcostal, apical, parasternal, and pleural windows [31]. In 2005, the rapid cardiac ultrasound was developed by clinicians with basic training, which only includes the subxiphoid window for

Table 1 5H's and 5 T's" checklist [8]

	H's	T's
Cardiac arrest	Hypovolemia[US] Hypothermia Hypoxia Hypo or hyperkalemia Hydrogen ion (acidosis)	-Cardiac tamponade[US] -Toxins -Tension pneumothorax[US] - Pulmonary thrombosis[US] Thrombosis coronary

US ultrasound

evaluation of primary findings [32]. The Focused echocardiographic evaluation in resuscitation management (FEER) protocol (FEEL) published by Breitkreutz et al., evaluated the subcostal, parasternal and apical window, which showed an improvement in the results [33], and later Prosen et al. published a modification of the FEER protocol [34]. The Cardiac arrest ultra-sound exam (CAUSE) [35] protocol published in 2008 evaluates the subcostal or parasternal or apical window added to the evaluation of the pulmonary window and has been widely disseminated in clinical practice. Testa's proposal of an integrated ultrasonographic approach into the ALS algorithm for cardiac arrest (PEA) protocol includes epigastric, pulmonary, and abdominal evaluation during CPR [36].

Dr. Lichtenstein proposes the Sequential Echographic Scanning Assessing Mechanism Or Origin of Severe Shock of Indistinct Cause (SESAME) protocol and suggests starting with a lung scan to rule out possible causes leading to cardiac arrest. First, pneumothorax must be ruled out. Second, a partial diagnosis of pulmonary embolism is made following the bedside lung ultrasonography (BLUE) protocol. Third, fluid therapy can be guided following the Fluid Administration Limited by Lung Sonography (FALLS) protocol. The SESAME protocol continues to scan the lower femoral veins to check for signs of deep vein thrombosis (DVT), followed by examining the abdomen for massive bleeding. The pericardium is then evaluated to exclude pericardial tamponade. Finally, a transthoracic cardiac ultrasound is performed to verify other (cardiac) causes that lead to cardiac arrest. The emphasis is on a holistic approach, where ultrasound can be the modern stethoscope to complete the physiological examination of critically unstable patients [37]. In 2017, a consensus of an expert panel was published and recommended the cardiac arrest protocol (CORE) at the time of POCUS and in specific clinical questions.

Central views are limited to cardiac views and should be performed during the rhythm check pause in chest compressions without causing a prolonged interruption in chest compressions. The best views are the subxiphoid (SUBX) and the apical four chambers (A4C), but the long axis parasternal window can be used if necessary. Other views include pulmonary windows (for the absence of lung sliding in pneumothorax or pleural fluid) and subcostal window for evaluation of the inferior vena cava (IVC). Either view should be used to search for pericardial fluid and examine ventricular shape (e.g., right heart pressure) and cardiac function (e.g., asystole versus organized cardiac activity).

Additional applications that may help during cardiac arrest include using POCUS for endotracheal tube confirmation, scanning of proximal leg veins for deep vein thrombosis (DVT), or searching for sources of blood loss (aortic artery evaluation, peritoneal or pelvic fluid).

These protocols represent a consensus on the prioritization of the examination for these critically ill patients, based on the probability of detecting the underlying pathology and the perceived impact on the patient's treatment [38].

Cardiac tamponade

Cardiac tamponade is one of the potentially reversible causes that can lead to cardiac arrest. Among the etiologies, they are known to be traumatic and non-traumatic in origin and, in general terms, acute pericardial effusions as small as 50 ml can cause tamponade. In contrast, under chronic conditions, the pericardium can slowly stretch to accommodate large effusions over time without causing tamponade. The most relevant echocardiographic findings that guide us towards cardiac tamponade are the presence of pericardial effusion visible in all windows, but the ideal ones are the subxiphoid, apical, and parasternal long axis, and it is relatively easy to recognize [39]. Pericardial effusion is generally recognized by a black or anechoic appearance (Additional file 4: Video S4). However, effusions resulting from an inflammatory or infectious condition may have a lighter or more echogenic gray appearance [40]. The traumatic pericardial effusion acquires a more hyperechoic appearance. To visualize the effusion, the reclining patient should be located as far as possible. In this position, the smallest effusions will be found in the posterior layer of the heart. As the effusions grow, they will surround the heart circumferentially and move into the anterior pericardial space [41]. Most effusions will flow freely into the pericardial sac, although loculated effusions may occasionally occur. Loculated or septate effusions generally occur in patients who have undergone cardiac surgery and in inflammatory conditions [39]. Spills are classified as minor, moderate, or large according to the following scale [40].

- Minor: Less than 1 cm deep, non-circumferential around the heart.
- Moderate: Less than 1 cm deep, circumferential around the heart.
- Large: More than 1 cm deep, circumferential around the heart.

It is essential to know how to differentiate pericardial effusion from pleural effusion; the pericardial effusion will be in front of the descending aorta and above the posterior pericardial reflection in the parasternal long axis view. In contrast, pleural effusions will be located behind the descending aorta and below posterior pericardial reflection [40]. The pericardial or epicardial fat pad can sometimes be mistaken for a pericardial effusion. The specific location of this structure is in the area just before the heart and below the anterior or near-field pericardial reflex, which is located within the pericardial sac. The pad has a classic appearance, with shiny or hyperechoic regions. In the parasternal window, an isolated anterior location suggests more a fat pad than an effusion. For an effusion to be visualized only on the anterior side of the pericardial sac, a circumferential effusion would generally be present. A downside to subxiphoid vision is that ascites can sometimes be mistaken for a pericardial effusion. Differentiation between the two is possible by noting that ascites will be located closer to the probe surrounding the liver within the abdominal cavity and outside the pericardial sac. A pericardial effusion will be found within the pericardial sac, below pericardial reflection near field and adjacent to the heart [40].

As mentioned, the presence of pericardial effusion does not make a diagnosis of cardiac tamponade [40], a competition of additional findings is required such as right atrial systolic collapse and right diastolic ventricular collapse (Additional file 5: Video S5). However, these signs are not seen in the patient with arrest, but they can occur prior to the arrest. In the patient before the arrest, the experts describe energetic cardiac movements as the "furiously contracting chamber," with hyperdynamic atrial contractions and exaggerated movements as tamponade progresses, making it challenging to assess systolic contraction for diastolic collapse (Additional file 1: Video S1). Although both right heart chambers must be evaluated, the diastolic collapse of the right ventricle is a more specific finding. This collapse is best understood as a spectrum of ultrasound findings of a subtle sudden deviation of the wall in diastole to complete compression of the chamber. In patients with pulmonary hypertension, the diastolic collapse of the right heart is a very late finding, so if you are in the context of a patient without underlying pathology, you must think of acute symptoms.

The inferior vena cava (IVC) can also be evaluated, which, if found plethoric, could indicate the increase in the atrial cavities (Fig. 3; Additional file 6: Video S6). These findings have a sensitivity of 96% and a specificity of 98% [40] (Fig. 4). Another more advanced finding includes changes in transvalvular flow velocity on the Doppler, which requires more training and evaluation time, which in the context of CPR may not be applicable, but if once the patient is evaluated at a stage of ROSC and hemodynamic stability [40].

In the patient with cardiac arrest presenting signs compatible with cardiac tamponade [41]· [42], ultrasound-guided pericardiocentesis can be performed emergently [43].

Pulmonary thromboembolism (PE)

Massive pulmonary thromboembolism can be detected by ultrasound with direct and indirect signs. The direct sign is the visualization of the clot, and the indirect ones include the acute dilation of the right ventricle (RV), exceeding the normal relationship with the left ventricle (LV), which must be 0.6: 1 in the apical four-chamber view, and that for it to be diagnostic of RV dilation should be a 1: 1 ratio Additional file 7: Video S7. The finding of the D-shaped RV in the parasternal short-axis window is another of the signs of RV dilatation [44]. In the pre-arrest patient, the deviation of the ventricular septum to the left side, paradoxical systolic septal movement, septal flattening in diastole, McConnell sign (although not exclusive to PE) can be seen [45] (Fig. 5; Additional file 8: Video S8). These ultrasound findings confirm the

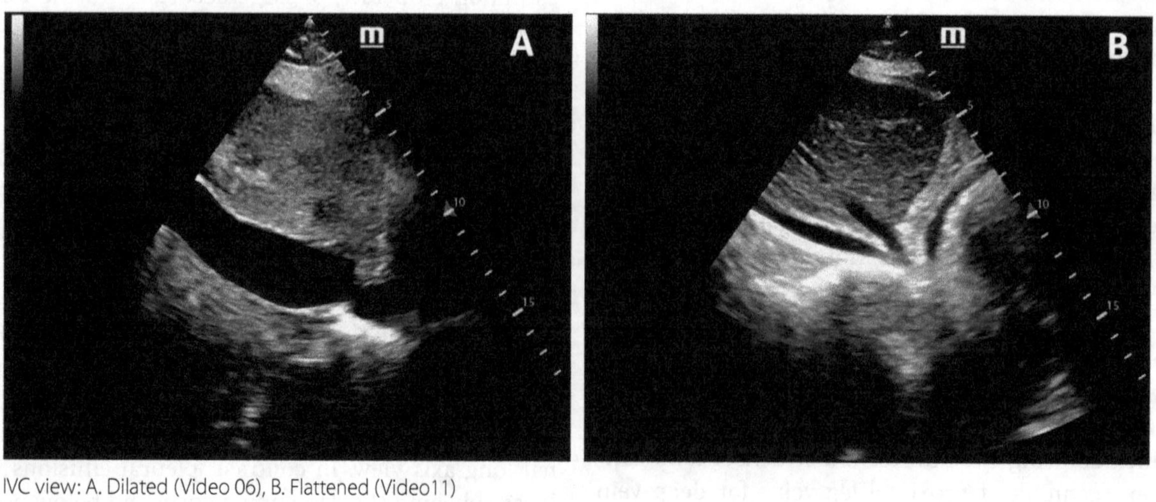

Fig. 3 IVC view: A. Dilated (Video 06), B. Flattened (Video11)

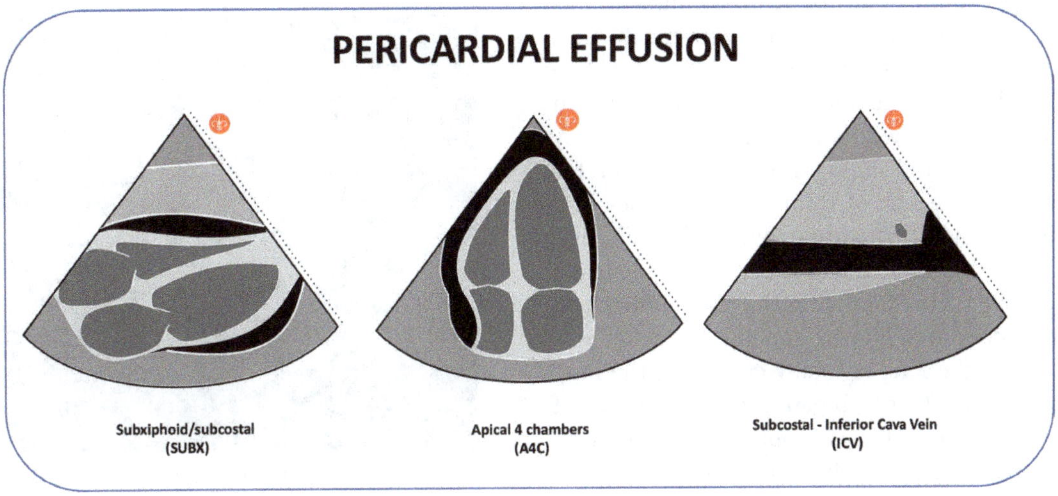

Fig. 4 Pericardial effusion and Cardiac tamponade findings

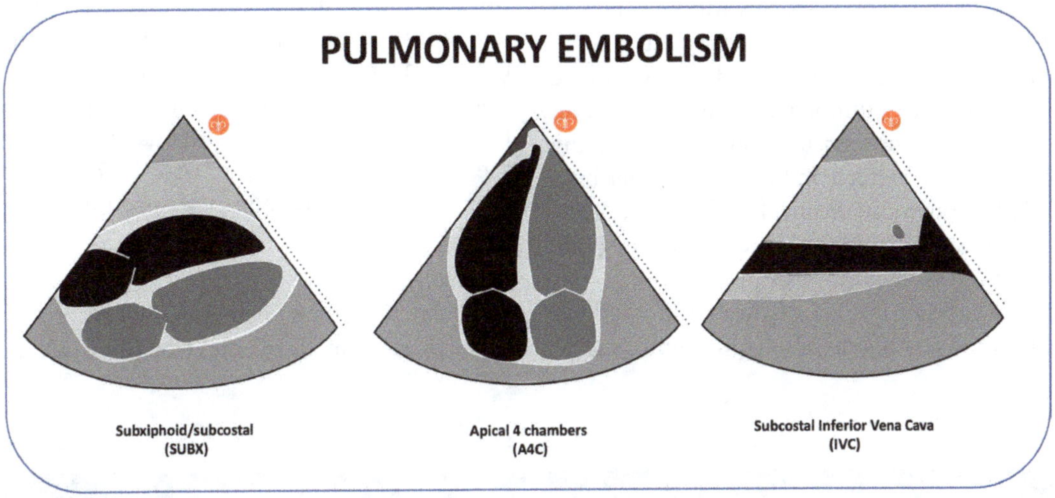

Fig. 5 Pulmonary embolism findings

right ventricular tension that can be observed in a severe pulmonary embolism. Right strain should be differentiated from chronic right heart pressure, which is generally seen in conditions of long-standing pulmonary arterial hypertension (such as primary pulmonary hypertension and cases of chronic pulmonary embolism); the right ventricular wall will compensate by hypertrophy, often larger than 5 mm. In acute right ventricular tension, the chamber will not have time to compensate for hypertrophy, and typically a thin wall measuring less than 5 mm will be seen [39]. The prominent trabecular architecture of the chamber and papillary muscles can also be recognized. When asked if the right ventricular chamber dilation is acute or chronic, the clinician can use these general rules to decide whether more emergent therapy, such as fibrinolysis, may be indicated. As previously mentioned, some protocols also include ultrasound signs of intraluminal thrombus in the deep veins" of the lower limbs for the diagnosis of pulmonary embolism (PE) during arrest [37]. The approach to confirm the diagnosis of deep venous thrombosis can be done more elaborately and more comprehensively (common femoral vein, calf veins, upper extremities) [37].

Tension pneumothorax

Tension pneumothorax is one of the leading causes of potentially reversible arrest in patients with traumatic etiology [46]. Acute decompression of pneumothorax is imperative to improve the patient's ventilatory mechanics and hemodynamics. Usually, the physical examination of tension pneumothorax may not be problematic in this context; however, in critically ill patients with mechanical ventilation, it may not be so easy to suspect [47]. Ultrasonographic findings of pneumothorax are visualized in the 4–5 intercostal space with a mid-clavicular line; they are the absence of pleural sliding, the sign of the stratosphere or barcode, the lack of B lines, and absence of a pulmonary pulse (Fig. 6). The lung point is the only sign that confirms pneumothorax, with very high specificity. However, extending the examination to the whole chest during a critical condition may be difficult.

Moreover, when the lung is totally collapsed, the lung point will be absent. The combination of the absence of sliding B-lines and pulse has the optimal sensitivity in ruling out pneumothorax. Their specificity is also high, but only in the critical scenario of a cardiac arrest [48]. A frequent pitfall is misunderstanding the physiological lung point sign or "mediastinal point sign" as if it were a pathological lung point. The mediastinal point sign is found in the 4th–5th intercostal space with the midclavicular line of the left hemithorax and is characterized by the lung sliding absence but with the underlying cardiac movements instead of the pulmonary A-line pattern and differs from the lung point sign that shows lung sliding absence but with A-line pattern and lack of another lung artifact sings (e.g., lung pulse, B lines) [49] (Fig. 7; Additional file 9: Video S9). Also, ultrasound can safely guide acute decompression of pneumotorax [40].

Hemothorax is another finding of the trauma patient, and if it is massive, it could generate hypovolemic shock, circulatory and pulmonary collapse. Ultrasonography can assess the volume and nature of effusion in addition to indicating the appropriate area for thoracentesis and thereby decrease the risk of complications. The volume calculation, in general, is done using the distance formula mm X 20; although this has not been validated in the patient with arrest, it could be considered once the patient stabilizes to define the need for intervention.

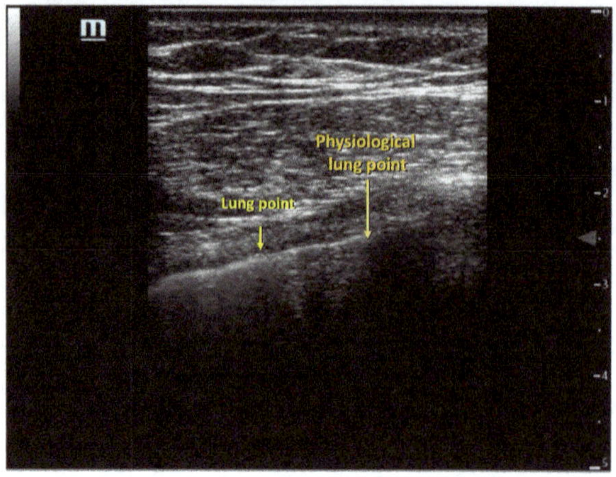

Fig. 7 Lung point sign and mediastinal point sign (Video 08)

Hypovolemia

The shock patient can rapidly progress to circulatory collapse. In the context of the trauma patient, the

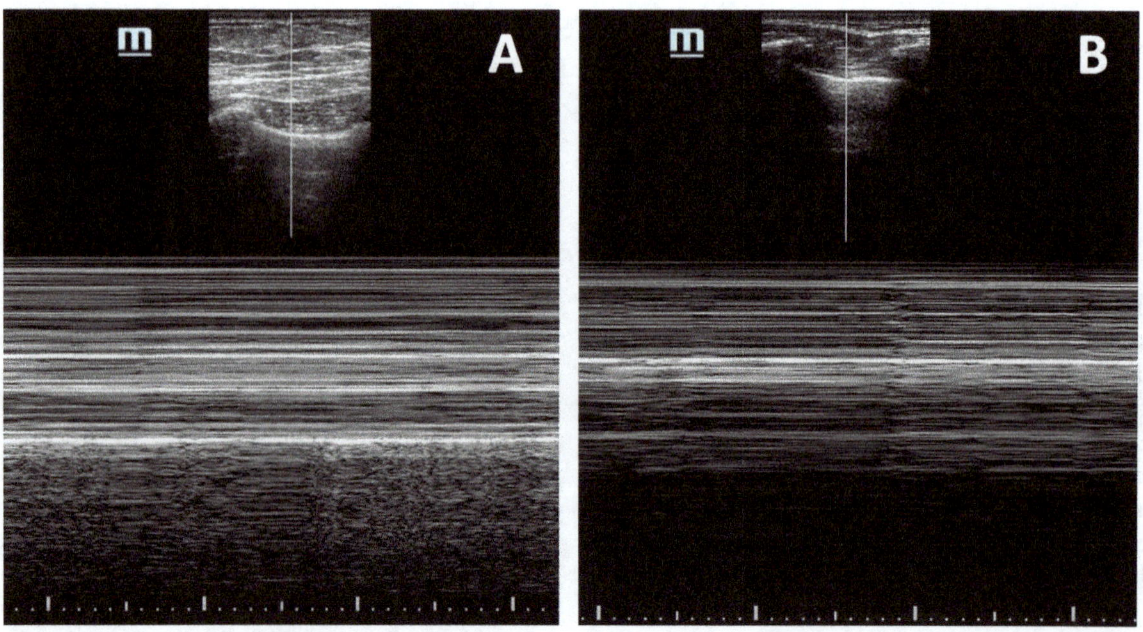

Fig. 6 Anterior pulmonary window (M mode). A) beach sign b) code bar sing

hemorrhagic hypovolemic shock should be considered initially, and the cardiogenic, distributive, or obstructive shock [50] should be considered in the medical patient, each profile with a different echocardiographic finding [51, 52], which can be evaluated using protocols such as RUSH [53, 54]. Hypovolemia in the patient with an pre-cardiac arrest can be assessed using sharable ultrasound findings with accelerated movements, hyperdynamic pattern, obliteration of the ventricles, small ventricular area at the end of systole and diastole (Additional file 10: Video S10; Additional file 11: Video S11), "kiss sign" in the Parasternal Short View, which is nothing more than the union of the ventricular walls and the papillary muscles in each beat due to the lack of intracavitary volume. The evaluation of the inferior vena cava (IVC) with the sign of "Empty tank" (diameter less than 2 cm, IVC collapse > 50% during inspiration); compatible with central venous pressure (PVC < 10cmH2O), is another of the signs that indicate hypovolemia [40]. In the patient with arrest, it can be visualized the obliteration of the ventricles and the collapsed inferior vena cava (IVC diameter < 2 cm), which added to the clinical course and other findings make us think of hypovolemia [53] (Fig. 8; Additional file 12: Video 12).

The RUSH protocol [53] allows an initial approach to the patient in shock by addressing three main parameters described as "pump, tank, and pipes", allowing the classification of the type of shock that the patient has according to the findings in each of the parameters, and facilitating the Etiological diagnosis of the clinical condition at the bedside in a fast and comprehensive way. The protocol simplifies the ultrasound evaluation into the physiological paradigm of "pump, tank, and pipes," allowing the clinician to remember the critical aspects of the exam components easily [55]. Although the RUSH protocol is helpful, it has limitations because of the lack of precision in the definitions of the findings and diagnostic patterns. In this sense, Volpicelli [56] et al. published a study in 2013 that enrolled 108 adult patients complaining of non-traumatic symptomatic hypotension of uncertain etiology. Patients received immediate point-of-care ultrasonography to determine the cardiac function and right/left ventricle diameter rate, inferior vena cava diameter, and collapsibility, pulmonary congestion, consolidations and sliding, as well as abdominal free fluid, aortic aneurysm, and deep venous thrombosis. The organ-oriented diagnoses were combined to formulate an ultrasound hypothesis of the cause of the hemodynamic instability. The ultrasound diagnosis was then compared with a final clinical diagnosis, obtaining as a result an adequate concordance between the point-of-care ultrasonography diagnosis and the definitive clinical diagnosis. In summary, the integration of a multiorgan ultrasonographic protocol in the diagnostic process of undifferentiated hypotension has great potential in guiding the first-line therapeutic approach [56].

Ultrasound allows the evaluation of signs of shock in the patient in pre-arrest and its evaluation during the post-arrest period to make etiological diagnoses that allow therapeutic decisions to be made once the patient is stable [12], for example, in the case of an acute myocardial infarction, a complete evaluation can be carried out on the left ventricular ejection fraction (LVEF), contractility disorders and anatomy of the papillary muscles to help determine the need for emergent cardiac catheterization, and in the case of massive pulmonary thromboembolism findings may guide thrombolysis. Ultrasound allows real-time evaluation of the response to

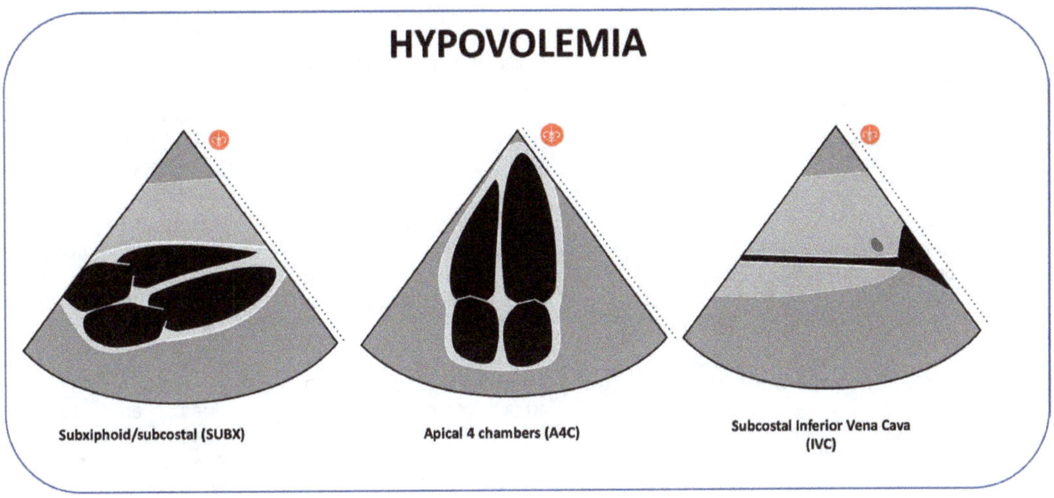

Fig. 8 Hypovolemia findings

interventions and allows to guide diagnostic procedures. The Ultrasound signs are found in (Table 2).

Evidence of ultrasound in arrest as a prognostic tool

Ultrasound in arrest has been studied in intrahospital and outpatient settings. As mentioned, there are multiple protocols to carry out the POCUS-CA, which require more extensive external validation, and so far, there is no study indicating which is superior; however, it is clear the more windows that are evaluated, the greater the success in collecting findings to integrate the information and make an adequate clinical interpretation, essential for decision-making that can modify the patient's prognostic course [17]. The POCUS-CA approach requires training, and some studies have concluded that the use of ultrasound in this setting can prolong the interruptions and the restart time of CPR and thus worsen the results. In 2018, a prospective study was published of 276 patients who underwent the CASA protocol (Cardiac Arrest Sonographic Assessment), a protocol that evaluates three main questions between each CPR cycle; cardiac tamponade, RV stress, and cardiac activity, with yes / no responses, and lasting less than 10 s. The protocol was carried out by residents of the university institution, and within the results, they found a reduction in the time of interruptions of 19.8–15.8s [57]. In 2019 the SHoC-ED group published a retrospective cohort study of 180 patients undergoing POCUS-CA; it concluded that POCUS-CA emergency department patients received more extended resuscitation with higher intervention rates than those with negative findings or when POCUS-CA was not performed. Patients with cardiac activity in POCUS-CA had improved clinical outcomes compared to patients who did not receive POCUS-CA and patients without activity in POCUS-CA [58]. A meta-analysis published in Resuscitation [59] of 15 studies with a total of 1695 patients concluded that POCUS-CA could be used to identify reversible causes and predict short-term outcomes in patients with cardiac arrest. In patients with a low prior probability of ROSC, the absence of spontaneous cardiac movements on echocardiography can predict a low chance of survival and guide the decision to end resuscitation. Another systematic review and meta-analysis of 10 studies with 1486 patients confirmed that cardiac activity in POCUS-CA was associated with better probabilities of ROSC and survival at discharge, in non-traumatic cardiac arrest, and with non-defibrillable rhythm [60]. The overall conclusion of the evidence is that the evaluation of cardiac motion on transthoracic echocardiography is a valuable tool in predicting short-term cardiac resuscitation outcomes. Given the safety and availability of ultrasound in the emergency department, it is reasonable to apply POCUS-CA to cardiopulmonary resuscitation if its use does not interrupt resuscitation [61]. Table 3 shows the different protocols described in the literature.

CPR techniques have evolved in the last decade in terms of implementing high-quality measures, early intervention in defibrillable rhythms for the impact of the electrical phase of arrest [62]. Still, it continues to

Table 2 Ultrasound signs for reversible causes

	View	Arrest signs	Peri-Arrest signs
Cardiac Tamponade	Subxiphoid View Apical 4 chambers Subcostal IVC Parasternal Long View*	Pericardial effusion Plethoric IVC	Pericardial effusion Plethoric IVC Systolic collapse of the right atrium Collapse of the right ventricle in diastole
Hypovolemia	Subxiphoid View Apical 4 chambers Subcostal IVC Parasternal views*	Obliteration of ventricles Inferior vena cava diameter <2 cm	Hyperdynamic Obliteration of ventricles Kiss sign "Empty tank" inferior vena cava (IVC diameter <2 cm collapse $>50\%$ during inspiration)
Pulmonary Embolism	Subxiphoid View Apical 4 chambers Subcostal IVC Parasternal views* Lower limb compression ultrasound*	Right heart thrombus Right ventricular dilation D sign of left ventricle Deep vein thrombosis	Pulmonary Hypertension Deep vein thrombosis Paradoxical septal systolic movement Septal flattening in diastole McConnell sign D sign of left ventricle
Tension pneumothorax	4th–5th intercostal space with midclavicular line	Absence lung sliding (during artificial ventilation) Stratosphere /barcode sign	Absence lung sliding Stratosphere /barcode sign Absence B lines Absence pulmonary pulse Lung point

*Optional

Table 3 Ultrasound protocols in cardiorespiratory arrest

2004. Jensen et al. [31]	FATE	1. Subcostal view 2. Apical view 3. Parasternal view 4. Pleural view
2005. Niendorff et al. [32]	Rapid Cardiac Ultrasound	1. Subcostal view
2007. Breitkreutz et al. [33]	FEER (FEEL)	1. Subcostal view 2. Parasternal view 3. Apical view
2008 Hernandez. [35]	CAUSE	1. Subcostal view or apical view or parasternal view 2. Lung view
2010 Prosen et al. [34]	Modified FEER	1. Subcostal view 2. Parasternal view 3. Apical view
2010 Testa et al. [36]	PEA	1. Epigastric scan 2. Pulmonary scan 3. Abdominal scan
2015. Lichtenstein. [37]	SESAME	1. Pulmonary view 2. Cardiac view 3. DVT detection at the V-point
2017 Arkinson et al. [38]	CORE	Consensus on the use of point of care ultrasound for undifferentiated hypotension and during cardiac arrest
2019 Arkinson et al. [56]	SHoc-ED	Sonography in Hypotension and Cardiac Arrest in the Emergency Department
2021. Ávila, Acevedo et al	POCUS-CA	1. Subcostal view 2. Apical view 3. Parasternal view 4. Pleural and pulmonar view 5. FAST-E

have unsuccessful results given the low rate and survival, influenced by multiple factors. Mechanical ventilation has physiological effects on the patient in cardiac arrest, and thus clinical challenges are posed on the mechanical ventilation strategy to be implemented during the arrest. Although there is still a lack of conclusive scientific evidence on the ventilatory mode and the parameters to be programmed in the ventilator during compressions in resuscitation, it is imperative further studies to determine the effects that mechanical ventilation has on ultrasound findings during cardiopulmonary resuscitation [63].

The intensivist involved may have information on the physiological conditions that led to the patient's arrest, but on some occasions, particularly in the emergency department patient, there is little information on the reason for cardiac arrest and the probability of survival. In this setting, bedside ultrasound shows promise as a critical tool in providing valuable information to help direct management. It is important to remember that the decision to end resuscitation should never be made based on ultrasound findings alone [21]. The POCUS in cardiac arrest is an excellent complementary tool in the hands of experienced providers. Although no current studies show an improvement in mortality, echocardiography is useful for diagnostic and prognostic purposes in cardiac arrest [12].

The cardiac activity present in the POCUS-CA is a finding of prognostic importance for ROSC and survival, as evidenced in multiple studies [23, 24, 64–76].

Conclusions

Ultrasound has become a safe and accurate diagnostic tool for critically ill patients in the intrahospital setting, prioritizing the emergency department and the ICU. Greater accessibility and portability have made ultrasound at the point of care an available tool for the intensivist [14]. The POCUS-CA in the hands of a trained clinician, allows the evaluation of the quality of the compressions, the rapid diagnosis of reversible causes of arrest with non-defibrillable rhythms, the monitoring of interventions in terms of response to treatment, and provides prognostic information regarding the possibility of ROSC and survival [9]. Given the importance that ultrasound has taken in this setting and its usefulness as a predictive tool, the importance of strengthening the available evidence through high-quality studies such as controlled clinical trials that allow integrating POCUS-CA into universal CPR algorithms is highlighted. In this sense, medical specialists must be intervened in ultrasound training to minimize the time necessary to obtain and interpret images in stressful situations [12]; the implementation of checklists could be carried out to allow rapid image acquisition and control of interruptions. [21].

Abbreviations

ACLS: Advanced cardiac life support; POCUS-CA: Point of care ultrasound in cardiac arrest; ROSC: Return to spontaneous circulation; CPR: Cardiopulmonary resuscitation; AHA: American Heart Association; TTE: Transthoracic echography; TEE: Transesophageal echography; VF: Ventricular fibrillation; PEA: Pulseless electrical activity; ICU: Intensive care unit; FAST-E: Extended Focused Assessment with Sonography in Trauma; FATE: Focus-Assessed transthoracic echocardiography; FEER: Focused echocardiographic evaluation in resuscitation management; CAUSE: Cardiac arrest ultra-sound exam; PEA: The proposal of an integrated ultrasonographic approach into the ALS algorithm for cardiac arrest; SESAME: Sequential Echographic Scanning Assessing Mechanism Or Origin of Severe Shock of Indistinct Cause; BLUE: The bedside lung ultrasonography; FALLS: Fluid Administration Limited by Lung Sonography; DVT: Deep vein thrombosis; CORE: Cardiac arrest protocol; SUBX: Subxiphoid; A4C: Apical 4 chambers; IVC: Inferior vena cava; PE: Pulmonary thromboembolism; RV: Right ventricle; LVEF: Left ventricular ejection fraction.

Supplementary Information

Additional file 1: Video S1. SUBX Pericardial efussion, right ventricule colapse.

Additional file 2: Video S2. PEA -Cardiac Activity.

Additional file 3: Video S3. PEA_Asytole non cardiac activity- dilated ICV.

Additional file 4: Video S4. Pericardial efussion A4C.

Additional file 5: Video S5. Pericardial efussion, right ventricule colapse SUBX.

Additional file 6: Video S6. Dilated ICV.

Additional file 7: Video S7. Pulmonar embolism—SUBX.

Additional file 8: Video S8. Pulmonar embolism—McConnell sign A4C.

Additional file 9: Video S9. Lung point and pelural poinrt (physiological lung point).

Additional file 10: Video S10. Hyperdinamic_ hypovolemic SUBX.

Additional file 11: Video S11. Hyperdinamic_ hypovolemic A4C.

Additional file 12: Video S12. Flattened ICV.

Acknowledgements

The authors thank Dr. Edgardo Quiñones Quiñones (Additional file 9: Video S9).

Authors' contributions

Study concept and design: DAR, AOAC, DREP, JFGG. Acquisition, analysis, and interpretation of data: DAR, AOAC. Drafting of the manuscript: DAR, AOAC, MAF, AGD. Original material and construction of images and videos: AOAC. Critical revision of the manuscript for important intellectual content: AOAC, DAR. Administrative, technical, and material support: DAR, AOAC, MAF, AGD. Study supervision: DAR, AOAC, DREP, JFGG. All authors submitted and agree to be accountable for all aspects of the work. All authors read and approved the final manuscript.

Author details

[1]Department of Critical Care Medicine, Universidad Tecnológica de Pereira, Grupo de Investigación Medicina Crítica Y Cuidados Intensivos (GIMCCI), Pereira, Colombia. [2]Department of Critical Care Medicine, Universidad Tecnológica de Pereira,, Pereira, Colombia. [3]Master en Ecocardiografía en Cuidados Intensivos, Sociedad Española de Imagen Cardíaca/Universidad Francisco de Vitoria, España, Pereira, Spain. [4]Department of Critical Care Medicine, Universidad Tecnológica de Pereira, Pereira, Colombia. [5]Grupo Investigación de Medicina Crítica Y Cuidados Intensivos (GIMCCI), Pereira, Colombia. [6]Department of Critical Care Medicine, Universidad Tecnológica de Pereira, Pereira, Colombia. [7]Department of Medicine, Universidad Tecnológica de Pereira, Pereira, Colombia.

References

1. Benjamin EM, Muntner P, Alonso A et al (2019) Heart Disease and Stroke Statistics—2019 Update. A Report from the American Heart Association. Circulation. 139:1
2. AHA Releases Latest Statistics on Sudden Cardiac Arrest. Available online at: https://www.sca-aware.org/sca-news/aha-releases-latest-statistics-on-sudden-cardiac-arrest. Accessed Jan 2, 2018
3. Mozaffarian D, Benjamin EJ, Go AS et al (2016) Heart disease and stroke statistics-2016 update: a report from the american heart association. Circulation 133(4):e38-360
4. Gazmuri R (2017) In-hospital cardiopulmonary resuscitation of the adult patient. Revista Med Clín Los Condes 28(2):228–238
5. Ashish RP, Berg KM, Hirsch K et al (2019) American Heart Association Focused Update on Advanced Cardiovascular Life Support: Use of Advanced Airways, Vasopressors, and Extracorporeal Cardiopulmonary Resuscitation During Cardiac Arrest: An Update to the American Heart Association Guidelines for Cardiopulmonary Resuscitation and Emergency Cardiovascular Care. Circulation. 140(24):e881–e894
6. Chardoli M, Heidari F, Rabiee H et al (2012) Echocardiography integrated ACLS protocol versus conventional cardiopulmonary resuscitation in patients with pulseless electrical activity cardiac arrest. Chin J Traumatol 15:284–287
7. Narasimhan M, Koenig SJ, Mayo PH (2014) Advanced echocardiography for the critical care physician: part 1. Chest 145:129–134
8. Link M, Berkow LC, Kudenchuk PJ et al (2015) 2015 American Heart Association Guidelines Update for Cardiopulmonary Resuscitation and Emergency Cardiovascular Care; Part 7: Adult Advanced Cardiovascular Life Support. Circulation 132:S444–S464
9. Blanco P, Buendía CM (2017) Point-of-care ultrasound in cardiopulmonary resuscitation: a concise review. J Ultrasound 20:193–198
10. Soar J, Nolan JP, Bottiger BW et al (2015) European resuscitation council guidelines for resuscitation 2015: section 3. Adult Advanced life support Resuscitation 95:100–147
11. Gaspari R, Weekes A, Adhikari S et al (2016) Emergency department point-of-care ultrasound in out-of-hospital and in-ED cardiac arrest. Resuscitation 109:33–39
12. Long B, Alerhand S, Maliel J, Koyfman A (2018) Echocardiography in cardiac arrest: An emergency medicine review. Am J Emerg Med 36(3):488–493
13. Blyth L, Atkinson P, Gadd K et al (2012) Bedside focused echocardiography as predictor of survival in cardiac arrest patients: a systematic review society for academic emergency medicine. Acad Emerg Med. 19(10):1119–26
14. Bakhru R, Schweickert W, Schmidt GA (2013) Intensive care ultrasound. Ann Am Thorac Soc 10(5):540–548
15. Randolph AG, Cook DJ, Gonzales CA et al (1996) Ultrasound guidance for placement of central venous catheters: a meta-analysis of the literature. Crit Care Med 24:2053–2058
16. Hind D, Calvert N, McWilliams R et al (2003) Ultrasonic locating devices for central venous cannulation: meta-analysis. BMJ 327:361
17. Maecken T, Grau T (2007) Ultrasound imaging in vascular access. Crit Care Med 35(5 Suppl):S178–S185
18. Ma I, Chun R, Kirkpatrick A (2015) Basics of Ultrasound. In: Ferrada P (ed) Ultrasonography in the ICU. Springer, Practical Applications. First Edition. Virginia, pp 1–36
19. Veld MA, Allison MG et al (2017) Ultrasound use during cardiopulmonary resuscitation is associated with delays in chest compressions. Resuscitation. 119:95–98
20. Clattenburg EJ, Wroe P, Brown S et al (2018) Point-of-care ultrasound use in patients with cardiac arrest is associated prolonged cardiopulmonary resuscitation pauses: a prospective cohort study. Resuscitation 122:65–68

21. Hussein L, Anzal M, Sajid R et al (2019) Bedside ultrasound in cardiac standstill: a clinical review. Ultrasound J. 11:35
22. Flato UA, Paiva EF, Carballo MT et al (2015) Echocardiography for prognostication during the resuscitation of intensive care unit patients with non-shock- able rhythm cardiac arrest. Resuscitation 92:1–6
23. Lien W, Hsu S, Kah-Meng C et al (2018) US-CAB protocol for ultrasonographic evaluation during cardiopulmonary resuscitation: validation and potential impact. Resuscitation. 127:125–131
24. Beckett N, Atkinson P, Fraser J et al (2019) Do combined ultrasound and electrocardiogram-rhythm findings predict survival in emergency department cardiac arrest patients? The Second Sonography in Hypotension and Cardiac Arrest in the Emergency Department (SHoC-ED2) study. CJEM 21(6):739–743
25. Hwang SO, Zhao PG, Choi HJ et al (2009) Compression of the left ventricular outflow tract during cardiopulmonary resuscitation. Acad Emerg Med 16(10):928–933
26. Shin J, Rhee JE, Kim K (2007) Is the inter-nipple line the correct hand position for effective chest compression in adult cardiopulmonary resuscitation? Resuscitation 75(2):305–310
27. Arntfield R, Pace J, Hewak M et al (2016) Focused transesophageal echocardiography by emergency physicians is feasible and clinically influential: observational results from a novel ultrasound program. J Emerg Med 50(2):286–294
28. ACEP Board of Directors. Guidelines for the Use of Transesophageal. Echocardiography (TEE) in the ED for Cardiac Arrest. Ann Emerg Med. 2017;70:442–445.
29. Parker B, Salerno A, Euerle B (2018) The use of transesophageal echocardiography during cardiac arrest resuscitarion. A Lierature Review. J Ultrasound Med 00:1–11
30. Williams S, Perera P, Gharahbaghian L (2014) The FAST and E-FAST in 2013: Trauma ultrasonography: overview, practical techniques, controversies, and new frontiers. Crit Care Clin 30(1):119–150
31. Jensen MB, Sloth E, Larsen KM et al (2004) Transthoracic echocardiography for cardiopulmonary monitoring in intensive care. Eur J Anaesthesiol 21(9):700–707
32. Niendorff DF, Rassias A, Palac R et al (2005) Rapid cardiac ultrasound of inpatients suffering PEA arrest performed by nonexpert sonographers. Resuscitation 67:81–87
33. Breitkreutz R, Walcher F, Seeger FH (2007) Focused echocardiographic evaluation in resuscitation management: concept of an advanced life support-conformed algorithm. Crit Care Med 35(5 Suppl):S150–S161
34. Prosen G, Krizmaric M, Zavrsnik J et al (2010) Impact of modified treatment in echocardiographically confirmed pseudo-pulseless electrical activity in out-of-hospital cardiac arrest patients with constant end-tidal carbon dioxide pressure during compression pauses. J Int Med Res. 38(4):1458–67
35. Hernandez C, Shuler K, Hannan H et al (2008) CAUSE: Cardiac arrest ultra-sound exam–a better approach to managing patients in primary non-arrhythmogenic cardiac arrest. Resuscitation 76(2):198–206
36. Testa A, Cibinel GA, Portale G et al (2010) The proposal of an integrated ultrasonographic approach into the ALS algorithm for cardiac arrest: the PEA protocol. Eur Rev Med Pharmacol Sci 14(2):77–88
37. Lichtenstein D, Malbrain ML (2015) Critical care ultrasound in cardiac arrest. Technological requirements for performing the SESAME-protocol–a holistic approach. Anaesthesiol Intensive Ther. 47(5):471–81
38. Atkinson P, Bowra J, Milne J et al (2017) International Federation for Emergency Medicine Consensus Statement: Sonography in hypotension and cardiac arrest (SHoC): An international consensus on the use of point of care ultrasound for undifferentiated hypotension and during cardiac arrest. Can Assoc Emerg Phys 2016:1–12
39. Grecu L (2012) Cardiac tamponade. Int Anesthesiol Clin Spring 50(2):59–77
40. Perera P, Lovo V, Williams SR et al (2014) Cardiac echocardiography. Crit Care Clin 30(1):47–92
41. Shabetai R (2004) Pericardial effusions: haemodynamic spectrum. Heart 90:255–256
42. Nagdev A, Stone MB (2011) Point-of-care ultrasound evaluation of pericardial effusions: does this patient have cardiac tamponade? Resuscitation 82(6):671–673
43. Glaser J, Conti B, Murthi S: Cardiac Ultrasound in the Intensive Care Unit: Point of Care Transthoracic and Transesophageal Echocardiography. I Ferrada P (Ed). *Ultrasonography in the ICU. Practical Applications*. First Edition. Virginia. Springer. 2015, Pp53–73.
44. Riley D, Hultgren A, Merino D et al (2011) Emergency department bedside echocar- diographic diagnosis of massive pulmonary embolism with direct visualization of thrombus in the pulmonary artery. Crit Ultrasound J 3(3):155–160
45. Walsh BM, Moore CL (2015) McConnell's sign is not specific for pulmonary embolism: case report and review of the literature. J Emerg Med 49(3):301–304
46. Stewart RM, Rotondo MF. Sharon H, *et al:* Advanced Trauma Life Support ATLS. American College of Surgeons. Tenth Edition. https://viaaerearcp.files.wordpress.com/2018/02/atls-2018.pdf . Accessed 2018
47. Yarmus L, Feller-Kopman D (2012) Pneumothorax in the critically ill patient. Chest 141(4):1098–1105
48. Lichtenstein DA (Ed). *Lung Ultrasound in the Critically Ill: The BLUE Protocol.* Pneumothorax and the A'- Profile. pp 97–108. Springer International Publishing Switzerland 2016.
49. Zhang Z, Chen L (2015) A physiological sign that mimics lung point in critical care ultrasonography. Crit Care 19(1):155
50. Vincent JL, De Backer D (2013) Circulatory Shock. N Engl J Med 369:1726–1734
51. Oren-Grinberg A, Talmor D, Brown S et al (2013) Focused critical care echocardiography. Crit Care Med 41(11):2618–2626
52. Spender KT (2015) Focused cardiac ultrasound: where do we stand? Curr Cardiol Rep 17(3):567
53. Perera P, Mailhot T, Riley D et al (2010) The RUSH exam: Rapid Ultrasound in SHock in the evaluation of the critically Ill. Emerg Med Clin North Am 28(1):29–56
54. Mohammad R, Mohammadhadi G, Ebrahimi A et al (2015) Accuracy of early rapid ultrasound in shock (RUSH) examination performed by emergency physician for diagnosis of shock etiology in critically ill patients. J Emerg Trauma Shock. 8(1):5–10
55. Perea P, Maihot T, Riley D, Examn The RUSH (2012) Rapid ultrasound in shock in the evaluation of the critically ill patient. Ultrasound Clin 7(2012):255–278. https://doi.org/10.1016/j.cult.2011.12.010
56. Volpicelli G, Lamorte A, Tullio M. Point-of-care multiorgan ultrasonography for the evaluation of undifferentiated hypotension in the emergency department. Intensive Care Med 2013;39(7):1290–8. doi: https://doi.org/10.1007/s00134-013-2919-7- and also -Crit Care Med. 2015;43(12):2562–9. doi: https://doi.org/10.1097/CCM.0000000000001285
57. Gardner KF, Clattenburg EJ, Wroe P et al (2018) The Cardiac Arrest Sonographic Assessment (CASA) exam - A standardized approach to the use of ultrasound in PEA. Am J Emerg Med 36(4):729–731
58. Atkinson P, Beckett N, French J et al (2019) Does Point-of-care Ultrasound Use Impact Resuscitation Length, Rates of Intervention, and Clinical Outcomes During Cardiac Arrest? A Study from the Sonography in Hypotension and Cardiac Arrest in the Emergency Department (SHoC-ED) Investigators. Cureus. 11(4):e4456
59. Tsou P-Y, Kurbedin J, Chen Y-S (2017) Accuracy of point-of-care focused echocardiography in predicting outcome of resuscitation in cardiac arrest patients: a systematic review and meta-analysis. Resuscitation 114:92–99
60. Lalande E, Burwash-Bernnan T, Buns K et al (2019) Is point-of-care ultrasound a reliable predictor of outcome during atraumatic, non-shockable cardiac arrest? A systematic review and meta-analysis from the SHoC investigators. Resuscitation. 139:159–166
61. Kedan I, Ciozda W, Palatinus J et al (2020) Prognostic value of point-of-care ultrasound during cardiac arrest: a systematic review. Cardiovasc Ultrasound 18:1
62. Weisfeldt ML, Becker LB (2002) Resuscitation after cardiac arrest: a 3-phase time-sensitive model. JAMA 288(23):3035–3038
63. Orso D et al (2021) Mechanical ventilation management during mechanical chest compressions. Respir Care 66(2):334–346. https://doi.org/10.4187/respcare.07775 (**Epub 2020 Sep 15 PMID: 32934100**)
64. Salen P, O'Connor R et al (2001) Can cardiac sonography and capnography be used independently and in combination to predict resuscitation outcomes? Acad Emerg Med. 8(6):610–5
65. Blaivas M, Fox JC (2001) Outcome in cardiac arrest patients found to have cardiac standstill on the bedside emergency department echocardiogram. Acad Emerg Med 8(6):616–621
66. Tayal VS, Kline J (2003) Emergency echocardiography to detect pericardial effusion in patients in PEA and near-PEA states. Resuscitation 59(3):315–318

67. Salen P, Melniker L, Chooljian C et al (2005) Does the presence or absence of sonographically identified cardiac activity predict resuscitation outcomes of cardiac arrest patients? Am J Emerg Med 23(4):459–462
68. Schuster KM, Lofthouse R, Moore C et al (2009) Pulseless electrical activity, focused abdominal sonography for trauma, and cardiac contractile activity as predictors of survival after trauma. J Trauma 67(6):1154–1157
69. Hayhurst C, Lebus C, Atkinson P et al (2011) An evaluation of echo in life support (ELS): is it feasible? What does it add? Emerg Med J 28(2):119–121
70. Cureton E, Yeung L, Kwan R et al (2012) The heart of the matter: Utility of ultrasound of cardiac activity during traumatic arrest. J Trauma Acute Care Surg 73(1):102–110
71. Tomruk O, Erdur B, Cetin G et al (2012) Assessment of Cardiac Ultrasonography in Predicting Outcome in Adult Cardiac Arrest. J Int Med Res 40(2):804–809
72. Cebicci H, Gurbuz S, Koyuncu S et al (2014) Benefit of cardiac sonography for estimating the early term survival of the cardiopulmonary arrest patients. Hippokratia 18(2):125–129
73. Ozen C, Salcin E, Akoglu H et al (2016) Assessment of ventricular wall motion with focused echocardiography during cardiac arrest to predict survival. Turk J Emerg Med 16(1):12–16
74. Zengin S, Yavuz E, Al B et al (2016) Benefits of cardiac sonography performed by a non-expert sonographer in patients with non-traumatic cardiopulmonary arrest. Resuscitation 102:105–109
75. Kim HB, Suh JY, Choi JH et al (2016) Can serial focussed echocardiographic evaluation in life support (FEEL) predict resuscitation outcome or termination of resuscitation (TOR)? A pilot study. Resuscitation 101:21–26
76. Bolbardi E, Mohsen S, Farzane R et al (2016) The prognostic value of using ultrasonography in cardiac resuscitation of patients with cardiac arrest. Int J Biomed Sci 12(3):110–114

18

Diagnosis at gut point: rapid identification of pneumoperitoneum via point-of-care ultrasound

Matthew A. Taylor[1], Christopher H. Merritt[1], Philip J. Riddle Jr.[2], Carter J. DeGennaro[3] and Keith R. Barron[2,4,5*]

Abstract

Undifferentiated abdominal pain is a common presentation often requiring immediate medical or surgical intervention. Providing an accurate diagnosis involves a detailed patient history and thorough physical exam. Point of care ultrasound is gaining acceptance as a rapid diagnostic tool that can be used to accurately detect life-threatening conditions while potentially avoiding unnecessary radiation exposure and facilitating rapid treatment. Detection of pneumoperitoneum with point-of-care ultrasound is a simple procedure that relies heavily on the experience of the investigating practitioner. Standard technique involves placing a high-frequency linear-array transducer in the right upper quadrant, where abdominal free air is most likely to accumulate. Detection of the 'gut point', which is the transition of abdominal wall sliding to lack thereof in a single image, is the pathognomonic finding of pneumoperitoneum. If visualization is difficult, moving the patient to the left lateral decubitus position or using the scissors technique can provide additional image views. This representative case report and review highlights the use of abdominal POCUS for the diagnosis of pneumoperitoneum. Ultrasound should continue to be explored by clinicians to narrow the differential diagnosis of acute abdominal pain.

Keywords: Ultrasound, Pneumoperitoneum, Free air, Intraperitoneal, Colonoscopy, Small bowel perforation

Background

Medical diagnosis, and undifferentiated abdominal pain in particular, is a complex, intricate, and multifactorial process that relies on years of experience and training. Physicians are often challenged to analyze a series of complicated, nonspecific symptoms, and expected to make a diagnostic conclusion. Undifferentiated abdominal pain is a symptom that points to a wide array of pathologies, ranging from benign to life-threatening conditions [1]. A recent study found that 64% of cases with diagnostic errors had undifferentiated chief complaints, such as abdominal pain [2]. Diagnostic errors may be attributed to a myriad of factors including variations in imaging interpretation, patient complexity, and increased case load [3]. These findings highlight the need for expansion of diagnostic methodologies for chief complaints with a broad differential diagnosis.

In patients with severe, acute abdominal pain, the preferred diagnostic tools are primarily multidetector Computed Tomography (MDCT) and abdominal radiography [4]. However, bedside ultrasonography use may be critical for assessment in certain patient populations where CT use should be limited; such as pregnant women, children, and patients with a previous exposure to high radiation [5, 6]. Recent advances in ultrasound technology allow for smaller, faster, and cheaper ultrasound machines to be used as part of the patient encounter at the bedside, termed point-of-care (POCUS) or bedside ultrasound. POCUS is increasingly being used, but investigation into its use in situations of undifferentiated abdominal pain are somewhat limited [7]. These limitations are largely due to the high skillset required to use

*Correspondence: Keith.Barron@uscmed.sc.edu
[5] Palmetto Health-USC Medical Group, 5 Medical Park Road, Columbia, SC 29203, USA
Full list of author information is available at the end of the article

and interpret ultrasound accurately as a diagnostic tool [8].

One potential etiology of undifferentiated abdominal pain is post-operative pneumoperitoneum, an often life-threatening condition that requires immediate surgical care to abrogate its high risk of mortality [9]. This case report and literature review will discuss the finding of intraperitoneal free air on POCUS led to the diagnosis of perforated small bowel following diagnostic colonoscopy. Then, the procedural technique and diagnostic criteria used to make the diagnosis will be reviewed, discussing how bedside ultrasound can best be used to complement CT and X-ray imaging in making a rapid diagnosis.

Case presentation

An 81-year-old woman presented to the emergency department with hematochezia. Although she had chronic nonspecific abdominal pain, she denied significant pain on presentation. She had no prior gastrointestinal bleeds, NSAID use, vaginal bleeding, or vaginal discharge. Remaining history was noncontributory. Physical examination was significant for diffuse abdominal tenderness and gross blood on digital rectal exam. Vital signs were unremarkable. Her hemoglobin was 9.9 g/dL, decreased relative to a known baseline of 14 g/dL. The patient was admitted to the hospitalist service for further evaluation of lower gastrointestinal bleeding.

The initial CT of the abdomen and pelvis only showed colonic diverticulosis without any findings of inflammation or free intraperitoneal air. During the first 24 h after admission, the patient required multiple transfusions of packed red blood cells. The gastroenterology team was consulted and ordered nuclear imaging given the large volume blood loss, which revealed no scintigraphic evidence of active GI bleeding. Esophagogastroduodenoscopy (EGD) was subsequently performed and was grossly unremarkable. A colonoscopy was then performed on hospital day 2, noting numerous diverticula, none of which appeared to be bleeding. The plan at that time was to monitor the patient given that she was hemodynamically stable, and her hemoglobin had stabilized without additional evidence of active bleeding.

The following day, the rounding hospitalist noted the patient had become acutely confused and complained of worsening abdominal pain. The hospitalist, who has received extensive POCUS training through completion of a primary care ultrasound fellowship [10], performed a bedside ultrasound of the abdomen and immediately noticed a diffuse A-line pattern without sliding of the visceral and parietal peritoneum; a "gut point" indicating a transition zone between free intraperitoneal air and abdominal contents was noted, strongly suggesting pneumoperitoneum (Fig. 1). A general surgeon was consulted,

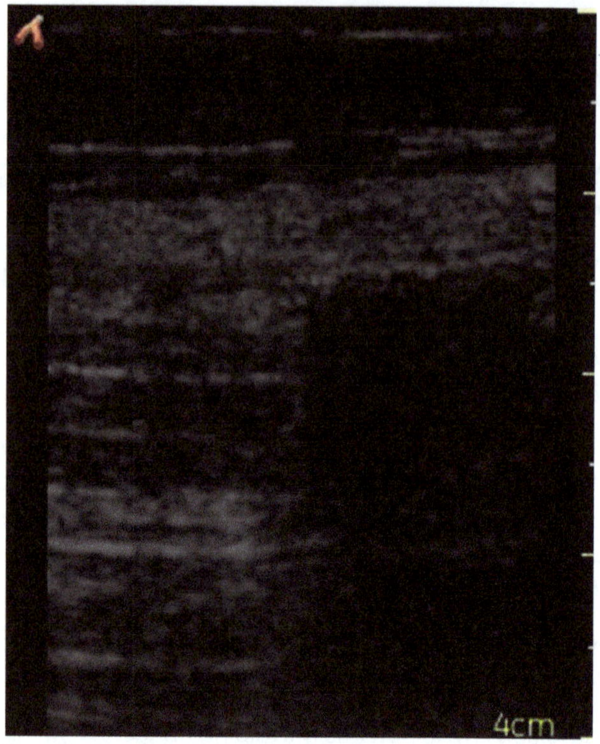

Fig. 1 The "gut point" is the transition zone between normal bowel artifact, that may normally contain A-lines, and the abnormal A-line pattern without sliding. Similar to pneumothorax, an absence of sliding with the presence of A-lines is a diagnostic indicator of pathologic free air

and a subsequent abdominal X-ray was ordered, showing significant free air throughout the abdomen as well as dilated prominent segments of the intestine, suggestive of ileus (Fig. 2). These findings were discussed with family, who wished to forego surgical intervention for probable iatrogenic colonic perforation and elected for conservative management.

Over the next hospital day, the patient had frequent episodes of hypotension and hypothermia and was transferred to the medical ICU, where she was started on vasopressors. She later developed persistent atrial fibrillation with rapid ventricular rate. The palliative care team was consulted, and comfort care was initiated. The patient died on hospital day 6.

Ultrasonographic identification of pneumoperitoneum

Technical background

A tissue–air interface acts as a strong reflector of ultrasound waves. Its strong acoustic reverberations are detected as bright repeating horizontal artifacts. In lung ultrasound, these repeating echogenic artifacts below the pleural line are often termed A-lines [11–13] (Fig. 3).

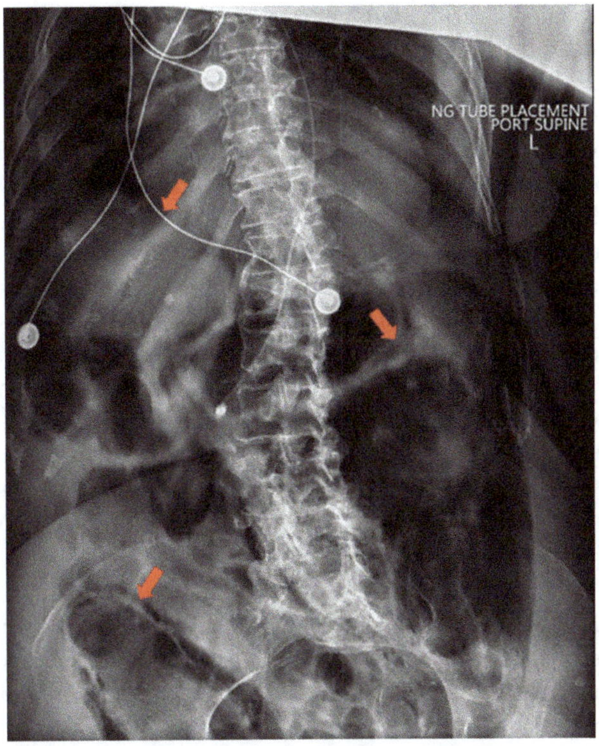

Fig. 2 Abdominal X-ray showing free intraperitoneal air due to a small bowl perforation. This image depicts suprahepatic accumulation of free air, which is considered a hallmark sign of pneumoperitoneum

In the abdomen, tissue–air interfaces are common, given the high air content within bowels in a normal patient, often resulting in multiple horizontal, repeating, echogenic artifacts, particularly over the colon. Thus, physiologic intra-intestinal air may easily be confused with pathologic free abdominal air. To differentiate between the two entities many authors have described different signs, although their varying descriptions may be somewhat confusing to novice ultrasound operators.

For example, intra-intestinal air will be seen moving with peristalsis or respiration. Intraperitoneal free air is generally located under the abdominal fascia and will not be affected by respiration [14]. Abdominal free air produces a strong linear echo with a pathognomonic peritoneal stripe sign [15]. Imaging consists of a single or double echogenic line posterior to the anterior abdominal wall [16]. Of note, visualization may be difficult in obese patients [17].

Standard technique

Patients should be placed in the supine position to allow free air to rise just beneath the anterior abdominal wall. Either a convex or linear transducer can be used, but the high-frequency (4–8 MHz) linear transducer is preferred. This will produce a shallow, but high-resolution image of anterior abdominal gas pockets while reducing interference of deep intestinal air [18]. Right upper

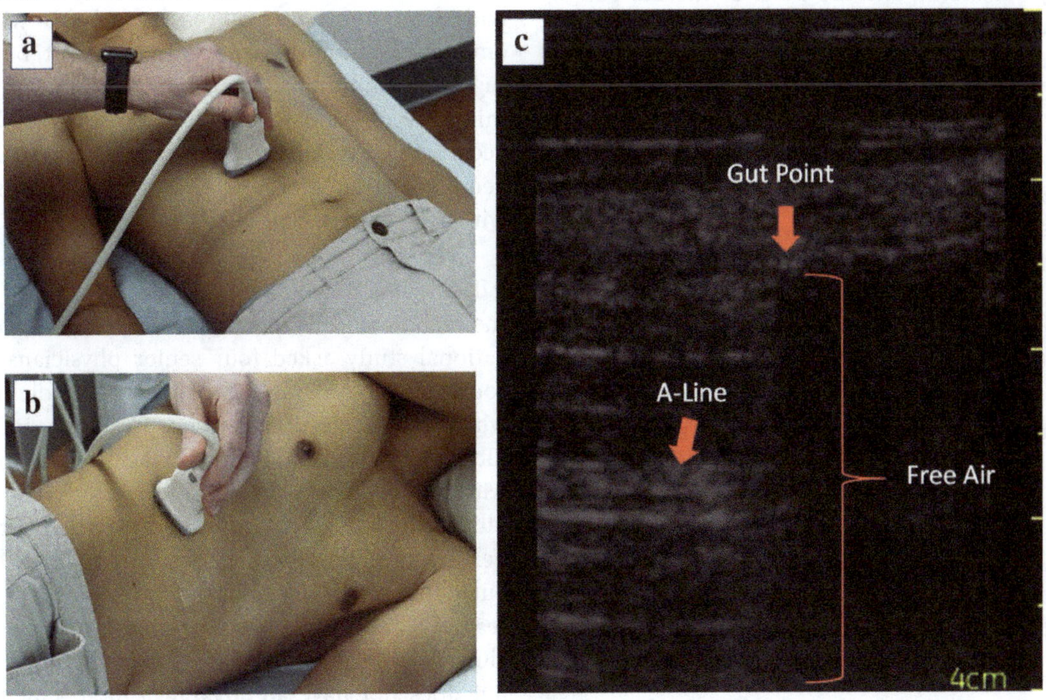

Fig. 3 **a** Patient placed in the supine position for an initial sonographic assessment for free intraperitoneal air. **b** Patient placed in the lateral decubitus position to allow free intraperitoneal air to accumulate anterior to the hepatic parenchyma. **c** Sonographic output of a patient with free intraperitoneal air. Air is a strong reflector of ultrasound waves. Reflection produces bright focal lines (A-lines, red arrow) with dark shadowing in between

quadrant imaging will provide the highest chance of detection, because free air will most likely accumulate anterior to the liver (Fig. 3a). It may be difficult to differentiate between intestinal air and abdominal free air due to similar appearing reverberation artifacts. If this is the case, the patient can be placed in the left lateral decubitus position for at least 2 min (Fig. 3b), encouraging free air to move to the area of least resistance and causing a shift of the reverberation artifacts. Any potential free air can be more easily seen around the hepatic parenchyma as hyperechoic reverberations that fluctuate with abdominal compression [19].

Abdominal sliding and "gut point"

For ultrasound operators familiar with lung ultrasound, a "gut point" may be thought of as analogous to a "lung point" found in pneumothorax [20]. In normal patients, a subtle sliding or shimmering is present along the peritoneal line, indicating apposition of the visceral and parietal peritoneum. The pathologic presence of intrabdominal air separates these structures, abolishing this artifact if free air abuts the peritoneum (Fig. 1) [11]. The presence of sliding allows the examiner to differentiate between pathologic abdominal free air and physiologic bowel gas, both of which generate repeating horizontal artifacts similar to A-lines. Sliding the probe laterally, a "gut point" may be seen at the transition point where both abdominal sliding and the absence thereof can be seen in a single ultrasound image (Figs. 1, 3c). Obtaining this image is a diagnostic hallmark of pneumoperitoneum [11] (Additional file 1: Video S1).

Scissors maneuver

The scissors maneuver can also be used to help detect intraperitoneal free air. It involves lightly placing a linear-array transducer parasagitally in the right epigastric region with the patient lying supine. The transducer should be lightly placed on the abdomen with careful consideration to not compress the skin surface. If reverberation artifacts are seen with a suspicion of abdominal free air, gently press the caudal end of the probe onto the abdomen. This should press the free air away from the anterior liver. The reverberation artifacts that were previously obstructing the liver should now be less prominent. Releasing the pressure from the probe should allow the free gas to return and make the reverberation artifacts more visible [21].

Discussion

Pneumoperitoneum arises from a variety of causes in both operative and non-operative settings. Exact patho physiology varies, but generally pneumoperitoneum is caused by a perforated hollow viscus in 85–90% of cases [22]. Recently, pneumoperitoneum has seen an increased incidence due to the greater utilization of minimally invasive endoscopies; leading to a bowel perforation in approximately 1.5 out every 1000 procedures (0.15%) [23]. The greatest independent risk factors include patients over 75 years old and those undergoing therapeutic colonoscopy [24, 25]. The differential diagnosis of non-operative causes of pneumoperitoneum is vast, including Crohn disease, diverticulitis, peptic ulcer disease, and malignancy [26–29]. Peptic ulcer disease and diverticulitis are the leading causes of gastrointestinal perforation (16%), followed by trauma (14%), malignancy (14%), and endoscopy (4%) [30]. Positive clinical outcomes are highly dependent on rapid identification and subsequent surgical intervention [31].

Most cases of suspected pneumoperitoneum are evaluated with CT or radiography [4]. CT is the gold standard for diagnosis but is often preceded by long wait times and unnecessary radiation exposure. A study by Chen and colleagues of 188 patients demonstrated that POCUS for identifying pneumoperitoneum can provide better sensitivity and diagnostic accuracy than abdominal radiography. Overall, ultrasound had improved sensitivity over radiography (92% vs. 78%) but similar specificity (both 53%). They found that both radiography and ultrasound had detection rates approaching 100% when a large amount of abdominal free air was present, but for detecting small amounts of free air originating from pathologic micro-perforations, ultrasound surpassed radiography in accuracy [12]. This can be attributed to the bright echogenic appearance of air on ultrasound that is detectable with air volumes as little as 1 mL [32].

The major downfall of POCUS is its heavy reliance on the technical skills of the operator. A prospective observational study asked four senior physicians with ultrasound experience and two internal medicine residents with no ultrasound experience to blindly interpret both ultrasound and radiographic images of patients with and without pneumoperitoneum. The study concluded that ultrasound had a higher sensitivity for detecting pneumoperitoneum compared to radiography (95.5% vs. 72.2%), but had a lower specificity (81.8% vs. 92.5%) [8]. These results are similar in comparison to previous studies concluding ultrasound surpasses radiography in sensitivity but does not have an advantage in specificity [12]. The diagnostic accuracy of internal medicine residents varied compared to senior physicians with ultrasound experience. Even though both cohorts did not have specific training in diagnosing pneumoperitoneum, senior physicians had a diagnostic accuracy of 89% compared to 68% accuracy by the residents. The authors emphasize that minimal ultrasound training can greatly improve a physician's diagnostic efficacy.

Many patients with risk factors for pneumoperitoneum may fall under medical, rather than surgical, care. This highlights the importance of not limiting pneumoperitoneum as a diagnostic consideration to surgical floors and emergency departments. Hospitalists and intensivists should consider pneumoperitoneum in patients presenting with undifferentiated abdominal pain with an additional history of abdominal pathology. To account for its low prevalence, ultrasound can be used as a rapid diagnostic tool to differentiate life-threatening pneumoperitoneum while also preventing unnecessary radiation exposure [5]. Such use of ultrasound may be particularly valuable in resource-poor settings, where access to more-advanced diagnostic imaging modalities may be limited.

Conclusion

Undifferentiated abdominal pain is a common diagnostic dilemma that may not always present with a clear answer. Understanding the basic technique of the abdominal ultrasound exam, along with the ability to differentiate between intestinal and free abdominal air provides clinicians with an additional imaging modality to rapidly detect life-threatening cases of acute pneumoperitoneum. Due to its high sensitivity, low cost, and safety profile, abdominal ultrasound should be considered a first-line imaging modality for diagnosing pneumoperitoneum, as demonstrated in the previously described case presentation. While already widely embraced by emergency medicine, improved ultrasound education in the primary care and surgical specialties will enable the confidence and proficiency to fully realize the scope of ultrasound as a powerful diagnostic tool.

Supplementary information

Additional file 1: Video S1. The "gut point" is the transition zone between normal bowel artifact, that may normally contain A-lines, and the abnormal A-line pattern without sliding. Similar to pneumothorax, an absence of sliding with the presence of A-lines is a diagnostic indicator of pathologic free air.

Acknowledgements

We would like to thank the University of South Carolina School of Medicine Ultrasound Institute and Prisma Health Richland Hospital, Columbia, SC.

Authors' contributions

Conceptualization: MT, CM, PR, CD, KB. Manuscript writing: MT, CM. Manuscript editing: PR, KB. Case analysis: MT, CD, KB. All authors read and approved the final manuscript.

Author details

[1] University of South Carolina School of Medicine, Columbia, SC 29209, USA. [2] Department of Internal Medicine, Prisma Health Midlands, University of South Carolina School of Medicine, Columbia, SC 29209, USA. [3] Department of Emergency Medicine, Prisma Health Midlands, University of South Carolina School of Medicine, Columbia, SC 29209, USA. [4] Ultrasound Institute, University of South Carolina School of Medicine, Columbia, SC 29209, USA. [5] Palmetto Health-USC Medical Group, 5 Medical Park Road, Columbia, SC 29203, USA.

References

1. Zhang Y, Padman R, Epner P, Bauer V, Solomonides A et al (2018) Identifying diagnostic paths for undifferentiated abdominal pain from electronic health record data. AMIA Summits Transl Sci Proc 2017:290–299
2. Zwaan L, De Bruijne M, Wagner C, Thijs A, Smits M et al (2010) Patient record review of the incidence, consequences, and causes of diagnostic adverse events. Arch Intern Med 170:1015–1021. https://doi.org/10.1001/archinternmed.2010.146
3. Mazzei MA, Volterrani L (2015) Errors in multidetector row computed tomography. Radiol Med 120:785–794. https://doi.org/10.1007/s11547-015-0558-5
4. Paolantonio P, Rengo M, Ferrari R, Laghi A (2016) Multidetector CT in emergency radiology: acute and generalized non-traumatic abdominal pain. Br J Radiol. https://doi.org/10.1259/bjr.20150859
5. Mazzei MA, Guerrini S, Squitieri NC, Cagini L, Macarini L et al (2013) The role of US examination in the management of acute abdomen. Crit Ultrasound J 5:1–9. https://doi.org/10.1186/2036-7902-5-S1-S6
6. Casciani E, De Vincentiis C, Mazzei MA, Masselli G, Guerrini S et al (2015) Errors in imaging the pregnant patient with acute abdomen. Abdom Imaging 40:2112–2126. https://doi.org/10.1007/s00261-015-0508-7
7. Moore CL, Copel JA (2011) Point-of-care ultrasonography. N Engl J Med 364:749–757. https://doi.org/10.1056/NEJMra0909487
8. Nazerian P, Tozzetti C, Vanni S, Bartolucci M, Gualtieri S et al (2015) Accuracy of abdominal ultrasound for the diagnosis of pneumoperitoneum in patients with acute abdominal pain: a pilot study. Crit Ultrasound J. https://doi.org/10.1186/s13089-015-0032-6
9. Langell JT, Mulvihill SJ (2008) Gastrointestinal perforation and the acute abdomen. Med Clin North Am 92:599–625. https://doi.org/10.1016/j.mcna.2007.12.004
10. Barron KR, Wagner MS, Hunt PS, Rao VV, Bell FE et al (2018) A primary care ultrasound fellowship: training for clinical practice and future educators. J Ultrasound Med. https://doi.org/10.1002/jum.14772
11. Bade BC, Callahan SP, Higuero JP, Pastis N, Huggins JT (2016) 83-year-old man with chronic kidney disease, fluid overload, and coronary artery disease develops altered mental status. Chest 149:e111–e114. https://doi.org/10.1016/j.chest.2015.11.032
12. Chen S-C, Yen Z-S, Wang H-P, Lin F-Y, Hsu C-Y et al (2002) Ultrasonography is superior to plain radiography in the diagnosis of pneumoperitoneum. Br J Surg 89:351–354. https://doi.org/10.1046/j.0007-1323.2001.02013.x
13. Goudie A (2013) Detection of intraperitoneal free gas by ultrasound. Australas J Ultrasound Med 16:56–61. https://doi.org/10.1002/j.2205-0140.2013.tb00166.x
14. Abu-Zidan FM, Cevik AA (2018) Diagnostic point-of-care ultrasound (POCUS) for gastrointestinal pathology: state of the art from basics to advanced. World J Emerg Surg 13:1–14. https://doi.org/10.1186/s13017-018-0209-y
15. Hoffmann B, Nürnberg D, Westergaard MC (2012) Focus on abnormal air: diagnostic ultrasonography for the acute abdomen. Eur J Emerg Med 19:284–291. https://doi.org/10.1097/MEJ.0b013e3283543cd3
16. Dahine J, Giard A, Chagnon DO, Denault A (2016) Ultrasound findings in critical care patients: the "liver sign" and other abnormal abdominal air patterns. Crit Ultrasound J. https://doi.org/10.1186/s13089-016-0039-7
17. Ghaffar A, Siddiqui TS, Haider H, Khatri H (2008) Postsurgical pneumoperitoneum—comparison of abdominal ultrasound findings with plain radiography. J Coll Physicians Surg Pak 18:477–480
18. Hefny AF, Abu-Zidan FM (2011) Sonographic diagnosis of intraperitoneal free air. J Emerg Trauma Shock 4:511–513. https://doi.org/10.4103/0974-2700.86649

19. Jones R (2007) Recognition of pneumoperitoneum using bedside ultrasound in critically ill patients presenting with acute abdominal pain. Am J Emerg Med 25:838–841. https://doi.org/10.1016/j.ajem.2007.02.004
20. Volpicelli G, Elbarbary M, Blaivas M, Lichtenstein DA, Mathis G et al (2012) International evidence-based recommendations for point-of-care lung ultrasound. Intensive Care Med 38:577–591. https://doi.org/10.1007/s00134-012-2513-4
21. Karahan OI, Kurt A, Yikilmaz A, Kahriman G (2004) New method for the detection of intraperitoneal free air by sonography: scissors maneuver. J Clin Ultrasound 32:381–385. https://doi.org/10.1002/jcu.20055
22. Tanner TN, Hall BR, Oran J (2018) Pneumoperitoneum. Surg Clin North Am 98:915–932. https://doi.org/10.1016/j.suc.2018.06.004
23. Paspatis GA, Dumonceau JM, Barthet M, Meisner S, Repici A et al (2014) Diagnosis and management of iatrogenic endoscopic perforations: European Society of Gastrointestinal Endoscopy (ESGE) position statement. Endoscopy 46:693–711
24. Lohsiriwat V, Sujarittanakarn S, Akaraviputh T, Lertakyamanee N, Lohsiriwat D et al (2009) What are the risk factors of colonoscopic perforation? BMC Gastroenterol 9:71. https://doi.org/10.1186/1471-230X-9-71
25. Joudeh LA, Newman MG (2018) Nonoperative management of pneumoperitoneum after colonoscopy. Baylor Univ Med Cent Proc 31:465–466. https://doi.org/10.1080/08998280.2018.1498722
26. Roy MK, Delicata RJ, Carey PD (1997) Crohn's disease presenting with acute colonic perforation. Postgrad Med J 73:645–646. https://doi.org/10.1136/pgmj.73.864.645
27. Paulson EK, Thompson WM (2015) Review of small-bowel obstruction: the diagnosis and when to worry. Radiology 275:332–342. https://doi.org/10.1148/radiol.15131519
28. Kothari K, Friedman B, Grimaldi GM, Hines JJ (2017) Nontraumatic large bowel perforation: spectrum of etiologies and CT findings. Abdom Radiol 42:2597–2608. https://doi.org/10.1007/s00261-017-1180-x
29. Mazzei MA, Squitieri NC, Guerrini S, Ianora AAS, Cagini L et al (2013) Sigmoid diverticulitis: US findings. Crit Ultrasound J 5:1–7. https://doi.org/10.1186/2036-7902-5-S1-S5
30. Kumar A, Muir MT, Cohn SM, Salhanick MA, Lankford DB et al (2012) The etiology of pneumoperitoneum in the 21st century. J Trauma Acute Care Surg 73:542–548. https://doi.org/10.1097/TA.0b013e31825c157f
31. An SB, Shin DW, Kim JY, Park SG, Lee BH et al (2016) Decision-making in the management of colonoscopic perforation: a multicentre retrospective study. Surg Endosc Other Interv Tech 30:2914–2921. https://doi.org/10.1007/s00464-015-4577-z
32. Seitz K, Reising KD (1982) Ultrasound detection of free air in the abdominal cavity. Ultraschall Med 3:4–6

The ultrasound competency assessment tool for four-view cardiac POCUS

Colin Bell[1,2*], Natalie Wagner[3], Andrew Hall[2,4,5,6], Joseph Newbigging[2], Louise Rang[2] and Conor McKaigney[1]

Abstract

Background: Point-of-care ultrasound (POCUS) has been recognized as an essential skill across medicine. However, a lack of reliable and streamlined POCUS assessment tools with demonstrated validity remains a significant barrier to widespread clinical integration. The ultrasound competency assessment tool (UCAT) was derived to be a simple, entrustment-based competency assessment tool applicable to multiple POCUS applications. When used to assess a FAST, the UCAT demonstrated high internal consistency and moderate-to-excellent inter-rater reliability. The objective of this study was to validate the UCAT for assessment of a four-view transthoracic cardiac POCUS.

Results: Twenty-two trainees performed a four-view transthoracic cardiac POCUS in a simulated environment while being assessed by two observers. When used to assess a four-view cardiac POCUS the UCAT retained its high internal consistency ($\alpha = 0.90$) and moderate-to-excellent inter-rater reliability (ICCs = 0.61–0.91; p's ≤ 0.01) across all domains. The regression analysis suggestion that level of training, previous number of focused cardiac ultrasound, previous number of total scans, self-rated entrustment, and intent to pursue certification statistically significantly predicted UCAT entrustment scores [$F(5,16) = 4.06$, $p = 0.01$; $R^2 = 0.56$].

Conclusion: This study confirms the UCAT is a valid assessment tool for four-view transthoracic cardiac POCUS. The findings from this work and previous studies on the UCAT demonstrate the utility and flexibility of the UCAT tool across multiple POCUS applications and present a promising way forward for POCUS competency assessment.

Keywords: POCUS, Medical education, Cardiac ultrasound, Assessment, Competency-based medical education, Focused echocardiography

Background

Point-of-care ultrasound (POCUS) has become an integral diagnostic and interventional tool within medicine [1]. For physicians from many specialty backgrounds, POCUS skills are recognized as vital to their practice of medicine. Furthermore, multiple medical societies have made strong recommendations about the inclusion of POCUS applications into bedside patient care, such as incorporating focused cardiac ultrasound into the initial assessment of patients with cardiopulmonary instability and undifferentiated shock [2]. While many trainees and faculty engage in POCUS training, and some POCUS assessment tools already exist [3–8], a lack of reliable and streamlined competency assessment processes with demonstrated validity remains a significant barrier to widespread clinical integration [9].

The Ultrasound Competency Assessment Tool (UCAT) [10], which utilizes a modern global entrustment scale [11] has recently been presented as an alternative to traditional checklist-based scales. The UCAT was expert derived using Delphi methodology to be a rapid and easy-to-use assessment tool relevant across most POCUS applications. While the initial UCAT study provided some validity evidence for its use in the evaluation of the focused assessment with sonography for trauma (FAST), demonstrating strong inter-rater reliability and

*Correspondence: Colinbell85@gmail.com
[1] Department of Emergency Medicine & Cumming School of Medicine, Emergency Physician, Calgary Zone, Alberta Health Services, University of Calgary, 7007 14th St. SW, Calgary, AB T2V1P9, Canada
Full list of author information is available at the end of the article

internal consistency, the UCAT was unable to discriminate between levels of training [10]. As the literature suggests that the FAST is a fairly simple POCUS assessment [12, 13], due to its large, accessible sonographic windows, it raises questions as to whether the lack of discriminatory ability was a result of the UCAT tool or the POCUS task itself. This limitation in the initial UCAT derivation study highlighted the need to explore the use of the UCAT with other POCUS applications [10].

A transthoracic cardiac POCUS, consisting of the cardinal four views (parasternal long, parasternal short, subxiphoid and apical four chamber), has a steeper learning curve than FAST and some other POCUS applications [12, 13]. Components of the four-view cardiac POCUS are regarded as more challenging due to smaller sonographic windows caused by intercostal spaces, variable location of the ideal interspace for cardiac visualization [14] and lung artifact. Occasionally changes in patient positioning and maneuvers coordinating image acquisition with the respiratory cycle are required. These factors can make image generation and image optimization more complex compared to other POCUS assessments such as the FAST. Thus, the objective of this study was to build on previous work and utilize the entrustment-based UCAT to assess POCUS competency for trainees performing a focused four-view cardiac ultrasound.

Methods

Study context

This study took place within the University of Calgary Emergency Medicine (EM) program. This program has two training streams with 20 trainees in the Royal College of Physicians and Surgeons specialist stream and 8 trainees in the Canadian College of Family Physicians enhanced skills Emergency Medicine stream. All trainees work in the same clinical environment and participate in shared academic days. In August 2019, trainees from both programs were invited to participate in this study during an existing academic day for oral exam practice. Informed consent was obtained from all trainees and participation in the study was voluntary. Performance had no impact on program academic standing. Ethics approval was provided by the University of Calgary (No. 18-0373) and Queen's University Health Science Research Ethics Board (No. 6023366).

Design

Prior to participating in the POCUS assessment, trainees completed a brief digital questionnaire on the Qualtrics survey platform (Provo, UT) quantifying their past ultrasound experience on different types of POCUS, including self-estimated previous number and types of POCUS scans performed, self-rated UCAT entrustment at POCUS (including all POCUS, and specifically FAST and four-view focused cardiac POCUS), intent to pursue ultrasound certification as a proxy for POCUS motivation, and previous exposure to ultrasound training.

Trainees were then assessed sequentially performing focused cardiac POCUS on a healthy, live simulated patient with suitable sonographic windows verified by one of the assessors (CM). Participants were first read a brief standardized stem by one of the assessors (CM), and then allowed 10 min to complete the station. The stem requested the examination of a previously healthy young male patient presenting with normal vital signs presenting and sudden onset acute dyspnea. The stem specifically requested the trainee perform and interpret a focused cardiac ultrasound consisting of the cardinal four two-dimensional (2D) views (parasternal long, parasternal short, subxiphoid and apical four chamber) and then articulate the subsequent investigations and management plan based on the POCUS results in the context of the stem and simulated patient. To standardize the assessment as much as possible, after completion of the scenario by each participant, the entire station including the POCUS machine placement and settings, bed position, and model positioning and draping were returned to their initial state. This was performed to blind the incoming trainee from actions performed by the previous participant. The focused cardiac ultrasound was selected because it has been demonstrated to be a more difficult POCUS application [12].

Two fellowship-trained sonographers watched each performance live (CB and CM), and independently assessed the trainees' POCUS competency using the UCAT. The UCAT was designed to be user-friendly and applicable to a broad range of POCUS applications. The UCAT consists of four domains (preparation, image acquisition, image optimization, and clinical integration), each with behavioral descriptors, as well as a single overall entrustment score (Additional file 1). A detailed description of the UCAT development and initial implementation can be found elsewhere [10]. Of the two raters, one assessor (CB) was from a different training site and had not previously interacted with the residents in a clinical or teaching environment making him blind to participants' previous POCUS experience.

Statistical analysis

Descriptive statistics were calculated on the questionnaire responses and UCAT scores for the focused cardiac ultrasound. A paired t-test compared participants self-rated entrustment on FAST versus cardiac POCUS. Two-way random, Intra-class Correlation Coefficients (ICC) were used to evaluate the inter-rater reliability across each performance domain. Cronbach's alpha was calculated to measure internal consistency, or agreement across performance domains. Raters' scores were then averaged for each domain and combined to create a composite score across all domains for each participant. A standard multiple regression analysis was used to explore the impact of postgraduate year (PGY), previous number of POCUS scans (total), previous number of focused cardiac ultrasound scans, self-reported entrustment on an advanced cardiac POCUS, and intent to pursue a POCUS certification on UCAT scores. The regression was run twice, once using the composite score as the UCAT performance outcome and once using the entrustment score alone, to evaluate whether the two indices provided similar information. All statistical analyses were conducted with SPSS Version 25 (IBM SPSS Statistics, Armonk, New York, USA). Statistical significance was considered at $p \leq 0.05$.

Results

A total of 22/28 (79%) of the Calgary EM trainees participated in our study. Participants represented PGY1 to PGY4 only, with PGY5 trainees unavailable due to their rotation and study schedules. Participants had variable experience doing FAST and focused cardiac ultrasound (Table 1). The paired t-test suggested that participants' self-rated entrustment for FAST was significantly higher than their self-rated entrustment for cardiac POCUS [$t(21)=6.5$, $p<0.001$). Participant self-ratings are also presented in Table 1.

Results of the intra-class correlation analyses suggested moderate-to-excellent inter-rater reliability across the UCAT domains, with ICC values of 0.61–0.91; $ps \leq 0.01$ (Table 2; ICC guidelines from Koo and Li 2016) [8]. In all cases when the raters varied, the variation was only by one point on the five-point scale. The results of the Cronbach's alpha suggested high internal consistency among performance categories in the UCAT ($\alpha = 0.90$).

Lastly, the multiple regression analysis suggested that PGY, previous number of focused cardiac ultrasound, previous number of total scans, self-rated entrustment, and intent to pursue certification statistically significantly predicted UCAT entrustment scores [$F(5,16)=4.06$, $p=0.01$; $R^2=0.56$]. While no variable was a statistically significant predictor on its own (Table 3), the factor that accounted for the most variance was self-rated entrustment on POCUS. When the analysis was run with UCAT composite scores as the outcome, the results were very similar (Table 3). Composite UCAT scores and entrustment scores alone are displayed by PGY in Fig. 1. Notably, while PGY was not a significant factor in the regression analysis, descriptive statistics suggest that the PGY4s UCAT scores were the highest among study participants, and that there was larger variation around the mean among PGY3s, compared to other cohorts (Fig. 1).

Table 1 Previous POCUS experience and self-rated entrustment

PGY	n	Previous number of scans: FAST		Previous number of scans: four-view cardiac		Previous number of scans: total		Self-rated entrustment (1 to 5)	
		Average (SD)	Range	Average (SD)	Range	Average (SD)	Range	FAST	Cardiac POCUS
PGY1	2/4	37 (5)	31–41	7 (7)	0–15	112 (11)	99–120	3.0 (0)	1.67 (0.6)
PGY2	4/4	82 (41)	57–144	58 (42)	2–101	355 (146)	234–560	3.75 (0.5)	2.0 (1.4)
PGY3	4/4	118 (39)	70–150	37 (19)	15–55	408 (90)	320–496	4.75 (0.5)	3.5 (1.3)
PGY4	3/4	171 (112)	97–300	35 (14)	23–50	572 (371)	348–1000	4.67 (0.6)	3.33 (0.6)
PGY5	0/4								
CCFP-EM	8/8	54 (52)	0–150	12 (14)	0–34	186 (173)	3–477	3.75 (1.4)	2.37 (1.1)

Table 2 Mean scores across raters and Intra-class Correlations Coefficients per domain

UCAT domain	Rater 1 (CB) Mean (SD)	Rater 1 (CB) Range	Rater 2 (CM) Mean (SD)	Rater 2 (CM) Range	Average of Two Raters	ICC (Absolute Agreement)	*p*-value
Preparation	2.45 (0.51)	2.0–3.0	2.60 (0.67)	1.0–3.0	2.52	0.71	0.003*
Image acquisition	1.64 (0.66)	1.0–3.0	1.77 (0.68)	1.0–3.0	1.70	0.86	<0.001*
Image optimization	1.64 (0.73)	1.0–3.0	1.91 (0.75)	1.0–3.0	1.78	0.61	0.01*
Clinical integration	2.14 (0.56)	1.0–3.0	2.32 (0.65)	1.0–3.0	2.23	0.68	0.005*
Entrustment	2.55 (1.14)	1.0–5.0	2.76 (1.09)	1.0–5.0	2.65	0.91	<0.001*

*Significance considered at $p \leq 0.05$

Table 3 Predictive factors for UCAT score

Factors	Entrustment scores beta coefficient	Entrustment scores t value	Entrustment scores *p*-values (sig.)	Composite scores beta coefficient	Composite scores t value	Composite scores *p*-values (sig.)
Number of total scans	0.43	1.46	0.16	0.32	1.02	0.32
PGY	− 0.11	− 0.40	0.70	− 1.08	− 0.36	0.73
Number of previous focused cardiac ultrasound scans	− 0.28	− 1.24	0.23	− 0.18	− 0.76	0.46
Intent to pursue POCUS certification	− 0.31	− 1.08	0.30	− 0.18	− 0.60	0.56
Self-rated entrustment focused cardiac ultrasound	0.47	1.97	0.07	0.54	2.15	0.05
All factors combined	R^2	F value (df)	*p*-value (sig)	R^2	F value (df)	*p*-value (sig)
	0.56	F (5,16) = 4.06	0.01	0.50	F (5,16) = 3.21	0.03

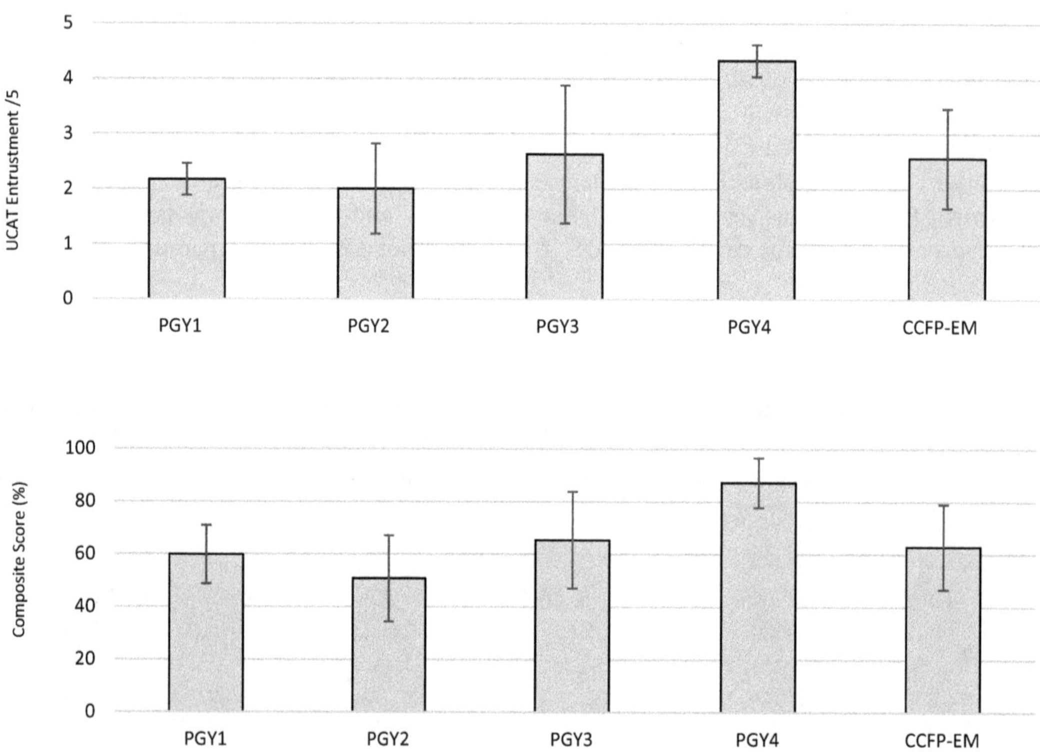

Fig. 1 UCAT score by postgraduate year (PGY)

Discussion

The UCAT was created to be a universally applicable, entrustment-based, POCUS competency assessment tool [10]. An early argument for validity of the UCAT for the assessment of FAST competency has been previously published as part of its derivation [10]. This current study sought to expand on previous work and explore the use of the UCAT with a more technically difficult application, the four-view cardiac POCUS. Using Messick's validity framework [15], we articulate how this study provides further validity evidence for the UCAT in the domains of internal structure validity (internal consistency, inter-rater reliability) and relations with other variables. We then propose how individuals and programs engaging in POCUS training and assessment can utilize the UCAT in their programs of assessment.

Internal structure validity

Our results suggest that the UCAT maintains high internal consistency ($\alpha = 0.90$) when used to assess cardiac POCUS, and that all four domains (preparation, image acquisition, image optimization, clinical integration) as well as the entrustment rating, captured relevant, but not redundant, information on POCUS competency. As per Koo and Li's (2016) Intra-Class Correlation (ICC) guidelines [16], the results of this study also demonstrate that the UCAT domains have moderate-to-excellent inter-rater reliability (ICCs=0.61–0.91). This level of agreement was achieved with one local rater who was aware of trainees' level and general ability, and one external rater who was blinded to the trainee's experience, which speaks to the strength of the tool. The inter-rater reliability and internal consistency findings are consistent with the UCAT results found when assessing a FAST [10], suggesting that the UCAT is a reliable POCUS assessment tool across multiple POCUS applications.

Consistent with previous literature [17, 18], the entrustment category had the highest Intra-class Correlation Coefficients (ICC=0.91). Global assessment of observable competencies using entrustment scales has become commonplace in postgraduate education, where the typical goal is to capture the assessors tacit capacity for judgement of the need for supervision of a trainee [19]. The UCAT both facilitates this global assessment of competency via an overall entrustment score and also provides individual domain scoring which may serve to facilitate feedback and coaching for improvement (or assessment *for* learning) [20]. The use of domain specific items and overall entrustment aligns with modern programs of assessment in North America, including the structure of entrustable professional activities and milestones in the Canadian Competency by Design framework [21], and milestones and sub-competencies in the ACGME Milestones Project [22]. Additionally, as our work identified similar validity evidence for the domain specific scores and the overall entrustment score, we believe both are critical and reliable features of the UCAT.

Correlations with other variables

The argument for the validity of the UCAT is further bolstered by its correlation with other variables that are traditionally used as indicators of POCUS competency, such as PGY, previous experience, intent to pursue POCUS certification, and self-rated entrustment or confidence. The results of this study suggest that together, these variables predicted UCAT scores [F (5,16)=4.06, p=0.01; R^2=0.56]. Although no variables were statistically significant predictors on their own, there were notable differences in mean UCAT scores based on PGY. Despite the PGY2-4 s having similar experience with POCUS scans (Table 1), the results of this study suggest that the PGY4 cohort outperformed the other trainees on the cardiac POCUS exam with a median entrustment score of ≥ 4 *out of* 5 on the UCAT. These results align with previous literature suggesting the number of previous scans and PGY year are not sufficiently reliable indicators of competency in isolation [12, 23–25], reinforcing the need for an assessment tool like the UCAT.

Moreover, in typical competency-based medical education frameworks, it is becoming widely recognized that a score of 4 (e.g., I needed to be there just in case) or above is often considered an acceptable indicator of competency for trainees. In this study, only the PGY4s had an average UCAT performance at 4 or higher. This is in sharp contrast to the initial FAST UCAT where all trainees who had previously completed the Canadian Association of Emergency Physicians POCUS curriculum [26] achieved a level of 4 or higher. This difference in entrustment scores between FAST and four-view cardiac assessments speaks to the discriminatory capacity of the tool. First, it aligns with the general relationship between expected trajectories of competency in FAST versus four-view cardiac. The difference in UCAT scores for FAST and four-view cardiac POCUS also aligns with prior research which suggests trainees are able to rapidly achieve competency with the FAST [12] and four-view cardiac POCUS requires more practice and training before competency is achieved [12, 27]. The results of the pre-session questionnaire in this study also support this, as trainees reported a high degree of FAST experience and self-rated entrustment, and a lower self-rated entrustment and experience with four-view cardiac POCUS. Taken together, these findings reinforce that a four-view cardiac POCUS is more difficult than FAST, and that the UCAT is able to capture differences in task difficulty.

UCAT implementation moving forward

POCUS is a core competency for graduating EM residents [22, 28], and practicing physicians. At present there is no consensus on which assessment tools are best to measure POCUS competency [3, 29]. This study shows that the UCAT can be used to effectively assess POCUS competency in a consistent manner, and, taken with previous work, that it is accurate across more than one POCUS study type. The UCAT's high inter-rater reliability and internal consistency means that it can be used as a direct observation tool for both low- and high-stakes assessments. Broad usage of the simple and adaptable UCAT would standardize the assessment of POCUS competency across EM and other specialties. This may simplify credentialling across institutions and professional associations.

Limitations

There are a number of limitations that must be mentioned with respect to the current study. This study occurred at a single center and was used with a small population of trainees who had largely undergone core ultrasound training emphasizing the subxiphoid cardiac view [26]. There were very few learners who had not had some exposure to the four-view cardiac POCUS, although most had only completed less than 30 studies. While this may be a limited exposure for this POCUS type, it is aligned with the findings on trainee experience from the previous UCAT study [10]. While all available trainees participated in the study, a post hoc power analysis suggested this study was underpowered (0.40), limiting our ability to identify individual predictors [30]. Moreover, the factors evaluated in the regression were treated as independent factors, and while there is some variability within and between PGY, number of studies completed, and entrustment, it is difficult to truly disentangle these measures. All background digital survey data were self-reported. Due to the charting and billing structure in this residency program, there was no way of verifying the quantity of POCUS studies previously performed by each resident. Both raters in this study were involved in the derivation and the FAST validation of the UCAT, thus further work is needed to confirm inter-rater reliability with assessors less familiar with the tool. Lastly, at present, assessments of the UCAT have taken place in a simulated environment. As a result, the documentation and comprehension components of the UCAT were assessed through the trainee's verbal articulation of their subsequent plan based on the findings from their POCUS study in the context of the stem rather than in a written medical record. Previously derived similar tools such as the Resuscitation Assessment Tool have shown a smooth transition from the simulated to the clinical environment [31], the UCAT should be trialed and evaluated in the clinical environment to ensure that it remains an effective evaluation tool for the assessment of POCUS competency.

Conclusions

The UCAT was created to be a universally applicable, simple, entrustment-based, POCUS competency assessment tool [10]. Previous work has demonstrated strong validity evidence in the use of the UCAT for assessing FAST [10]. This study has expanded on this work, replicating and confirming the UCAT's validity evidence with respect to inter-rater reliability, internal consistency, and comparison with other variables such as PGY, previous number of four-view cardiac POCUS, previous number of total scans, self-rated entrustment, and intent to pursue certification together. Further, this study has expanded the evidence for its discriminatory capacity through a demonstration of its performance characteristics in the more difficult four-view cardiac POCUS examination when compared to FAST. Taken together, the findings from this work and previous studies on the UCAT demonstrate the utility and flexibility of the UCAT tool across multiple POCUS applications and present a promising way forward for measuring trainee POCUS competency.

Abbreviations

POCUS: Point-of-care ultrasound; UCAT: Ultrasound competency assessment tool; FAST: Focused assessment with sonography in trauma.

Supplementary Information

Additional file 1: The Ultrasound Comptency Assessment Tool.

Acknowledgements

Not applicable

Authors' contributions

CB, AH and CM conceived and designed the study, and supervised the conduct of the study. CB, CM, JN, LR and AH obtained funding for the project. CB and CM obtained the data. CB, NW and AH analyzed and interpreted the data. CB, NW, JN, LR and AH drafted the manuscript. All authors read and approved the final manuscript.

Author details

[1]Department of Emergency Medicine & Cumming School of Medicine, Emergency Physician, Calgary Zone, Alberta Health Services, University of Calgary, 7007 14th St. SW, Calgary, AB T2V1P9, Canada. [2]Department of Emergency Medicine, Queen's University, 76 Stuart St Kingston, Kingston, ON K7L2V7, Canada. [3]Department of Biomedical & Molecular Sciences, Queen's University, 74 Union St Kingston, Kingston, ON K7L3N6, Canada. [4]Office of Professional Development & Educational Scholarship, Queen's University, 68 Barrie St Kingston, Kingston, ON K7L3N6, Canada. [5]Royal College of Physicians and Surgeons Canada, 774 Echo Drive, Ottawa, ON K1S5N8, Canada. [6]Department of Emergency Medicine, The Ottawa Hospital and University of Ottawa, 1053 Carling Ave, E-Main, Room EM-206, Box 227, Ottawa, ON K1Y4E9, Canada.

References

1. Solomon SD, Saldana F (2014) Point-of-care ultrasound in medical education—stop listening and look. N Engl J Med 370(12):1083–1085
2. Via G, Hussain A, Wells M, Reardon R, ElBarbary M, Noble VE, Oren-Grinberg A (2014) International evidence-based recommendations for focused cardiac ultrasound. J Am Soc Echocardiogr 27(7):683-e681
3. Damewood SC, Leo M, Bailitz J, Gottlieb M, Liu R, Hoffmann B, Gaspari RJ (2020) Tools for measuring clinical ultrasound competency: recommendations from the ultrasound competency work group. AEM Educ Train 4:S106–S112
4. Lewiss RE, Pearl M, Nomura JT, Baty G, Bengiamin R, Duprey K, Akhtar S (2013) CORD–AEUS: consensus document for the emergency ultrasound milestone project. Acad Emerg Med 20(7):740–745

5. Hofer M, Kamper L, Sadlo M, Sievers K, Heussen N (2011) Evaluation of an OSCE assessment tool for abdominal ultrasound courses. Ultraschall Med 32(02):184–190
6. Dashi G, Hall A, Newbigging J, Rang L, La Rocque C, McKaigney C (2016) The development and evaluation of an assessment tool for competency in point-of-care ultrasound in emergency medicine: 636. Acad Emerg Med 23:263
7. Ma IWY, Desy J, Woo MY, Kirkpatrick AW, Noble VE (2020) Consensus-based expert development of critical items for direct observation of point-of-care ultrasound skills. J Grad Med Educ 12(2):176–184
8. Boniface KS, Ogle K, Aalam A, LeSaux M, Pyle M, Mandoorah S, Shokoohi H (2019) Direct observation assessment of ultrasound competency using a mobile standardized direct observation tool application with comparison to asynchronous quality assurance evaluation. AEM Educ Train 3(2):172–178
9. Stowell JR, Kessler R, Lewiss RE, Barjaktarevic I, Bhattarai B, Ayutyanont N, Kendall JL (2018) Critical care ultrasound: a national survey across specialties. J Clin Ultrasound 46(3):167–177
10 Bell C, Hall AK, Wagner N, Rang L, Newbigging J, McKaigney C (2021) The Ultrasound competency assessment tool (UCAT): development and evaluation of a novel competency-based assessment tool for point of care ultrasound. AEM Educ Train. https://doi.org/10.1002/aet2.10520
11. Gofton WT, Dudek NL, Wood TJ, Balaa F, Hamstra SJ (2012) The Ottawa surgical competency operating room evaluation (O-SCORE): a tool to assess surgical competence. Acad Med 87(10):1401–1407
12. Blehar DJ, Barton B, Gaspari RJ (2015) Learning curves in emergency ultrasound education. Acad Emerg Med 22(5):574–582
13. Kwan C, Pusic M, Pecaric M, Weerdenburg K, Tessaro M, Boutis K (2020) The variable journey in learning to interpret pediatric point-of-care ultrasound images: a multicenter prospective cohort study. AEM Educ Train 4(2):111–122
14. Olszynski PA, Bryce R, Hussain Q, Dunn S, Blondeau B, Atkinson P, Woods R (2021) A novel anatomic landmark to target the left ventricle during chest compressions in cardiac arrest. Cureus. https://doi.org/10.7759/cureus.13652
15. Messick S (1989) Validity, 3rd edn. Macmillian Publishing Company, New York
16. Koo TK, Li MY (2016) A guideline of selecting and reporting intraclass correlation coefficients for reliability research. J Chiropr Med 15(2):155–163
17. Saliken D, Dudek N, Wood TJ, MacEwan M, Gofton WT (2019) Comparison of the Ottawa Surgical Competency Operating Room Evaluation (O-SCORE) to a single-item performance score. Teach Learn Med 31(2):146–153
18. MacEwan MJ, Dudek NL, Wood TJ, Gofton WT (2016) Continued validation of the O-SCORE (Ottawa Surgical Competency Operating Room Evaluation): use in the simulated environment. Teach Learn Med 28(1):72–79
19. Rekman J, Gofton W, Dudek N, Gofton T, Hamstra SJ (2016) Entrustability scales: outlining their usefulness for competency-based clinical assessment. Acad Med 91(2):186–190
20. Lockyer J, Carraccio C, Chan M-K, Hart D, Smee S, Touchie C, Collaborators ICME (2017) Core principles of assessment in competency-based medical education. Med Teach 39(6):609–616
21. Royal College of Physicians and Surgeons Canada (2018). Competency by Design. Retrieved from https://www.royalcollege.ca/rcsite/cbd/competence-by-design-cbd-e Accessed 24 Jun 2021
22. Holmboe ES, Edgar L, Hamstra S (2016) The milestones guidebook. Accreditation Council for Graduate Medical Education, Chicago
23. Duanmu Y, Henwood PC, Takhar SS, Chan W, Rempell JS, Liteplo AS, Kimberly HH (2019) Correlation of OSCE performance and point-of-care ultrasound scan numbers among a cohort of emergency medicine residents. Ultrasound J 11(1):1–5
24. Gaspari RJ, Dickman E, Blehar D (2009) Learning curve of bedside ultrasound of the gallbladder. J Emerg Med 37(1):51–56
25. Peyrony O, Legay L, Morra I, Verrat A, Milacic H, Franchitti J, Elezi A (2018) Monitoring personalized learning curves for emergency ultrasound with risk-adjusted learning-curve cumulative summation method. AEM Educ Train 2(1):10–14
26. Olszynski P, Kim DJ, Chenkin J, Rang L, CAEP EUC Curriculum Working Group (2018) The CAEP emergency ultrasound curriculum-objectives and recommendations for implementation in postgraduate training: executive summary. Can J Emerg Med 20(5):736–738
27. Nair P, Siu SC, Sloggett CE, Biclar L, Sidhu RS, Eric HC (2006) The assessment of technical and interpretative proficiency in echocardiography. J Am Soc Echocardiogr 19(7):924–931
28. Royal College of Physicians and Surgeons Canada. (2017). Emergency Medicine Competencies. Retrieved from https://www.royalcollege.ca/rcsite/ibd-search-e?N=10000033+10000034+4294967050&label=Emergency%20Medicine Accessed 24 Jun 2021
29. Schmidt JN, Kendall J, Smalley C (2015) Competency assessment in senior emergency medicine residents for core ultrasound skills. West J Emerg Med 16(6):923
30. Faul F, Erdfelder E, Buchner A, Lang A-G (2009) Statistical power analyses using G* Power 3.1: tests for correlation and regression analyses. Behav Res Methods 41(4):1149–1160
31. Weersink K, Hall AK, Rich J, Szulewski A, Dagnone JD (2019) Simulation versus real-world performance: a direct comparison of emergency medicine resident resuscitation entrustment scoring. Adv Simul 4(1):1–10

20

First diagnosis of multisystem inflammatory syndrome in children (MIS- C): an analysis of PoCUS findings in the ED

Angelo G. Delmonaco[1], Andrea Carpino[2*], Irene Raffaldi[1], Giulia Pruccoli[3], Emanuela Garrone[1], Francesco Del Monte[2], Lorenzo Riboldi[2], Francesco Licciardi[3], Antonio F. Urbino[1] and Emilia Parodi[3]

Abstract

Children with multisystem inflammatory syndrome (MIS-C) tend to develop a clinical condition of fluid overload due both to contractile cardiac pump deficit and to endotheliitis with subsequent capillary leak syndrome. In this context, the ability of point-of-care ultrasound (PoCUS) to simultaneously explore multiple systems and detect polyserositis could promote adequate therapeutic management of fluid balance. We describe the PoCUS findings in a case-series of MIS-C patients admitted to the Emergency Department. At admission 10/11 patients showed satisfactory clinical condition without signs and symptoms suggestive for cardiovascular impairment/shock, but PoCUS showed pathological findings in 11/11 (100%). In particular, according to Rapid Ultrasound in SHock (RUSH) protocol, cardiac hypokinesis was detected in 5/11 (45%) and inferior vena cava dilatation in 3/11 (27%). Peritoneal fluid was reported in 6/11 cases (54%). Lung ultrasound (LUS) evaluation revealed an interstitial syndrome in 11/11 (100%), mainly localized in posterior basal lung segments. We suggest PoCUS as a useful tool in the first evaluation of children with suspected MIS-C for the initial therapeutic management and the following monitoring of possible cardiovascular deterioration.

Keywords: SARS-CoV-2 infection, MIS-C, Children, PoCUS, LUS

Introduction

Multisystem inflammatory syndrome (MIS-C) is a newly defined severe pediatric illness related to previous SARS-CoV-2 infection [1]. The clinical presentation is usually nonspecific and features of MIS-C overlap with those of many other pediatric conditions. Most children present to the Emergency Department (ED) with common symptoms, such as fever and abdominal pain, in some cases associated with Kawasaki-like signs [2]. Nevertheless, MIS-C is a severe disease and prominent cardiac involvement has been reported in a high proportion of patients affected, requiring an intensive level of care in more than 50% of patients [3, 4]. For this reason, the prompt recognition of potential cardiovascular instability in the ED is crucial for patient care.

The usefulness of point-of-care ultrasound (PoCUS) in assessing adult and pediatric shock has already been reported [5, 6]. During the recent pandemic, PoCUS performed by pediatricians in ED has also been demonstrated as a useful method to detect lung abnormalities in children with MIS-C and COVID-19 [7, 8].

Herein, we describe the PoCUS findings in a case-series of MIS-C patients at ED admission.

Materials and methods

In the ED of our Tertiary Care Pediatric Hospital (Regina Margherita Children's Hospital -OIRM-, Turin, Italy), bedside PoCUS is routinely performed in high-risk children by experienced pediatricians. Our internal standard PoCUS protocol is derived from Copetti protocol [9, 10] for lung evaluation and from Rapid

*Correspondence: andrea.carpino@unito.it
[2] Postgraduate School of Pediatrics, University of Turin, Piazza Polonia 94, 10126 Turin, Italy
Full list of author information is available at the end of the article

Ultrasound in SHock (RUSH) protocol [6] for cardiac and abdominal evaluation. Lung evaluation was performed with a linear or curvilinear probe (5–10 MHz) placed perpendicular, oblique and parallel to the ribs in the anterior, lateral and posterior (lower and upper) thorax and sitting positions were used to scan the posterior thorax. For RUSH protocol a curvilinear (2–5 MHz) and a phased array probe (2–8 MHz) were used (MyLab Seven; Esaote, Genoa, Italy).

On the 10th of January 2021, we performed a retrospective analysis of charts of all patients admitted to our ED with symptoms consistent with a presumptive diagnosis of MIS-C and subsequently discharged with a confirmed diagnosis between the 1st of April 2020 and the 31st of December 2020. The diagnosis of MIS-C at admission to the ED is presumptive. The current CDC case definition requires clinical, laboratory and anamnestic findings, without considering imaging features [1, 2].

Data of children who underwent PoCUS within the first 24 h from the admission were collected and retrospectively analyzed.

Archived PoCUS images were blind reviewed by three trained pediatricians with more than 5 years experience in bedside US, and then collegially discussed according to our internal protocol. Regarding lung, the presence of "pleural line irregularities", "vertical artifacts", "white lung" and "interstitial syndrome", "consolidation" and "pleural effusion" was assessed. The interstitial syndrome is characterized by B-lines, arising from one point of the pleural line and from peripheral consolidations spreading down until the edge of the screen without fading [11, 12]. The pattern considered pathologic is the presence of multiple B-lines (at least three between two ribs in one longitudinal scan) fanning out from the lung–wall interface [9, 10, 13]. Regarding cardiac evaluation, we defined "cardiac kinetic alteration" the presence of an abnormal size or contractility status of the left ventricle and/or a relative increase of the size of right ventricle (i.e., hypocontractile hearth) compared to the left ventricle. Both B mode and M-Mode tracing were used to evaluate systolic fractional shortening, according to RUSH protocol [6]. The pericardial sac was visualized to assess the presence of "pericardial effusion".

The evaluation of inferior caval vein positioning the probe in the epigastric area in a long-axis configuration was used in order to estimate the intravascular volume. A reduced compliance to respiratory cycles (i.e., IVC Sniff Test) was defined as "IVC dilatation".

Data regarding reasons for ED admission, clinical features including signs and symptoms of cardiovascular involvement and/or shock (capillary refill time > 2 s, cold extremities, hypotension, shortness of breath, severe tachycardia), laboratory data and X-ray imaging findings were collected, too.

The statistical analysis was performed using IBM SPSS statistics package 27.0. A descriptive analysis of the variables was conducted. The data were reported as absolute numbers and percentages for categorical variables while as medians and range for continuous variables.

Results

Between the 1st of April and the 31th December 2020, 40 patients presented to our ED with a high suspicion of MIS-C disease with fever for more than 24 h and presence of laboratory evidence of inflammation or SARS-CoV-2 infection. Twenty-four/40 received alternative diagnosis during hospitalization. The remaining 16 were subsequently discharged with a confirmed diagnosis according to CDC case definition; of these, 11 (69%) underwent PoCUS in the first 24 h from admission in the ED and were enrolled in the study (see Fig. 1).

Eleven/11 (100%) presented to ED for fever, associated with abdominal pain in 8/11 (73%), vomiting in 6/11 (55%), and Kawasaki-like signs (i.e., mucositis and conjunctivitis) in 3/11 (27%). At admission 10/11 (91%) showed good clinical condition without signs and symptoms suggestive for cardiovascular impairment/shock, with the exception of the only child appearing in critical condition, presenting severe hypotension and requiring admission to intensive care unit. PoCUS showed pathological findings in 11/11 (100%). According to RUSH protocol, cardiac hypokinesis was detected in 5/11 (45%) and inferior vena cava dilatation in 3/11 (27%). Peritoneal fluid was reported in 6/11 cases (54%). Lung ultrasound (LUS) evaluation revealed an interstitial syndrome in 11/11 (100%), mainly localized in posterior basal lung segments. One child appearing in critical condition at admission showed alteration both at LUS and RUSH protocol (Table 1, patient number 3).

During hospitalization all children developed cardiac injury with a median NT-pro BNP level of more than 8500 ng/l and pathological findings at echocardiogram. Detailed PoCUS and chest X-ray findings, as well as the first detection of N-terminal pro B-type natriuretic peptide (NT-pro BNP), are reported in Table 1. The five patients (Patient Number 3,4,5,7 and 9, Table 1) with kinetic cardiac alteration displayed a hypocontractile heart confirmed by the ejection fraction measurement at subsequent echocardiogram. Peculiar imaging findings at chest X-ray, LUS and RUSH exam are shown in Fig. 2.

Discussion

Even though the radiographic features of COVID-19 in children have been thoroughly reported [9], data describing imaging findings in MIS-C are limited. Recently, a

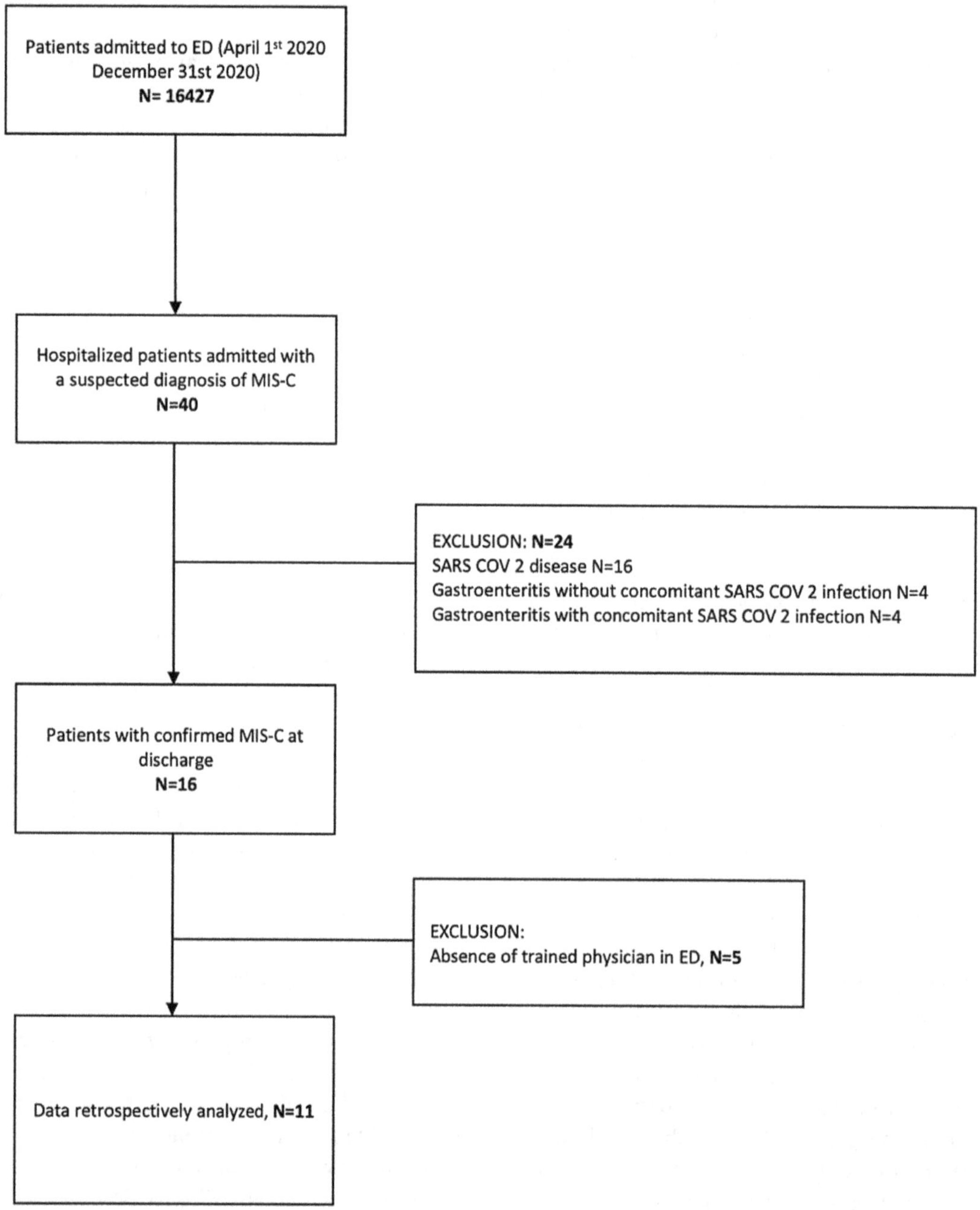

Fig. 1 Flowchart of patient enrollment and exclusion criteria

prospective observational study summarizing chest and abdominal imaging findings has been published [14].

To the best of our knowledge, for the first time we report here a detailed analysis on the PoCUS findings in the ED patients with confirmed MIS-C [7].

In our case-series, PoCUS was performed in 11 children with MIS-C within 24 h from hospitalization. Most patients presented to the ED for fever and abdominal pain in good clinical condition. However, the development of cardiac injury in all children during hospitalization (median NT-pro BNP level of more than 8500 ng/l) is consistent with the already reported clinical instability of MIS-C patients, who are at risk for sudden cardiovascular worsening [4]. For this reason a strict clinical, laboratory and imaging monitoring is strongly recommended.

In our case-series, despite initial fair clinical condition, PoCUS revealed early cardiac hypokinesis in almost half of our patients and IVC dilatation in three [15]. As a consequence, PoCUS allowed early identification of cardiopulmonary involvement, even before the

Table 1 PoCUS and X-rays findings, reason for ED admission and NT-pro BNP value at admission in children with MIS-C

	Patient 1	Patient 2	Patient 3	Patient 4	Patient 5	Patient 6	Patient 7	Patient 8	Patient 9	Patient 10	Patient 11
Reason for ED admission	Fever, abdominal pain	Fever, abdominal pain, vomiting and diarrhea	Fever, abdominal pain, vomiting	Fever, abdominal pain, vomiting, conjunctivitis	Fever, headache, abdominal pain, vomiting and diarrhea	Fever, abdominal pain, vomiting and diarrhea	Fever, abdominal pain, vomiting and diarrhea, rash, conjunctivitis	Fever, conjunctivitis	Fever, neck and scrotal pain, headache, fatigue	Fever, cough, abdominal pain, rash	Fever, headache, chest pain
NT-proBNP value (ng/L)	NA	NA	12,571	31,820	9211	557	976	1050	10,097	15,284	1452

PoCUS	All	Patient 1	Patient 2	Patient 3	Patient 4	Patient 5	Patient 6	Patient 7	Patient 8	Patient 9	Patient 10	Patient 11
Copetti LUS protocol												
Pleural line irregularities	11/11 (100%)	Bilateral	Bilateral	Bilateral	Bilateral	Bilatateral	Bilateral	Bilateral	Bilateral	Bilateral	Bilateral	Bilateral
Vertical artifacts	11/11 (100%)	Yes	Yes	Yes	Yes	Yes	Yes	Yes	Yes	Yes	Yes	Yes
White lung	2/11 (18%)	No	No	Yes	No	No	No	No	No	Yes	No	No
Consolidation	4/11 (36%)	No	No	Yes	Yes	Yes	No	No	No	Yes	No	No
Pleural effusion	6/11 (54%)	No	No	Yes	Yes	No	Yes	No	No	Yes	Yes	Yes
RUSH protocol												
Cardiac Kinetic alteration	5/11 (45%)	No	No	Yes	Yes	Yes	No	Yes	No	Yes	No	No
Pericardial effusion	3/11 (27%)	No	No	Yes	No	No	No	Yes	No	Yes	No	No
IVC dilatation	3/11 (27%)	No	No	Yes	No	Yes	No	No	No	Yes	No	No
Peritoneal fluid	6/11 (54%)	No	Yes	Yes	Yes	Yes	No	No	No	Yes	No	Yes
Chest X Ray		Normal	Normal	Perihilar interstitial thickening, cardiomegaly	Consolidation, perihilar interstitial thickening, cardiomegaly	Normal	NA	NA	Atelectasis	Normal	Normal	Pleural effusion, cardiomegaly

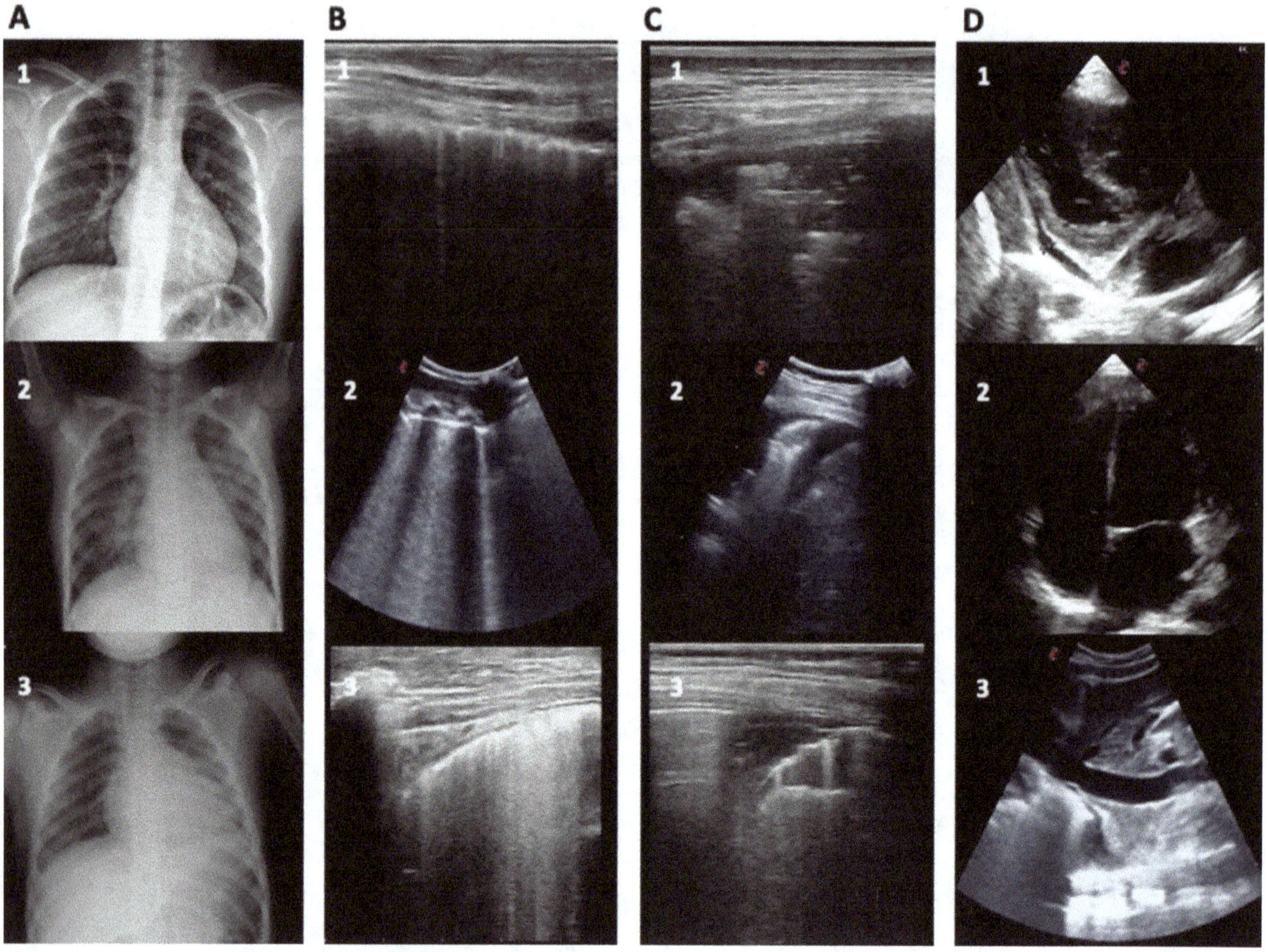

Fig. 2 Imaging findings: **A** chest X-ray findings; **B** LUS exam: **B1** initial interstitial pattern, **B2** vertical artifacts, **B3** white lung; **C** LUS exam: **C1** lung consolidations; **C2, C3** lung consolidations with pleural effusion; **D** RUSH exam: **D1** pericardial effusion, **D2** dilated cardiac chambers, **D3** plethoric IVC

patients developed symptoms suggestive for cardiovascular impairment/shock.

The PoCUS findings also showed abdominal free fluid in more than half of our patients, confirming the frequent involvement of gastrointestinal tract previously described [2, 14].

Children with MIS-C tend to develop a clinical condition of fluid overload due both to contractile cardiac pump deficit and to endotheliitis with subsequent capillary leak syndrome. In this context, the ability of PoCUS to simultaneously explore multiple systems and detect polyserositis promotes adequate therapeutic management of fluid balance.

Finally, all our patients presented at least one alteration at LUS examination, with the predominance of the interstitial pattern, underlying an inflammatory and edemigenous genesis [16]. Furthermore, pathological findings in the X-ray were reported in only 3/11 cases (27%), suggesting its marginal role in the initial evaluation (Fig. 2) [17].

PoCUS has unquestionable advantages: the ability to explore at a first sight the multi-organ involvement typical of MIS-C; the possibility of being performed at any moment by a pediatrician in the ED; and the opportunity to be repeated without any risk during the follow-up.

We are aware of the limits of our study (i.e., the retrospective nature of the analysis and the small sample size). However, if our data will be confirmed by further research on larger samples, PoCUS might be considered as a useful and non-invasive tool in the first evaluation of children with suspected MIS-C, although a specific MIS-C-correlated ultrasound pattern has not been identified. Moreover, it could play a key role to help physicians also in the therapeutic management of fluid balance, as well as in the following monitoring of these pediatric patients, at risk for cardiovascular deterioration.

Abbreviations

ED: Emergency department; IVC: Inferior vena cava; LUS: Lung US; MIS-C: Multisystem inflammatory syndrome in children; NT-pro BNP: N-terminal pro B-type natriuretic peptide; PoCUS: Point-of-care ultrasound; RUSH: Rapid Ultrasound in SHock; RT-PCR: Real-time polymerase chain reaction; US: Ultrasound.

Authors' contributions

Dr GAD, Dr AC and Dr IR substantially contributed to conception and design, collected data, drafted the article, reviewed and revised the manuscript. Dr GP contributed to conception and design, collected data, and reviewed and revised the manuscript. Dr FDM and Dr LR collected data, reviewed and revised the manuscript. Dr FL, Dr AFU and Dr EG supervised data collection and critically reviewed and revised the manuscript. Dr EM substantially contributed to conception and design, coordinated and supervised data collection, drafted the article and critically reviewed and revised the manuscript. All authors read and approved the final manuscript.

Author details

[1]Department of Pediatric Emergency, Regina Margherita Children's Hospital, A.O.U. Città Della Salute E Della Scienza Di Torino, Turin, Italy. [2]Postgraduate School of Pediatrics, University of Turin, Piazza Polonia 94, 10126 Turin, Italy. [3]Department of Pediatric and Public Health Sciences, Regina Margherita Children's Hospital, A.O.U. Città Della Salute E Della Scienza Di Torino, University of Turin, Turin, Italy.

References

1. CDC Health Alert Network. Multisystem inflammatory syndrome in children (MIS-C) associated with coronavirus disease 2019 (COVID-19) 1. HAN archive—00432. Health Alert Network (HAN). https://emergency.cdc.gov/han/2020/han00432.asp. Accessed 24 Aug 2021.
2. Nakra NA, Blumberg DA, Herrera-Guerra A, Lakshminrusimha S (2020) Multi-system inflammatory syndrome in children (MIS-C) following SARS-CoV-2 infection: review of clinical presentation, hypothetical pathogenesis, and proposed management. Children 7:69. https://doi.org/10.3390/children7070069
3. Capone CA, Subramony A, Sweberg T, Schneider J, Shah S, Rubin L et al (2020) Characteristics, cardiac involvement, and outcomes of multisystem inflammatory syndrome of childhood associated with severe acute respiratory syndrome coronavirus 2 infection. J Pediatr 224:141–145. https://doi.org/10.1016/j.jpeds.2020.06.044
4. Valverde I, Singh Y, Sanchez-de-Toledo J, Theocharis P, Chikermane A, Di Filippo S et al (2021) Acute cardiovascular manifestations in 286 children with multisystem inflammatory syndrome associated with COVID-19 infection in Europe. Circulation 143:21–32. https://doi.org/10.1161/CIRCULATIONAHA.120.050065
5. Park DB, Presley BC, Cook T, Hayden GE (2015) Point-of-care ultrasound for pediatric shock. Pediatr Emerg Care 31:591–601. https://doi.org/10.1097/PEC.0000000000000519
6. Perera P, Mailhot T, Riley D, Mandavia D (2010) The RUSH exam: Rapid Ultrasound in SHock in the evaluation of the critically Ill. Emerg Med Clin North Am 28:29–56. https://doi.org/10.1016/j.emc.2009.09.010
7. Kennedy TM, Dessie A, Kessler DO, Malia L, Rabiner JE, Firnberg MT, Ng L (2021) Point-of-care ultrasound findings in multisystem inflammatory syndrome in children: a cross-sectional study. Pediatr Emerg Care 37(6):334–339. https://doi.org/10.1097/PEC.0000000000002410
8. Giorno EPC, De Paulis M, Sameshima YT, Weerdenburg K, Savoia P, Nanbu DY et al (2020) Point-of-care lung ultrasound imaging in pediatric COVID-19. Ultrasound J. https://doi.org/10.1186/s13089-020-00198-z
9. Copetti R, Cattarossi L (2008) Ultrasound diagnosis of pneumonia in children. Radiol Medica 113:190–198. https://doi.org/10.1007/s11547-008-0247-8
10. Soldati G, Copetti R, Sher S (2009) Sonographic interstitial syndrome: the sound of lung water. J Ultrasound Med 28(2):163–174
11. Volpicelli G, Gargani L (2020) Sonographic signs and patterns of COVID-19 pneumonia. Ultrasound J 12(1):22. https://doi.org/10.1186/s13089-020-00171-w
12. Volpicelli G, Gargani L, Perlini S, Spinelli S, Barbieri G, Lanotte A, Casasola GG, Nogué-Bou R, Lamorte A, Agricola E, Villén T, Deol PS, Nazerian P, Corradi F, Stefanone V, Fraga DN, Navalesi P, Ferre R, Boero E, Martinelli G, Cristoni L, Perani C, Vetrugno L, McDermott C, Miralles-Aguiar F, Secco G, Zattera C, Salinaro F, Grignaschi A, Boccatonda A, Giostra F, Infante MN, Covella M, Ingallina G, Burkert J, Frumento P, Forfori F, Ghiadoni L, on behalf of the International Multicenter Study Group on LUS in COVID-19 (2021) Lung ultrasound for the early diagnosis of COVID-19 pneumonia: an international multicenter study. Intensive Care Med 47(4):444–454. https://doi.org/10.1007/s00134-021-06373-7
13. Volpicelli G, Elbarbary M, Blaivas M, Lichtenstein DA, Mathis G, Kirkpatrick AW, Melniker L, Gargani L, Noble VE, Via G, Dean A, Tsung JW, Soldati G, Copetti R, Bouhemad B, Reissig A, Agricola E, Rouby JJ, Arbelot C, Liteplo A, Sargsyan A, Silva F, Hoppmann R, Breitkreutz R, Seibel A, Neri L, Storti E, Petrovic T, International Liaison Committee on Lung Ultrasound (ILC-LUS) for International Consensus Conference on Lung Ultrasound (ICC-LUS) (2012) International evidence-based recommendations for point-of-care lung ultrasound. Intensive Care Med 38(4):577–591. https://doi.org/10.1007/s00134-012-2513-4
14. Hameed S, Elbaaly H, Reid CEL, Santos RMF, Shivamurthy V, Wong J et al (2020) Spectrum of imaging findings at chest radiography, US, CT, and MRI in multisystem inflammatory syndrome in children associated with COVID-19. Radiology 298:E1–E10. https://doi.org/10.1148/RADIOL.2020202543
15. Labovitz AJ, Noble VE, Bierig M, Goldstein SA, Jones R, Kort S et al (2010) Focused cardiac ultrasound in the emergent setting: a consensus statement of the American society of Echocardiography and American College of Emergency Physicians. J Am Soc Echocardiogr 23:1225–1230. https://doi.org/10.1016/j.echo.2010.10.005
16. Salehi S, Abedi A, Balakrishnan S, Gholamrezanezhad A (2020) Coronavirus disease 2019 (COVID-19): a systematic review of imaging findings in 919 patients. Am J Roentgenol 215:87–93. https://doi.org/10.2214/AJR.20.23034
17. Rostad BS, Shah JH, Rostad CA, Jaggi P, Richer EJ, Linam LE et al (2021) Chest radiograph features of multisystem inflammatory syndrome in children (MIS-C) compared to pediatric COVID-19. Pediatr Radiol. https://doi.org/10.1007/s00247-020-04921-9

21

Diagnostic accuracy of lung ultrasound for SARS-CoV-2: a retrospective cohort study

Daniel S. Brenner[1*], Gigi Y. Liu[2*], Rodney Omron[1], Olive Tang[3], Brian T. Garibaldi[4] and Tiffany C. Fong[1]

Abstract

Background: As medical infrastructures are strained by SARS-CoV-2, rapid and accurate screening tools are essential. In portions of the world, reverse transcription polymerase chain reaction (RT-PCR) testing remains slow and in limited supply, and computed tomography is expensive, inefficient, and involves exposure to ionizing radiation. Multiple studies evaluating the efficiency of lung point-of-care ultrasound (POCUS) have been published recently, but include relatively small cohorts and often focus on characteristics associated with severe illness rather than screening efficacy. This study utilizes a retrospective cohort to evaluate the test characteristics (sensitivity, specificity, likelihood ratios, predictive values) of lung POCUS in the diagnosis of SARS-CoV-2, and to determine lung score cutoffs that maximize performance for use as a screening tool.

Results: Lung POCUS examinations had sensitivity 86%, specificity 71.6%, NPV 81.7%, and PPV 77.7%. The Lung Ultrasound Score had an area under the curve of 0.84 (95% CI 0.78, 0.90). When including only complete examinations visualizing 12 lung fields, lung POCUS had sensitivity 90.9% and specificity 75.6%, with NPV 87.2% and PPV 82.0% and an area under the curve of 0.89 (95% CI 0.83, 0.96). Lung POCUS was less accurate in patients with a history of interstitial lung disease, severe emphysema, and heart failure.

Conclusions: When applied in the appropriate patient population, lung POCUS is an inexpensive and reliable tool for rapid screening and diagnosis of SARS-CoV-2 in symptomatic patients with influenza-like illness. Adoption of lung POCUS screening for SARS-CoV-2 may identify patients who do not require additional testing and reduce the need for RT-PCR testing in resource-limited environments and during surge periods.

Keywords: POCUS, Ultrasound, COVID-19, SARS-CoV-2, Triage, Diagnosis, RT-PCR

Introduction

A pandemic of severe acute respiratory syndrome coronavirus 2 (SARS-CoV-2), which causes the syndrome known as COVID-19 has led to over 75 million infections and over 1 million deaths as of December 2020 [1]. Early diagnosis is vital to enable early isolation, reduce ongoing transmission, and facilitate clinical decision-making. SARS-CoV-2 RT-PCR is the current diagnostic gold standard but has an estimated sensitivity of 75% [2, 3], and may take multiple days to result in some high-demand areas [4]. In the absence of sufficient RT-PCR availability, thoracic computed tomography (CT) has been used to detect the characteristic peripheral ground-glass opacities of COVID-19 pneumonia [5–8]. However, CT is not an optimal screening tool as it exposes patients to ionizing radiation, requires extensive decontamination, and is not readily available in many resource-limited situations [9–11].

Lung point-of-care-ultrasound (POCUS) has been proposed as a screening tool for COVID-19, and may offer several advantages. For non-SARS-CoV-2 interstitial syndromes, lung ultrasound has better sensitivity and specificity than chest radiograph and CT [5, 12,

*Correspondence: dbrenne7@jhmi.edu; Gliu12@jhmi.edu
[1] Department of Emergency Medicine, Johns Hopkins School of Medicine, 1830 East Monument St Suite 6-100, Baltimore, MD 21287, USA
[2] Hospitalist Program, Division of General Internal Medicine, Department of Medicine, Johns Hopkins School of Medicine, Baltimore, MD, USA
Full list of author information is available at the end of the article

13]. In confirmed cases of SARS-CoV-2 infection, lung POCUS evaluation of disease severity has correlated well with CT chest [14]. In addition to superior performance, lung POCUS is cost-effective [15, 16], portable, provides real-time data, and does not require ionizing radiation. POCUS supports infection control efforts by minimizing the number of healthcare workers exposed to patients under investigation (PUI) for COVID-19, and decontamination of ultrasound machines is relatively quick and easy compared with other imaging modalities [17]. Thus, if proven reliable, lung POCUS would allow for expedited and cost-efficient diagnosis of COVID-19 in hospitals, in the community, in resource-limited settings, and in surge situations when RT-PCR or CT chest availability is limited.

Preliminary studies have prompted the World Health Organization (WHO) to endorse ultrasound for use in the diagnosis of COVID-19, although this endorsement is noted as being based on weak preliminary evidence [18–20]. Characteristic findings of the COVID-19 syndrome on lung POCUS include a thickened or irregular pleural line, confluent B-lines, and subpleural consolidations [19, 21–23]. These findings correlate closely with those observed on CT [22], and demonstrate promise in trending clinical progression from onset to peak to resolution [21, 24]. Descriptive studies [25–31] have revealed the potential utility of lung POCUS but are limited by small sample sizes, lack of in-depth statistical analysis, and limited evaluation of patient characteristics that impact the utility of lung POCUS. To facilitate optimal application of lung POCUS for the diagnosis of COVID-19, we report the diagnostic accuracy of lung POCUS compared the criterion standard of SARS-CoV-2 RT-PCR test.

Materials and methods

A convenience sample of COVID-19 PUI > 18 years old evaluated between March 16, 2020 and May 16, 2020 who had lung POCUS recorded as part of their routine emergency department or inpatient care were included in this retrospective cohort study conducted at two urban academic tertiary care centers. PUI designation was identified by the presence of a SARS-CoV-2 RT-PCR order by the treating physician. Criteria for SARS-CoV-2 testing during the study period included either exposure to COVID-19 or report of at least two of the following symptoms: fever, acute cough, sore throat, dyspnea, myalgias, or loss of taste or smell. Details of all patients included in the study as well as alternate diagnoses are in Additional file 1: Figure S1. This study was performed in accordance with the Declaration of Helsinki. This human study was approved by Johns Hopkins Institutional Review Board—approval: IRB00255571. Adult participant consent was not required because this was a retrospective study.

The institutional POCUS database (Qpath Ultrasound Manager, Telexy Healthcare, Blaine WA) was queried to identify all lung POCUS examinations performed on COVID-19 PUI during the study period. All lung examinations performed during routine evaluation for COVID-19 by residents and faculty credentialed in the use of lung POCUS in the departments of Emergency Medicine and Internal Medicine were included. Study team members performed 89.1% of ultrasound studies, and all studies were evaluated for image adequacy by study team members blinded to clinical information. No dedicated training in lung POCUS or COVID-19-specific ultrasound was provided. A 12-field protocol was encouraged for POCUS users across the institution, including views of the bilateral anterior lung (L1–L2/R1–R2), lateral lung (L3–L4/R3–R4), and posterior lung (L5–L6/R5–R6) (Fig. 1). Ultrasound scans were acquired using equipment from Sonosite (Bothell WA), GE Healthcare (Waukesha WA), Philips (Bothell WA), and EchoNous (Redmond WA) (Additional file 2: Table S1).

Demographic characteristics including age, gender, race, duration of symptoms before POCUS examination, duration of symptoms before RT-PCR, RT-PCR result, body mass index (BMI), and history of comorbid conditions were recorded in a REDCap database (Vanderbilt University, Nashville TN). Two study team members credentialed in lung POCUS and blinded to all clinical information interpreted the lung POCUS studies. Reviewers did not evaluate POCUS examinations that they acquired. The blinded reviewers recorded their assessments in a separate REDCap tool based on a Lung Ultrasound Score described for use in COVID-19 pneumonia [21]. Each lung field was assessed for abnormal findings including pleural irregularity (0 points), multiple discrete B-lines (1 point), confluent B-lines (2 points), subpleural consolidations (3 points), and pleural effusion (0 points). Examples of these findings are presented in Additional file 3: Video S1, Additional file 4: Video S2, Additional file 5: Video S3, Additional file 6: Video S4, Additional file 7: Video S5, Additional file 8: Video S6. The reviewers also provided a summary assessment of whether the POCUS examination was consistent with COVID-19. A third blinded reviewer adjudicated any disagreements between reviewers. The reviewer whose ultrasound COVID-19 determination was concordant with the adjudicator was retained in the analysis.

The test characteristics and discriminative power of the Lung Ultrasound Score relative to the SARS-CoV-2 RT-PCR result were calculated. The point totals for all lung fields were summed to yield a total Lung Ultrasound Score for each reviewer. Mean Lung Ultrasound

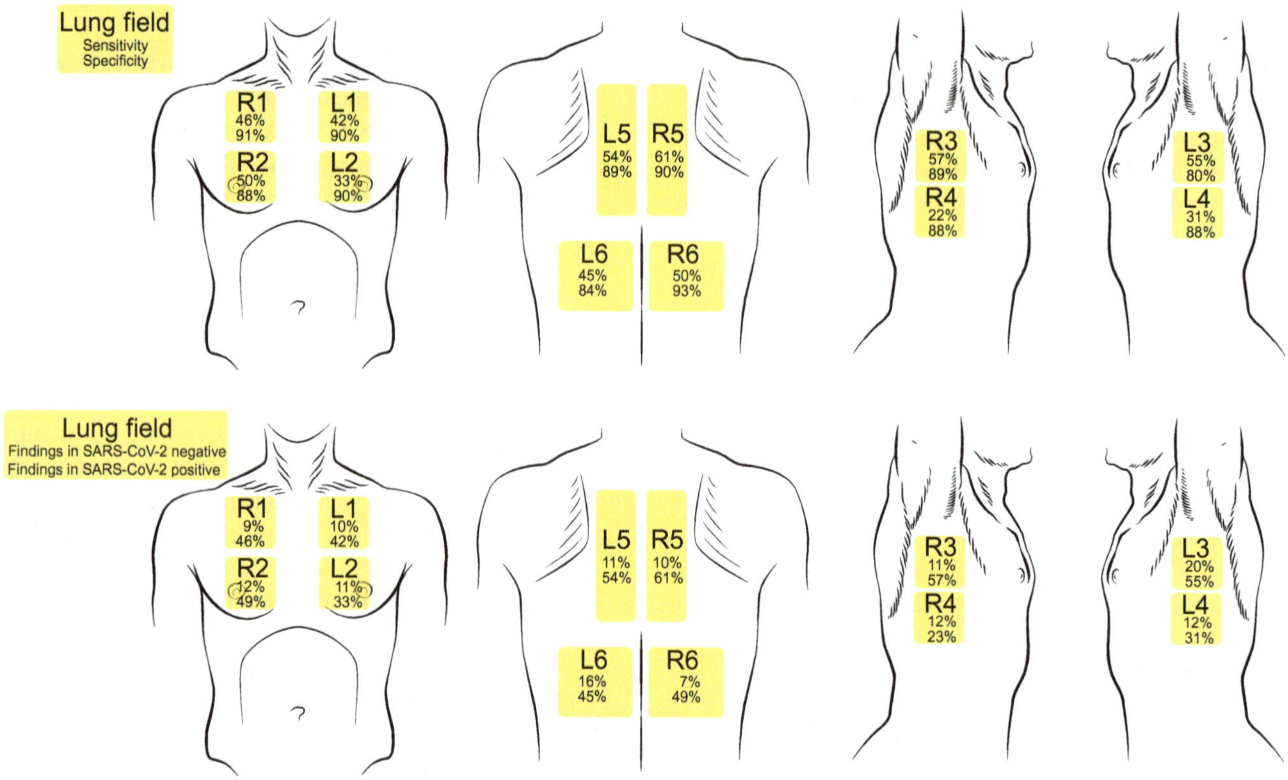

Fig. 1 Test characteristics and distribution of findings in lung POCUS for the evaluation of SARS-CoV-2. Upper panels: Lung fields are labeled in yellow across the thorax. Green numbers represent the sensitivity and black numbers represent the specificity for SARS-CoV-2 infection of each lung field. Lower panels: Green numbers represent the percentage of patients with negative RT-PCR test for SARS-CoV-2 who had abnormal findings in each lung window. Black numbers represent the percentage of patients with positive RT-PCR test for SARS-CoV-2 who had abnormal findings in each lung window

Score was calculated as the mean score between the two ultrasound reviewers. POCUS examinations were compared with the institutional gold standard RT-PCR test. A secondary analysis of complete examinations (12 acquired lung fields) was also performed. Means and proportions were compared using Student's *T* test and Chi-squared testing. Inter-rater reliability of lung POCUS interpretation was assessed using percent agreement, percent positive agreement, and kappa statistics. The sensitivity, specificity, negative predictive value, and positive predictive value associated with overall COVID-19 status determination by ultrasound and individual lung fields were also calculated. Agreement between SARS-CoV-2 RT-PCR testing and lung POCUS was evaluated using kappa statistics. The area under the receiver operator curve was then calculated for the Lung Ultrasound Score, and a cutoff proposed based on the Youden J statistic [32]. Scoring frameworks assigning negative points for pleural effusions were assessed, and the framework with the highest discriminative power (pleural effusion − 3 points) was included for analysis.

Results

Patients included in the cohort ($n = 174$) had mean age of 53.1 years, were 52.9% male, and 53% had positive RT-PCR testing for SARS-CoV-2 (Table 1). 77% were admitted to the hospital, 26.4% were admitted to the intensive care unit, 5.7% required high-flow nasal cannula oxygen support, and 14.4% required intubation (Table 1, Additional file 2: Table S2). Other details of hospital admission and level of care are reported in Additional file 2: Table S2. Pathological lung findings were identified more frequently in all lung fields in patients who tested positive for SARS-CoV-2 RNA compared to those who tested negative ($p < 0.001$). Bilateral lung involvement was more common among those with a positive RT-PCR result (78%), compared to those with a negative RT-PCR result (26%).

Test characteristics for lung POCUS in the diagnosis of COVID-19 are detailed in Table 2. Compared to the standard of RT-PCR testing, lung POCUS had a sensitivity 86.0% and specificity 71.6%, with negative predictive value (NPV) 81.7% and positive predictive value (PPV) 77.7%. Test characteristics for the involvement of more

Table 1 Baseline characteristics by SARS-CoV-2 RT-PCR results, *N* = 174

	Overall	RT-PCR result		*p* value
		Negative	Positive	
N	174	81	93	
Age, mean (SD)	53.1 (16.8)	51.9 (19.2)	54.2 (14.3)	0.37
Male, no. (%)	92 (53%)	40 (49%)	52 (56%)	0.39
Race, no. (%)				< 0.001
Caucasian	66 (38%)	36 (44%)	30 (32%)	
African American	33 (19%)	4 (5%)	29 (31%)	
Hispanic or Asian	75 (43%)	41 (51%)	34 (37%)	
Body mass index, kg/m^2, mean (SD)[a]	29.1 (7.2)	28.1 (7.8)	30.0 (6.6)	0.098
Number of comorbidities, no. (%)				0.013
0	101 (58.0%)	37 (46%)	64 (69%)	
1	53 (30.5%)	30 (37%)	23 (25%)	
2	15 (8.6%)	10 (12%)	5 (5%)	
3	5 (2.9%)	4 (5%)	1 (1%)	
Interventions needed, no. (%)				
High-flow nasal cannula oxygen	10 (5.7%)	1 (1%)	9 (10%)	0.017
Intubation	25 (14.4%)	5 (6%)	20 (22%)	0.004
Comorbidities, no. (%)				
Interstitial lung disease	7 (4%)	6 (7%)	1 (1%)	0.034
Asthma	20 (12%)	8 (10%)	12 (13%)	0.53
COPD	12 (7%)	9 (11%)	3 (3%)	0.041
Heart failure	39 (22%)	27 (33%)	12 (13%)	0.001
EF ≤ 35%	11 (6%)	9 (11%)	2 (2%)	0.015
HIV/AIDS CD4 < 200	5 (3%)	4 (5%)	1 (1%)	0.13
Immunosuppression	10 (6%)	5 (6%)	5 (5%)	0.82
ESRD	5 (3%)	3 (4%)	2 (2%)	0.54
Lung Ultrasound Score, mean (SD)	6.2(5.7)	2.6 (3.2)	9.4 (5.5)	< 0.001
Positive findings by lung field, no. (%)				
L1	47 (27%)	8 (10%)	39 (42%)	< 0.001
L2	40 (23%)	9 (11%)	31 (33%)	< 0.001
L3	67 (39%)	16 (20%)	51 (55%)	< 0.001
L4	39 (22%)	10 (12%)	29 (31%)	0.003
L5	59 (34%)	9 (11%)	50 (54%)	< 0.001
L6	55 (32%)	13 (16%)	42 (45%)	< 0.001
R1	50 (29%)	7 (9%)	43 (46%)	< 0.001
R2	56 (32%)	10 (12%)	46 (49%)	< 0.001
R3	62 (36%)	9 (11%)	53 (57%)	< 0.001
R4	31 (18%)	10 (12%)	21 (23%)	0.078
R5	65 (37%)	8 (10%)	57 (61%)	< 0.001
R6	52 (30%)	6 (7%)	46 (49%)	< 0.001
Days between symptom onset and test				
RT-PCR, median (IQR)	3 (2, 7)	3 (2, 5)	5, (3, 7)	< 0.001
POCUS, median (IQR)	6 (3, 10)	3 (2, 6)	8 (6, 14)	< 0.001
Extent of lung findings, no. (%)				
No findings	53 (31%)	42 (52%)	11 (12%)	< 0.001
Single field involvement	16 (9%)	102 (15%)	4 (4%)	
Multiple unilateral field involvement	11 (6%)	6 (7%)	5 (5%)	
Bilateral field involvement	94 (54%)	21 (26%)	73 (78%)	

EF ejection fraction, *HIV/AIDS* human immunodeficiency virus/acquired immunodeficiency syndrome, *ESRD* end-stage renal disease, *IQR* interquartile range

[a] 6.9% missing

Table 2 Sensitivity, specificity, negative predictive value (NPV), positive predictive value (PPV), and kappa statistics associated with lung ultrasound findings compared to SARS-CoV-2 RT-PCR testing

	Sensitivity	Specificity	NPV	PPV	Kappa
All ultrasounds, $N=174$					
Ultrasound SARS-CoV-2 diagnosis	86.0	71.6	81.7	77.7	0.58
Multiple field involvement	83.9	66.7	78.3	74.3	0.51
Posterior field involvement	71.0	70.4	67.9	73.3	0.41
Bilateral lung involvement	78.5	74.1	75.0	77.7	0.53
Bilateral posterior field involvement	57.0	91.4	64.9	88.3	0.47
Any discrete B-lines	86.0	54.3	77.2	68.4	0.41
Any confluent B-lines	43.0	98.8	60.2	97.6	0.40
Any pleural thickening or irregularity	86.0	51.9	76.4	67.2	0.39
No pathologic lung findings	11.8	48.1	32.2	20.8	-0.39
Ultrasound SARS-CoV-2 diagnosis					
No ILD, $N=167$	87.0	77.3	82.9	82.5	0.65
No ILD, no HF EF $\leq 35\%$, $N=158$	85.4	82.4	83.6	86.8	0.70
No ILD, no HF EF $\leq 35\%$, no immunosuppression, $N=144$	89.3	83.3	84.7	88.2	0.73
Complete ultrasounds, $N=174$	90.9	75.6	87.2	82.0	0.67

ILD interstitial lung disease, *EF* ejection fraction, *HIV/AIDS* human immunodeficiency virus/acquired immunodeficiency syndrome, *ESRD* end-stage renal disease

than one lung field, posterior lung field involvement, and bilateral lung field involvement are also reported in Table 2. Examinations with multiple discrete B-lines had a sensitivity 86.0%, specificity 54.3%, NPV 77.2%, and PPV 68.4% while examinations with confluent B-lines had a sensitivity 43.0%, specificity 98.8%, NPV 60.2%, PPV 97.6%. Lung POCUS was more accurate in patients with more significant oxygen requirement or requiring higher level of care (Table 3).

Patients with positive SARS-CoV-2 RT-PCR testing had higher Lung Ultrasound Scores than those with negative tests (9.4 ± 5.5 versus 2.6 ± 3.2). There was high discrimination (AUC 0.84, 95% CI 0.78, 0.90) of the Lung Ultrasound Score for COVID-19 syndrome (Fig. 2). The test characteristics associated with various cutoff points are reported in Fig. 2. A Lung Ultrasound Score of 2 points maximized sensitivity (sensitivity 88%, specificity 55%, positive likelihood ratio (+ LR) 1.98, negative likelihood ratio (− LR) 0.21, PPV 80.4%, NPV 69.5%). A Lung Ultrasound Score of 8 points maximized specificity (sensitivity 59%, specificity 91%, +LR 6.84, − LR 0.45, PPV 66.1%, NPV 88.7%). A Lung Ultrasound Score of 6 points optimized a balance of sensitivity and specificity (sensitivity 77%, specificity 84%, +LR 4.82, −LR 0.27, PPV 76.4%, NPV 84.7%) are also reported in Fig. 2. A grey zone analysis in Fig. 3 demonstrates that Lung Ultrasound Scores under 4 have sensitivity over 90% of SARS-CoV-2 infection, and that scores over 6 have over 90% specificity for the detection of SARS-CoV-2 infection. A modified version of the Lung Ultrasound Score that

Table 3 Sensitivity, specificity, negative predictive value (NPV), positive predictive value (PPV), and kappa statistics by disposition and oxygen requirement

	Sensitivity	Specificity	NPV	PPV	Kappa
Disposition					
Discharged from ED, $N=41$	76.9	89.3	89.3	76.9	0.66
Floor/IMC, $N=86$	82.9	64.4	80.6	68.0	0.47
ICU, $N=46$	92.1	50.0	57.1	89.7	0.44
Oxygen requirement					
None or nasal canula, $N=139$	84.4	73.3	84.6	73.0	0.57
HFNC, $N=10$	88.9	100.0	50.0	100.0	0.62
Intubation, $N=25$	90.0	40.0	50.0	85.7	0.32

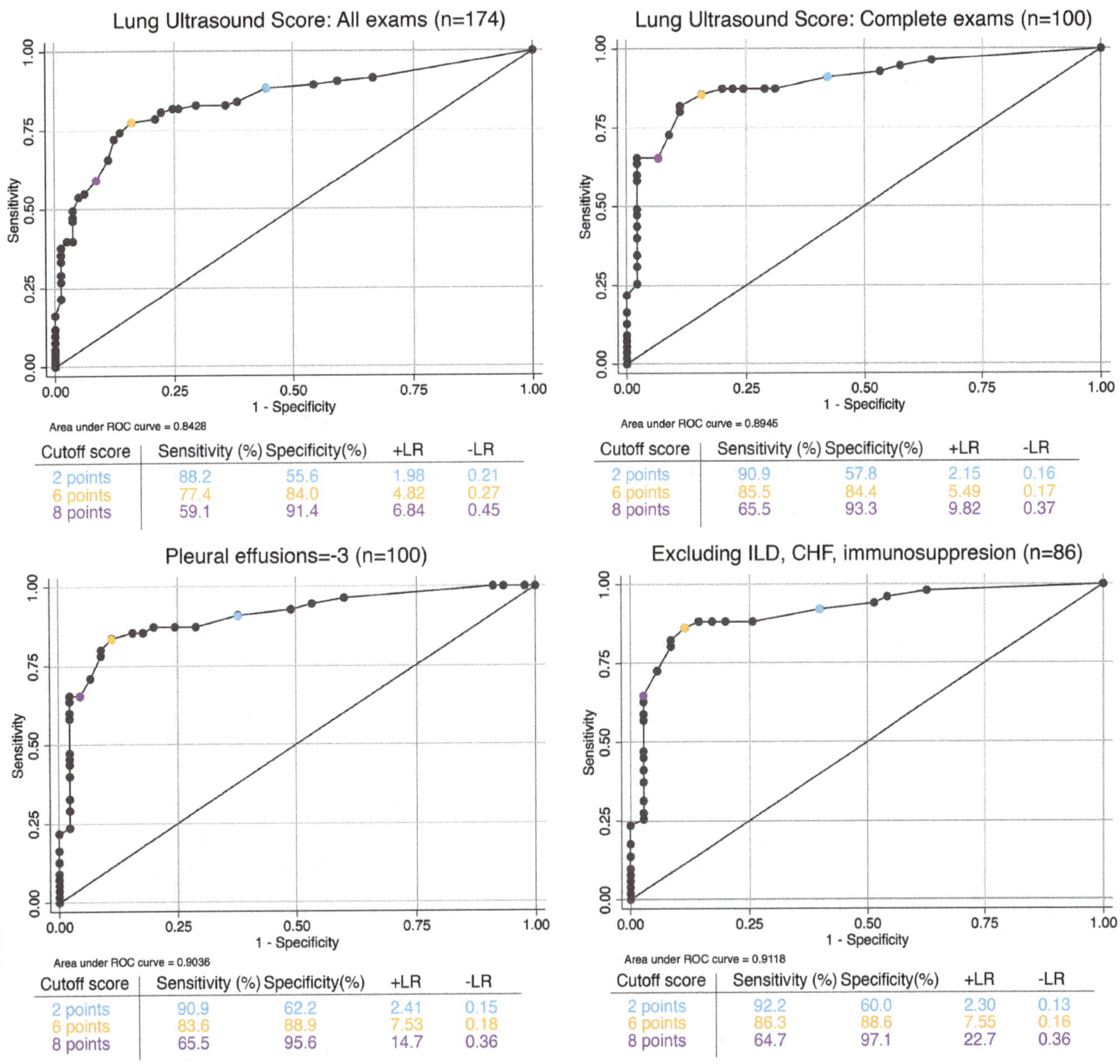

Lung Ultrasound Score: All exams (n=174)

Cutoff score	Sensitivity (%)	Specificity(%)	+LR	-LR
2 points	88.2	55.6	1.98	0.21
6 points	77.4	84.0	4.82	0.27
8 points	59.1	91.4	6.84	0.45

Lung Ultrasound Score: Complete exams (n=100)

Cutoff score	Sensitivity (%)	Specificity(%)	+LR	-LR
2 points	90.9	57.8	2.15	0.16
6 points	85.5	84.4	5.49	0.17
8 points	65.5	93.3	9.82	0.37

Pleural effusions=-3 (n=100)

Cutoff score	Sensitivity (%)	Specificity(%)	+LR	-LR
2 points	90.9	62.2	2.41	0.15
6 points	83.6	88.9	7.53	0.18
8 points	65.5	95.6	14.7	0.36

Excluding ILD, CHF, immunosuppresion (n=86)

Cutoff score	Sensitivity (%)	Specificity(%)	+LR	-LR
2 points	92.2	60.0	2.30	0.13
6 points	86.3	88.6	7.55	0.16
8 points	64.7	97.1	22.7	0.36

Fig. 2 Receiver operator curves for Lung Ultrasound Score for all examinations (top left), examinations with all 12 views (top right), examinations with 12 views including pleural effusions as a negative prognostic factor for SARS-CoV-2 diagnosis (bottom left), and excluding confounding pre-existing comorbidities (bottom right)

scored the presence of pleural effusion as −3 points had improved discrimination compared to the standard Lung Ultrasound Score (Fig. 2; AUC 0.90, 95% CI 0.84, 0.96), and improved test characteristics (Fig. 2). Using pleural effusions as a negative prognostic factor improved the performance of the Lung Ultrasound Score in the grey zone analysis, narrowing the area of uncertain diagnosis (Fig. 3).

Patient-related factors associated with decreased lung POCUS accuracy were also investigated. Patients with false-negative lung POCUS scans ($n=13$) had higher average BMI compared to patients with true-positive scans (36.5 kg/m$^2\pm$9.4 versus 29.3 kg/m$^2\pm$8.1; $p<0.001$) (Table 4). Patients with false-positive lung POCUS scans ($n=23$) were more likely to have pre-existing ILD than patients with true negative scans (26% versus 0%, $p<0.001$; Table 4). Patients with false-positive lung POCUS scans were also more likely to have systolic heart failure (57% versus 24% $p<0.001$) and heart failure with ejection fraction (EF) under 35% (30% vs 3% $p<0.001$; Table 4). There was no difference in the prevalence of asthma, COPD, HIV with

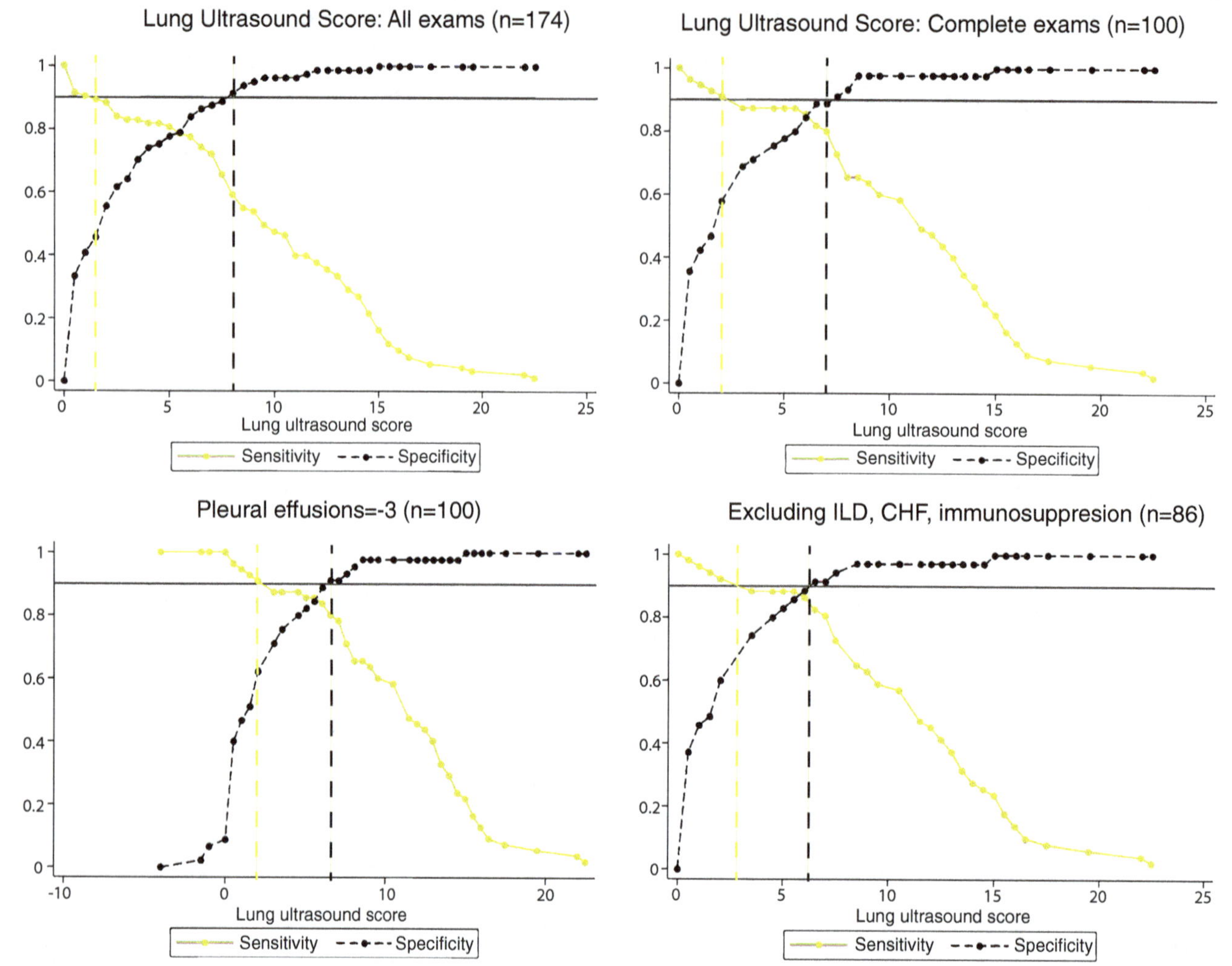

Fig. 3 Grey zone analysis for Lung Ultrasound Score for all examinations (top left), examinations with all 12 views (top right), examinations with 12 views including pleural effusions as a negative prognostic factor for SARS-CoV-2 diagnosis (bottom left), and excluding confounding pre-existing comorbidities (bottom right)

CD4 < 200, immunosuppression, or end-stage renal disease in patients with discordance between lung POCUS and RT-PCR result (Table 4).

Exclusion of patients with these comorbid conditions associated improved the diagnostic performance of lung POCUS for COVID-19 (Table 2). In patients without these confounding conditions, the sensitivity was 89.3%, specificity was 83.3%, NPV 84.7%, and PPV 88.2%. These exclusions also improved the discriminative ability of the Lung Ultrasound Score (Fig. 2; AUC 0.91, 95% CI 0.85, 0.98) and narrowed the grey zone area of uncertain diagnosis (Fig. 3). The test characteristics associated with cutoff points maximizing sensitivity (2 points: PPV 84.0%), specificity (8 points: NPV 97.1%), or statistically optimizing a balance of sensitivity and specificity (6 points: PPV 81.6%, NPV 91.7%) are also reported in Fig. 2.

A secondary analysis including only complete lung POCUS examinations with all 12 lung fields was performed. Participants with complete POCUS lung evaluation ($n = 100$) had a mean age of 51.3 years, were 54% male, and 55% had positive RT-PCR testing for SARS-CoV-2 (Additional file 2: Table S3). Complete examinations had improved test characteristics and better discriminative ability (Additional file 9: Figure S2) compared to examinations that did not include all lung fields (AUC 0.89, 95% CI 0.83, 0.96. Sensitivity 90.9%, specificity 75.6%, NPV 87.2%, PPV 82.0%) (Fig. 2).

Table 4 Factors associated with concordance or discordance between SARS-CoV-2 RT-PCR and POCUS diagnosis of SARS-CoV-2

SARS-CoV-2 RT-PCR POCUS SARS-CoV-2	Negative Negative	Positive Negative	Negative Positive	Positive Positive	*p* value
N	58	13	23	80	
Body mass index, kg/m², mean (SD)[a]	29.3 (8.1)	36.5 (9.4)	25.4 (6.3)	29.1 (5.6)	<0.001
Number of lung fields visualized, median (IQR)	12 (8, 12)	11 (10, 12)	11 (9, 12)	12 (10, 12)	0.38
Lung Ultrasound Score, mean (SD)	1.1 (1.6)	0.6 (0.9)	6.3 (3.2)	10.8 (4.5)	<0.001
Days between symptom onset and test					
POCUS, median (IQR)	3 (2, 5)	6 (4, 8)	3 (2, 6)	9.0 (6.0, 14.0)	<0.001
RT-PCR, median (IQR)	0 (0, 0)	3.0 (0, 5)	0 (0, 1)	2 (0, 6)	<0.001
Number of comorbidities, no (%)					
0	32 (55%)	7 (54%)	5 (22%)	57 (71%)	0.041
1	19 (33%)	4 (31%)	11 (48%)	19 (24%)	
2	7 (12%)	1 (8%)	3 (13%)	4 (5%)	
3	0 (0%)	1 (8%)	4 (17%)	0 (0%)	
Comorbidities, no (%)					
Interstitial lung disease	0 (0%)	1 (8%)	6 (26%)	0 (0%)	<0.001
Asthma	6 (10%)	1 (8%)	2 (9%)	11 (14%)	0.84
COPD (without severe emphysematous changes)	6 (10%)	1 (8%)	3 (13%)	2 (2%)	0.18
Heart failure	14 (24%)	4 (31%)	13 (57%)	8 (10%)	<0.001
EF ≤ 35%	2 (3%)	1 (8%)	27 (30%)	1 (1%)	<0.001
HIV/AIDS CD4 < 200	2 (3%)	0 (0%)	2 (9%)	1 (1%)	0.26
Immunosuppression	4 (7%)	2 (15%)	1 (4%)	3 (4%)	0.39
ESRD	1 (2%)	0 (0%)	2 (9%)	2 (2%)	0.32

EF ejection fraction, *HIV/AIDS* human immunodeficiency virus/acquired immunodeficiency syndrome, *ESRD* end-stage renal disease, *IQR* interquartile range

[a] 7% missing

Discussion

These data demonstrate that lung POCUS provides rapid information regarding COVID-19 status that is consistent with results of the current gold standard RT-PCR test. In our patient cohort, there was also anecdotal evidence that lung POCUS could outperform the RT-PCR test. At least three patients in this study with initially negative RT-PCR testing but lung POCUS examinations suggestive of COVID-19 were subsequently diagnosed with SARS-CoV-2 infection through more invasive testing.

While descriptive studies of lung POCUS findings in COVID-19 are numerous [19, 22, 25], this is most thorough investigation of a quantitative lung POCUS score to diagnose COVID-19 with data allowing maximization of sensitivity, specificity, and discriminative ability. Other studies do provide information on the test characteristics of lung POCUS in the diagnosis of COVID-19, but are limited by much smaller cohorts and unable to demonstrate the performance in populations with various comorbidities [26, 27, 29, 31]. The present study provides a more comprehensive assessment of the diagnostic power of lung POCUS in a large heterogenous population, and provides vital information for properly applying lung POCUS in the diagnosis of COVID-19.

These data suggest that a Lung Ultrasound Score cutoff of 2 points maximizes sensitivity for use in screening of symptomatic patients. Using this approach, any POCUS examination with three or more discrete B-lines in two distinct lung fields, or any examination with confluent B-lines or subpleural consolidation in any single lung field is concerning for COVID-19, requires isolation, and may benefit from additional testing. Any lung POCUS examination with a Lung Ultrasound Score of 0 points or 1 point is very unlikely to be associated with COVID-19, and can be triaged out of PUI workflows and investigated for other etiologies of their symptoms. At any point during the examination, if the cumulative Lung Ultrasound Score is equal to or greater than 2 points, the clinician can stop and order confirmatory testing, and move on to the next patient. This approach deliberately maximizes the sensitivity and negative predictive value at the expense of the specificity and positive predictive value, and will need to be externally validated. Additionally, while this approach may be advantageous for efficiency, the secondary analysis strongly suggests that complete examinations with 12 lung fields have improved diagnostic power compared to abbreviated examinations. Other cutoffs maximizing specificity (8 points) or balancing between sensitivity and specificity (6 points) can be considered in the appropriate clinical contexts.

The accuracy of lung POCUS may be impacted by patient factors. Elevated BMI reduced the sensitivity of lung POCUS for COVID-19, consistent with prior studies that have reported similar effects of obesity [33]. Pre-existing interstitial lung disease reduced the specificity of lung POCUS for COVID-19. This confounder may be due to the pre-existing pathology of interstitial inflammation, scarring, and thickening leading to a similar ultrasonographic appearance. It is also challenging to differentiate between pulmonary edema due to heart failure [34] or end-stage renal disease and the interstitial inflammation caused by COVID-19. In patients with B-lines on lung POCUS, a concurrent cardiac POCUS may help differentiate between COVID-19 and cardiac etiologies [35]. Other tools such as M-mode evaluation for pleural irregularities [35] and the presence of "spared areas" [36] have been used to differentiate interstitial syndrome from pulmonary edema in the past, but have not been validated for use with COVID-19. Avoiding the use of lung POCUS in patients with these confounding comorbidities (morbid obesity, interstitial lung disease, heart failure) improves the diagnostic performance for COVID-19.

Study limitations

The retrospective design predisposes to recruitment bias. This study is somewhat insulated from this limitation since the RT-PCR testing often had not resulted when the POCUS images were acquired and when the patients were identified for inclusion in the review. The inclusion of patients with variable duration of symptoms and illness severity as well as in different practice environments raises concerns for spectrum bias, but also demonstrates the accuracy that can be expected with real-world application of this diagnostic test.

The majority (77%) of the patients evaluated in this study were admitted to the hospital, which may limit the applicability of these findings in patients who do not require hospitalization. Several factors contribute to this bias, including triage of less severe, outpatient-appropriate patients to a treatment tent without ultrasound equipment, absence of clear guidelines for safe discharge early in the pandemic, and the nature of the tertiary hospital study site as a transfer center for care of the majority of admitted COVID-19 patients in the health system. Despite the preponderance of hospitalized patients, the variable lengths of stay (interquartile range 1–11 days) hint at a wide spectrum of illness severity and resource requirement and suggest that the lung POCUS findings may be broadly generalizable.

Another limitation is the dependence on POCUS operator skill and experience. Less-experienced point-of-care ultrasonographers tended to more aggressively label mild abnormalities in a single lung field as evidence COVID-19 even though the data suggest that most patients with positive SARS-CoV-2 RT-PCR tests have bilateral pathological findings. Undergained or overgained images could also lead to false-negative or false-positive POCUS interpretations, although all images for this study were assessed for quality prior to inclusion. Mimics such as Z-lines (short, comet-tail artifacts arising from the pleural line that do not reach the distal end of the screen or erase A-lines) [37] and E-lines (long comet-tail artifacts that do erase A-lines but arise from the subcutaneous tissue rather than the pleura) [37] can easily be confused with B-lines and lead to false-positive diagnoses. The development of training resources will be crucial for widespread implementation of lung POCUS as a screening tool for COVID-19.

As this study only included PUI for COVID-19, it is unknown whether lung POCUS can be used as a screening tool for asymptomatic SARS-CoV-2 carriers. It is also unclear whether lung POCUS can be used for the diagnosis of COVID-19 in patients with primarily gastrointestinal [38] or neurological [39] symptoms. Additional studies will be necessary before lung POCUS can be applied for the screening and diagnosis of COVID-19 in these situations.

The results of this study are also applicable only during the current clinical environment, with high prevalence of SARS-CoV-2. In future periods with lower prevalence, lung POCUS may not perform well enough to use as a screening tool.

Finally, the use of RT-PCR as the reference standard is a significant limitation. Although RT-PCR is currently the gold standard for diagnosis, its sensitivity is known to be relatively limited [2]. Future, prospective studies will be needed to test whether lung POCUS provides improved sensitivity over RT-PCR testing in certain circumstances.

Conclusions

Lung POCUS is a rapid, inexpensive tool that provides results that are concordant with RT-PCR testing in patients under investigation for COVID-19. The low cost, rapid assessment, lack of ionizing radiation, and applicability to a variety of practice environments make it an appealing option for use when other diagnostic tests such RT-PCR or CT chest are unavailable.

Supplementary Information

Additional file 1: Figure S1. Flowsheet of patients that were included, results of testing, and associated confounding factors.

Additional file 2: Table S1. Ultrasound machines, probes, and parameters. **Table S2**. Disposition of included patients. **Table S3**. Characteristics of ultrasound cohort with complete examinations ($N = 100$). **Table S4.** Characteristics of ultrasound cohort with complete examinations ($N = 100$) by ultrasound and RT-PCR SARS-CoV-2 diagnosis.

Additional file 3: Video S1. Normal lung POCUS findings.

Additional file 4: Video S2. Lung POCUS findings from a patient diagnosed with COVID-19, including discrete B-lines, confluent B-lines, irregular pleural line, and small subpleural consolidations

Additional file 5: Video S3. Lung POCUS findings from a patient diagnosed with COVID-19, including subpleural consolidation.

Additional file 6: Video S4. Lung POCUS findings from a patient with CHF consistent with cardiogenic pulmonary edema. These findings lead to a false-positive lung POCUS interpretation.

Additional file 7: Video S5. Lung POCUS findings demonstrating a large pleural effusion from a patient with heart failure.

Additional file 8: Video S6. Lung POCUS findings from a patient with interstitial lung disease. These findings lead to a false-positive lung POCUS interpretation.

Additional file 9: Figure S2. Test characteristics and distribution of findings in complete 12-field lung POCUS examinations for the evaluation of SARS-CoV-2. Upper panels: Lung fields are labeled in yellow across the thorax. Green numbers represent the sensitivity and black numbers represent the specificity for SARS-CoV-2 infection of each lung field. Lower panels: Green numbers represent the percentage of patients with negative RT-PCR test for SARS-CoV-2 who had abnormal findings in each lung window. Black numbers represent the percentage of patients with positive RT-PCR test for SARS-CoV-2 who had abnormal findings in each lung window.

Abbreviations
POCUS: Point of care ultrasound; SARS-CoV-2: Severe Acute Respiratory Syndrome Coronavirus 2; RT-PCR: Reverse transcription polymerase chain reaction; CT: Computed tomography; PUI: Patient under investigation; +LR: Positive likelihood ratio; -LR: Negative likelihood ratio; PPV: Positive predictive value; NPV: Negative predictive value; AUC: Area under the curve; HIV: Human immunodeficiency virus; BMI: Body mass index; COPD: Chronic obstructive pulmonary disease; ESRD: End stage renal disease.

Acknowledgements
We thank Matthew Sullivan for the use of his artwork.

Authors' contributions
DB: Conceptualization, methodology, validation, investigation, writing—original draft, writing—review and editing, visualization, supervision, and project administration. GL: Conceptualization, methodology, investigation, writing—review and editing, and supervision. TF: Conceptualization, methodology, investigation, writing—review and editing, and supervision. OT: Formal analysis and writing—review and editing. BG and RO: Conceptualization, methodology, investigation, and writing—review and editing. All authors read and approved the final manuscript.

Author details
[1] Department of Emergency Medicine, Johns Hopkins School of Medicine, 1830 East Monument St Suite 6-100, Baltimore, MD 21287, USA. [2] Hospitalist Program, Division of General Internal Medicine, Department of Medicine, Johns Hopkins School of Medicine, Baltimore, MD, USA. [3] Medical Scientist Training Program, Johns Hopkins School of Medicine, Baltimore, MD, USA. [4] Department of Pulmonary and Critical Care Medicine, Johns Hopkins Hospital, Baltimore, MD, USA.

References

1. Dong E, Du H, Gardner L (2020) An interactive web-based dashboard to track COVID-19 in real time. Lancet Infect Dis 20:533–534. https://doi.org/10.1016/S1473-3099(20)30120-1
2. Woloshin S, Patel N, Kesselheim AS (2020) False negative tests for SARS-CoV-2 infection—challenges and implications. N Engl J Med. 382:e38. https://doi.org/10.1056/NEJMp2015897
3. Feng H, Liu Y, Lv M, Zhong J (2020) A case report of COVID-19 with false negative RT-PCR test: necessity of chest CT. Jpn J Radiol 38:409–410. https://doi.org/10.1007/s11604-020-00967-9
4. Goldstein J, McKinley J (2020) 9-Day waits for test results threaten N.Y.C.'s ability to contain virus. The New York Times A1
5. Zhao W, Zhong Z, Xie X et al (2020) Relation between chest CT findings and clinical conditions of coronavirus disease (Covid-19) pneumonia: a multicenter study. Am J Roentgenol 214:1072–1077. https://doi.org/10.2214/AJR.20.22976
6. Ai T, Yang Z, Xia L (2020) Correlation of chest CT and RT-PCR testing in coronavirus disease. Radiology. https://doi.org/10.14358/PERS.80.2.000
7. Caruso D, Zerunian M, Polici M et al (2020) Chest CT features of COVID-19 in Rome. Italy Radiol 77:201237. https://doi.org/10.1148/radiol.2020201237
8. Li B, Li X, Wang Y et al (2020) Diagnostic value and key features of computed tomography in Coronavirus Disease 2019. Emerg Microbes Infect 9:787–793. https://doi.org/10.1080/22221751.2020.1750307
9. Organization WH Computed tomography (CT) units per million. https://www.who.int/diagnostic_imaging/collaboration/ctpermill_14.jpg?ua=1
10. Sippel S, Muruganandan K, Levine A, Shah S (2011) Review article: Use of ultrasound in the developing world. Int J Emerg Med 4:1–11. https://doi.org/10.1186/1865-1380-4-72
11. Peyrony O, Marbeuf-Gueye C, Truong V et al (2020) Accuracy of Emergency Department clinical findings for diagnostic of coronavirus disease-2019. Ann Emerg Med. https://doi.org/10.1016/j.annemergmed.2020.05.022
12. Lichtenstein D, Goldstein I, Mourgeon E et al (2004) Comparative diagnostic performances of auscultation, chest radiography, and lung ultrasonography in acute respiratory distress syndrome. Anesthesiology 100:9–15. https://doi.org/10.1097/00000542-200401000-00006
13. Tierney DM, Huelster JS, Overgaard JD et al (2020) Comparative performance of pulmonary ultrasound, chest radiograph, and CT among patients with acute respiratory failure. Crit Care Med. https://doi.org/10.1097/CCM.0000000000004124
14. Zieleskiewicz L, Markarian T, Lopez A et al (2020) Comparative study of lung ultrasound and chest computed tomography scan in the assessment of severity of confirmed COVID-19 pneumonia. Intensive Care Med 46:1707–1713. https://doi.org/10.1007/s00134-020-06186-0
15. Zieleskiewicz L, Cornesse A, Hammad E et al (2015) Implementation of lung ultrasound in polyvalent intensive care unit: impact on irradiation and medical cost. Anaesth Crit Care Pain Med 34:41–44. https://doi.org/10.1016/j.accpm.2015.01.002
16. Jones BP, Tay ET, Elikashvili I et al (2016) Feasibility and safety of substituting lung ultrasonography for chest radiography when diagnosing pneumonia in children: a randomized controlled trial. Chest 150:131–138. https://doi.org/10.1016/j.chest.2016.02.643
17. Wimalasena Y, Kocierz L, Strong D et al (2018) Lung ultrasound: a useful tool in the assessment of the dyspnoeic patient in the emergency department. Fact or fiction? Emerg Med J 35:258–266. https://doi.org/10.1136/emermed-2016-205937
18. Poggiali E, Dacrema A, Bastoni D et al (2020) Can lung US help critical care clinicians in the early diagnosis of novel coronavirus (COVID-19) pneumonia? Radiology 295:E6–E6. https://doi.org/10.1148/radiol.2020200847
19. Peng Q-Y, Wang X-T, Zhang L-N (2020) Findings of lung ultrasonography of novel corona virus pneumonia during the 2019–2020 epidemic. Intensive Care Med. https://doi.org/10.1007/s00134-020-05996-6
20. Akl EA, Blazic I, Yaacoub S et al (2020) Use of chest imaging in the diagnosis and management of COVID-19: a WHO rapid advice guide. Radiology. https://doi.org/10.1148/radiol.2020203173
21. Volpicelli G, Lamorte A, Villén T (2020) What's new in lung ultrasound during the COVID-19 pandemic. Intensive Care Med. https://doi.org/10.1007/s00134-020-06048-9

22. Huang Y, Wang S, Liu Y, et al (2020) A preliminary study on the ultrasonic manifestations of peripulmonary lesions of non-critical novel coronavirus pneumonia (COVID-19). SSRN
23. Volpicelli G, Gargani L (2020) Sonographic signs and patterns of COVID-19 pneumonia. Ultrasound J 12:20–22. https://doi.org/10.1186/s13089-020-00171-w
24. Duggan NM, Shokoohi H, Liteplo AS et al (2020) Best practice recommendations for point-of-care lung ultrasound in patients with suspected COVID-19. J Emerg Med 59:515–520. https://doi.org/10.1016/j.jemermed.2020.06.033
25. Mohamed MFH, Al-Shokri S, Yousaf Z et al (2020) Frequency of abnormalities detected by point-of-care lung ultrasound in symptomatic COVID-19 patients: systematic review and meta-analysis. Am J Trop Med Hyg. https://doi.org/10.4269/ajtmh.20-0371
26. Bar S, Lecourtois A, Diouf M et al (2020) The association of lung ultrasound images with COVID-19 infection in an emergency room cohort. Anaesthesia. https://doi.org/10.1111/anae.15175
27. Favot M, Malik A, Rowland J et al (2020) Point-of-care lung ultrasound for detecting severe presentations of coronavirus disease 2019 in the emergency department: a retrospective analysis. Crit Care Explor 2:e0176. https://doi.org/10.1097/cce.0000000000000176
28. Alharthy A, Faqihi F, Abuhamdah M et al (2020) Prospective longitudinal evaluation of point-of-care lung ultrasound in critically ill patients with severe COVID-19 pneumonia. J Ultrasound Med. https://doi.org/10.1002/jum.15417
29. Deng Q, Zhang Y, Wang H et al (2020) Semiquantitative lung ultrasound scores in the evaluation and follow-up of critically ill patients with COVID-19: a single-center study. Acad Radiol. https://doi.org/10.1016/j.acra.2020.07.002
30. Perrone T, Soldati G, Padovini L et al (2020) A new lung ultrasound protocol able to predict worsening in patients affected by severe acute respiratory syndrome coronavirus 2 pneumonia. J Ultrasound Med 2:1–9. https://doi.org/10.1002/jum.15548
31. Sahu AK, Mathew R, Bhoi S et al (2020) Lung sonographic findings in COVID-19 patients. Am J Emerg Med. https://doi.org/10.1016/j.ajem.2020.08.080
32. Youden WJ (1950) Index for rating diagnostic tests. Cancer 3:32–35. https://doi.org/10.1002/1097-0142(1950)3:1%3c32::aid-cncr2820030106%3e3.0.co;2-3
33. Brainin P, Claggett B, Lewis EF et al (2020) Body mass index and B-lines on lung ultrasonography in chronic and acute heart failure. ESC Heart Fail. https://doi.org/10.1002/ehf2.12640
34. Maw AM, Hassanin A, Ho PM et al (2019) Diagnostic accuracy of point-of-care lung ultrasonography and chest radiography in adults with symptoms suggestive of acute decompensated heart failure: a systematic review and meta-analysis. JAMA Netw Open 2:e190703. https://doi.org/10.1001/jamanetworkopen.2019.0703
35. Singh AK, Mayo PH, Koenig S et al (2018) The use of M-Mode ultrasonography to differentiate the causes of B lines. Chest 153:689–696. https://doi.org/10.1016/j.chest.2017.10.019
36. Copetti R, Soldati G, Copetti P (2008) Chest sonography: a useful tool to differentiate acute cardiogenic pulmonary edema from acute respiratory distress syndrome. Cardiovasc Ultrasound 6:1–10. https://doi.org/10.1186/1476-7120-6-16
37. Lee FCY (2016) Lung ultrasound-a primary survey of the acutely dyspneic patient. J Intensive Care. https://doi.org/10.1186/s40560-016-0180-1
38. D'Amico F, Baumgart DC, Danese S, Peyrin-Biroulet L (2020) Diarrhea during COVID-19 infection: pathogenesis, epidemiology, prevention, and management. Clin Gastroenterol Hepatol 18:1663–1672. https://doi.org/10.1016/j.cgh.2020.04.001
39. Helms J, Kremer S, Merdji H et al (2020) Neurologic features in severe SARS-CoV-2 infection. N Engl J Med. https://doi.org/10.1056/NEJMc2008597

22

ACUTE ABDOMEN systemic sonographic approach to acute abdomen in emergency department

Maryam Al Ali[1*], Sarah Jabbour[2] and Salma Alrajaby[1]

Abstract

Background: Acute abdomen is a medical emergency with a wide spectrum of etiologies. Point-of-care ultrasound (POCUS) can help in early identification and management of the causes. The ACUTE–ABDOMEN protocol was created by the authors to aid in the evaluation of acute abdominal pain using a systematic sonographic approach, integrating the same core ultrasound techniques already in use—into one mnemonic. This mnemonic ACUTE means: A: abdominal aortic aneurysm; C: collapsed inferior vena cava; U: ulcer (perforated viscus); T: trauma (free fluid); E: ectopic pregnancy, followed by ABDOMEN which stands: A: appendicitis; B: biliary tract; D: distended bowel loop; O: obstructive uropathy; Men: testicular torsion/Women: ovarian torsion. The article discusses two cases of abdominal pain the diagnosis and management of which were directed and expedited as a result of using the ACUTE–ABDOMEN protocol. The first case was of a 33-year-old male, who presented with a 3-day history of abdominal pain, vomiting and constipation. Physical exam revealed a soft abdomen with generalized tenderness and normal bowel sounds. Laboratory tests were normal. A bedside ultrasound done using the ACUTE–ABDOMEN protocol showed signs of intussusception. This was confirmed by CT-abdomen. The second case was of a 70-year-old female, a known case of diabetes and hypertension, who presented with a 3-hour history of abdominal pain, vomiting and diarrhea. She had a normal physical exam and laboratory studies. Her symptoms mimicking simple gastroenteritis had improved. However, bedside ultrasound, using the ACUTE–ABDOMEN protocol showed localized free fluid with dilated small bowel loop in right lower quadrant with absent peristalsis. A CT abdomen confirmed a diagnosis of intestinal obstruction. These two cases demonstrate that the usefulness of applying POCUS in a systematic method—like the "ACUTE–ABDOMEN" approach—can aid in patient diagnosis and management.

Case presentation: We are presenting two cases of undifferentiated acute abdomen pain, where ACUTE ABDOMEN sonographic approach was applied and facilitated the accurate patient management and disposition.

Conclusion: ACUTE ABDOMEN sonographic approach in acute abdomen can play an important role in ruling out critical diagnosis, and can guide emergency physician or any critical care physician in patient management.

Keywords: Acute abdomen, POCUS, Emergency ultrasound, Critical ultrasound

Background

The use of bedside ultrasound by physicians has become increasingly popular in the last two decades, even more so in critically ill patients. In emergency medicine, point of care ultrasound (POCUS) is being used as a diagnostic modality, given its easy accessibility and non-invasive nature. It is used as an adjunct, directing physicians on further testing modalities and treatment plans.

However, there has always been the question of reliability of ultrasound being performed by non-radiologists. In a study involving 651 patients complaining of renal colic, emergency physicians were found to have moderate to high sensitivity for identifying hydronephrosis on POCUS when compared with the consensus

*Correspondence: Maryamsaif86@gmail.com
[1] Arab Board in Emergency Medicine, Rashid Hospital Trauma Center, Dubai Health Authority, oud metha, Dubai, United Arab Emirates
Full list of author information is available at the end of the article

interpretation of the same studies by emergency radiologists [1].

Emergency ultrasound is now considered a core skill for emergency physician. American College of Emergency Physicians has introduced Emergency Ultrasound Guidelines that were introduced in 2008 and revisited in 2016, acknowledging that emergency ultrasound is a part of patient assessment within different clinical categories.

Given the time constraint and critical conditions of patients in the emergency, ultrasound approach in the ED should be focused, systemic and specific to patient symptom. Thus, the different protocols for different patient symptom came into practice. These fall under ACEP's functional clinical category of "symptom or sign-based ultrasound". To mention a few, FAST ultrasound for the trauma patient, RUSH protocol for the hypotensive patient, and BLUE protocol for the dyspneic patient [2].

Similarly, the ACUTE ABDOMEN protocol [3] was created by the authors to aid in the evaluation of acute abdominal pain using a systematic sonographic approach, integrating the same core ultrasound techniques already in use, into one mnemonic. This novel approach to the patient with abdominal pain systematically assesses the five critical causes—in the first part of the mnemonic "ACUTE" followed by scanning for other surgical causes in the second part of the mnemonic "ABDOMEN".

The mnemonic ACUTE stands for—A: abdominal aortic aneurysm, C: collapsed inferior vena cava, U: ulcer (perforated viscus), T: trauma (free fluid), E: ectopic pregnancy, followed by ABDOMEN which stands for—A: appendicitis, B: biliary tract, D: distended bowel loop, O: obstructive uropathy, Men: testicular torsion, Women: ovarian torsion.

This might seem quite overwhelming and time consuming for an already busy ER, but if done in the proposed systemic approach, it can, on the contrary, provide pertinent information in a short time. An example of how the ACUTE ABDOMEN protocol directed the patient management is demonstrated in the two cases discussed below.

Case presentation

Case 1

A 33-year-old male of Asian (Pakistani) origin was presented to Rashid Emergency and Trauma Center with a complaint of sudden non-radiating epigastric abdominal pain. The pain was associated with vomiting and constipation for 3 days. There was no chest pain, diarrhea, fever or melena.

The patient had similar presentation in his country 4 years ago and was managed conservatively.

Vital signs were normal. Abdomen was soft with generalized tenderness and normal bowel sounds.

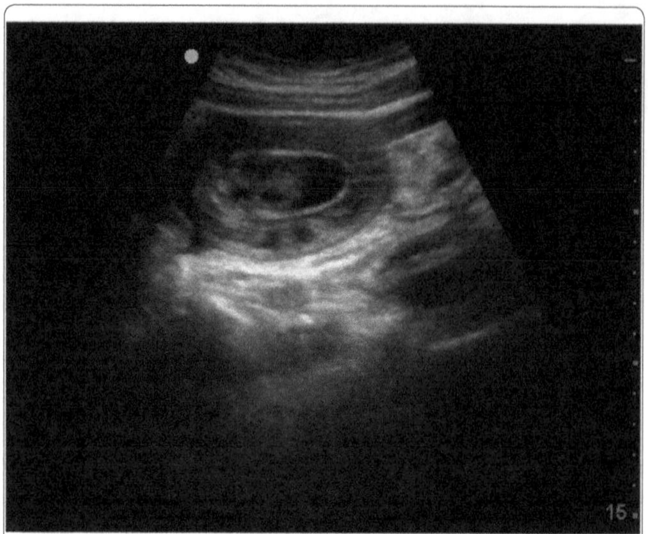

Fig. 1 Point of care ultrasound for acute abdomen (ACUTE approach) showed localized free fluid with doughnut sign edematous bowel loop wall

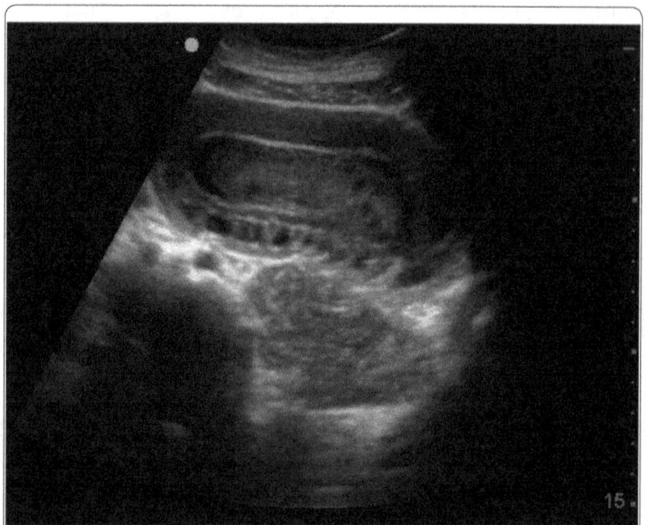

Fig. 2 Point of care ultrasound for acute abdomen (ACUTE approach) showed bowel telescoping inside itself with edematous bowel loop wall (long axis)

Laboratory studies were normal.

Point of care ultrasound for acute abdomen (ACUTE approach) showed:

A: normal aortic diameter
C: collapsed IVC > 50%,
U: no free air
T: localized free fluid with doughnut sign (Fig. 1), and long axis of the segment showed bowel telescoping inside itself with oedematous bowel loop wall (Fig. 2).

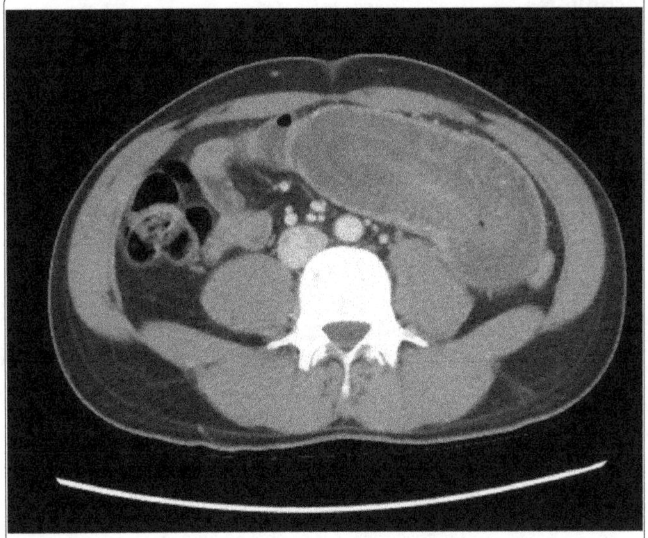

Fig. 3 CT scan abdomen with contrast showed a long segment entero-enteric (jejuno-jejunal) intussusception seen mainly in the left side of the abdomen

Abdominal X-ray was normal

After ultrasound finding, we decided to perform urgent CT scan of the abdomen which showed the evidence of long segment entero-enteric (jejuno-jejunal) intussusception seen mainly in the left side of the abdomen, with relatively collapsed intussusceptum segment. Mild amount of intraperitoneal free fluid was seen in the jejunal mesentery next to the involved segments as well as in the pelvic peritoneal pouches (Fig. 3).

Surgical consultation was obtained; however, the patient preferred to continue the medical care in his country.

Case 2

A 70-year-old female diabetic and hypertensive was presented to Rashid Emergency and Trauma Center with generalized abdominal pain for 3 h after food which was associated with vomiting and diarrhea twice. There was no urinary complaint, chest pain or fever.

Vital signs were normal. Abdomen was soft with mild tenderness in the right lower abdomen, without peritonitis clinical sign. Laboratory test was insignificant, except for leukocytosis $17.2{\cdot}10^3/\mu L$ ($3.6–11.0{\cdot}10^3/\mu L$) and plasma lactic acid 3.7 mmol/L (0.5–2.2 mmol/L).

Point of care ultrasound for acute abdomen (ACUTE approach) showed:

A: normal aortic diameter
C: normal IVC
U: no free air
T: localized free fluid with dilated small bowel loop in right lower quadrant with absent peristalsis (Fig. 4).

CT abdomen showed evidence of significantly dilated small bowel loops in the right side of the lower abdomen and pelvis with a short segment critical stenosis measuring about 2.3 cm. It also showed an evidence suggestive

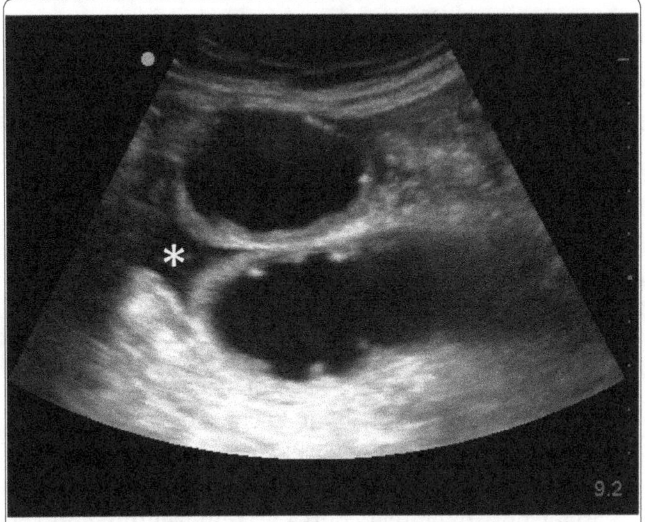

Fig. 4 Point of care ultrasound for acute abdomen showed localized free fluid * with dilated small bowel loop in right lower quadrant with absent peristalsis

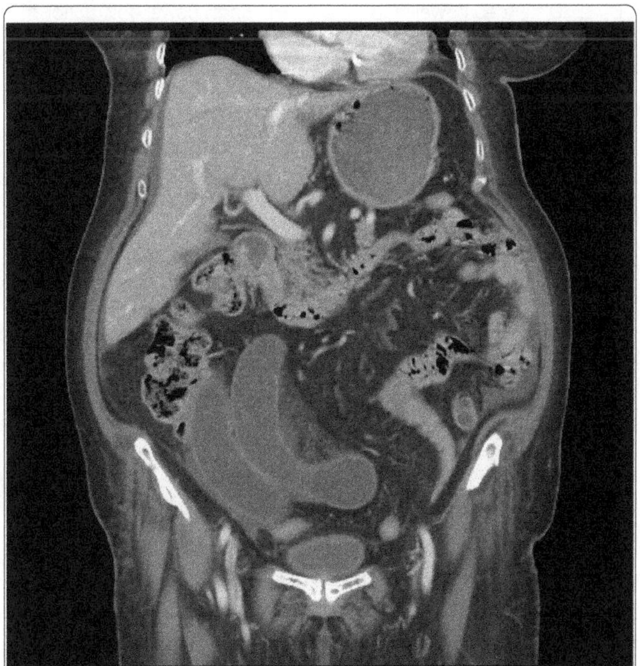

Fig. 5 CT abdomen with contrast showed dilated small bowel loops in the right side of the lower abdomen and pelvis with a short segment critical stenosis measuring about 2.3 cm

Table 1 ACUTE ABDOMEN sonographic aproach: findings and techniques

	Pathology	Finding	Technique
A. ACUTE			
A	Abdominal aortic aneurysm	Abdominal aortic > 3 cm?	Probe: curvilinear or phased array Scan: long axis and short axis from epigastric till the bifurcation of common iliac
C	Collapsed inferior vena cave (assessment of patient's volume status)	IVC collapsing > 50%?	Probe: curvilinear or phased array Scan: subxiphoid long axis, assessing the respiratory dynamics of the IVC
U	Ulcer (perforated viscus)	Pneumoperitoneum? Direct sign: Increased echogenicity of peritoneal stripe Presence of A lines Indirect sign: Intraperitoneal free fluid Air bubbles in ascetic fluid Thickened bowel loop Bowel or gallbladder thickened wall with ileus	Probe: curvilinear or high frequency linear Scan: epigastrium through the right upper quadrant (RUQ) along the transverse and longitudinal axes
T	Trauma (free fluid)	Intraperitoneal hypoechoic fluid?	Probe: curvilinear or phased array Scan: right upper quadrant, left upper quadrant, suprapubic Localized free fluid: scan right and left paracolic gutter
E	Ectopic pregnancy (empty uterus)	Intraperitoneal hypoechoic fluid, empty uterus or extra-uterine gestational sac?	Probe: curvilinear Scan suprapubic long and short axis
B. ABDOMEN			
A	Appendicitis	Non compressible Diameter > 6 mm	Probe: high frequency linear Scan: right lower abdomen
B	Biliary tract	Cholecystitis: Precystic fluid Sonographic murphy Gallbladder calculi Choledocholithiasis CBD > 6 mm	Probe: curvilinear or phased array Scan: right upper abdomen
D	Distended bowel loop	Small bowel obstruction? Dilated small bowel loop > 3 cm Back-and-forth movement of spot echoes inside fluid-filled bowel Decrease bowel peristalsis	Probe: curvilinear or high frequency linear Scan: epigastrium, bilateral colic gutters, and suprapubic regions
O	Obstructive uropathy	Hydronephrosis? Dilated renal calyces Renal stone: acoustic echogenic foci urterovesical junction.	Probe: curvilinear Scan: Longitudinal view Lower intercostal, right: mid axillary line, left: posterior axillary line.
MEN	Men: testicular torsion	Hypoechoic testis compare to normal Reduce or no perfusion	Probe: high frequency linear Scan: scrotal transverse and longitudinal Doppler
	Women: ovarian torsion	Adnexal mass > 4 cm Pelvic free fluid Reduced blood flow on Doppler	Probe: curvilinear Scan: suprapubic, sagittal and transverse identify uterus, then move right and left

of internal herniation with dilated loops of bowel. Jejunal loops and distal ileum appear collapsed. Free fluid was seen in the abdomen and pelvis (Fig. 5).

Urgent surgical consultation was obtained and the patient had undergone laparotomy which was conclusive of an omental band adherent to the small bowel mesentery.

About 150 cm proximal to ileo cecal juction producing congestion with punctuate haemorrhages and dilatation of the proximal bowel of about 30 cm. After the band was released; the color of the bowel changed to normal with good peristalsis. No bowel resection was needed.

Patient post-operative course was uneventful, and she was discharged home after 5 days.

Patient symptoms that mimicked simple gastroenteritis had improved, but because of our ultrasound finding that suggested intestinal obstruction, it was decided to perform a CT abdomen. If not for our preliminary ultrasound findings, this patient would have been discharged without further imaging.

Discussion

POCUS approaches have been published in multiple critical care conditions such as Bedside Lung Ultrasound in Emergency (BLUE) protocol in respiratory failure which concluded that lung ultrasound immediately provided the diagnosis of acute respiratory failure in 90.5% of cases. The BLUE protocol focused on lung ultrasound only [4]; however, the RUSH protocol demonstrated that initial integration of bedside ultrasound into the evaluation of the patient with shock results in a more accurate initial diagnosis with an improved patient care plan [5].

In this case series, we presented two cases where ACUTE ABDOMEN played an important role in their management, POCUS can play an important role in acute abdomen, by early recognition and diagnosing critical conditions. Instead of relying only on physical examination which might have very low sensitivity in comparison to ultrasound, for example in physical examination can identify 38% of patients with AAA [6], ultrasound by emergency physician can detect AAA in 93% to 100% of cases, with specificities approaching 100% [7–9].

In other pathologies like pneumoperitoneum, X-ray is more frequently used, but ultrasound is superior to upright chest and lateral decubitus X-ray where the sensitivity is 92% versus 78% for X-ray [10].

The two cases presented with undifferentiated acute abdomen, in which bedside ultrasound was started with ACUTE approach after history and physical examination, (Table 1A) [11] showed unexpected finding, which needed further radiological evaluation by CT scan with contrast and early referral to surgical team.

For the second part of the approach, ABDOMEN (Table 1B) [11] usually will be a secondary survey and will focus the assessment with guide of the history and examination.

Conclusions

ACUTE and ABDOMEN sonographic approach in acute abdomen can play an important role in ruling out critical diagnosis, and can guide emergency physician or any critical care physician in patient management.

Further prospective studies are warranted.

Abbreviations

POCUS: point of care ultrasound; BLUE: bedside lung ultrasound in emergency; RUSH: rapid ultrasound in shock; AAA: abdominal aortic aneurysm; IVC: inferior vena cava.

Acknowledgements

None.

Authors' contributions

SJ: presentation of the cases, MAA and SA: discussion of the case. All authors read and approved the final manuscript.

Author details

[1] Arab Board in Emergency Medicine, Rashid Hospital Trauma Center, Dubai Health Authority, oud metha, Dubai, United Arab Emirates. [2] Emergency Medicine Resident, Rashid Hospital Trauma Center, Dubai Health Authority, oud metha, Dubai, United Arab Emirates.

References

1. Pathan S, Mitra B, Mirza S, Momin U, Ahmed Z, Andraous L et al (2018) Emergency physician interpretation of point-of-care ultrasound for identifying and grading of hydronephrosis in renal colic compared with consensus interpretation by emergency radiologists. Acad Emerg Med 25(10):1129–1137
2. Ultrasound Guidelines: emergency, point-of -care, and clinical ultrasound guidelines in medicine. Acep.org (2019). https://acep.org/patient-care/policy-statements/ultrasound-guidelines-emergency-point-of–care-andclinical-ultrasound-guidelines-in-medicine/. Accessed 14 Mar 2019
3. Abdominal Pain in ED (2017) Using a novel sonographic approach Maryam Al Ali and Salma Alrajaby Emergency Department, Rashid Hospital, Dubai, United Arab Emirates. Eur J Emerg Med. 24:e1–e15
4. Lichtenstein D, Mezière G (2008) Relevance of lung ultrasound in the diagnosis of acute respiratory failure: the BLUE Protocol. Chest 134(1):117–125
5. Perera P, Mailhot T, Riley D, Mandavia D (2012) The RUSH Exam 2012: rapid ultrasound in shock in the evaluation of the critically ill patient. Ultrasound Clin 7(2):255–278
6. Chervu A, Clagett G, Valentine R, Myers S, Rossi P (1995) Role of physical examination in detection of abdominal aortic aneurysms. Surgery 117(4):454–457
7. Dent B, Kendall RJ, Boyle AA et al (2007) Emergency ultrasound of the abdominal aorta by UK emergency physicians: a prospective cohort study. Emerg Med J 24:547–549
8. Costantino TG, Bruno EC, Handly N et al (2005) Accuracy of emergency medicine ultrasound in the evaluation of abdominal aortic aneurysm. J Emerg Med 29:455–460
9. Tayal VS, Graf CD, Gibbs MA (2003) Prospective study of accuracy and outcome of emergency ultrasound for abdominal aortic aneurysm over two years. Acad Emerg Med 10:867–871
10. Chen S, Yen Z, Wang H, Lin F, Hsu C, Chen W (2002) Ultrasonography is superior to plain radiography in the diagnosis of pneumoperitoneum. Br J Surg 89(3):351–354
11. Case Report: POCUS to FOCUS–POCUS Journal. Pocusjournal.com (2018). http://pocusjournal.com/article/2018-03-01p15-17/. Accessed 28 Aug 2018

Renal resistive index is associated with acute kidney injury in COVID-19 patients treated in the intensive care unit

Mårten Renberg[1,2*], Olof Jonmarker[3], Naima Kilhamn[1], Claire Rimes-Stigare[1,2], Max Bell[1,2] and Daniel Hertzberg[1,2]

Abstract

Background: Renal resistive index (RRI) is a promising tool for the assessment of acute kidney injury (AKI) in critically ill patients in general, but its role and association to AKI among patients with Coronavirus disease 2019 (COVID-19) is not known.

Objective: The aim of this study was to describe the pattern of RRI in relation to AKI in patients with COVID-19 treated in the intensive care unit.

Methods: In this observational cohort study, RRI was measured in COVID-19 patients in six intensive care units at two sites of a Swedish University Hospital. AKI was defined by the creatinine criteria in the Kidney Disease Improving Global Outcomes classification. We investigated the association between RRI and AKI diagnosis, different AKI stages and urine output.

Results: RRI was measured in 51 patients, of which 23 patients (45%) had AKI at the time of measurement. Median RRI in patients with AKI was 0.80 (IQR 0.71–0.85) compared to 0.72 (IQR 0.67–0.78) in patients without AKI ($p=0.004$). Compared to patients without AKI, RRI was higher in patients with AKI stage 3 (median 0.83, IQR 0.71–0.85, $p=0.006$) but not in patients with AKI stage 1 (median 0.76, IQR 0.71–0.83, $p=0.347$) or AKI stage 2 (median 0.79, min/max 0.79/0.80, $n=2$, $p=0.134$). RRI was higher in patients with an ongoing AKI episode compared to patients who never developed AKI (median 0.72, IQR 0.69–0.78, $p=0.015$) or patients who developed AKI but had recovered at the time of measurement (median 0.68, IQR 0.67–0.81, $p=0.021$). Oliguric patients had higher RRI (median 0.84, IQR 0.83–0.85) compared to non-oliguric patients (median 0.74, IQR 0.69–0.81) ($p=0.009$). After multivariable adjustment, RRI was independently associated with AKI (OR for 0.01 increments of RRI 1.22, 95% CI 1.07–1.41).

Conclusions: Critically ill COVID-19 patients with AKI have higher RRI compared to those without AKI, and elevated RRI may have a role in identifying severe and oliguric AKI at the bedside in these patients.

Keywords: Renal resistive index, Point-of-care ultrasound, Ultrasonography, Renal Doppler, Acute kidney injury, COVID-19

Background

The Coronavirus disease 2019 (COVID-19) pandemic is causing great suffering and is placing strain on health care systems worldwide. Acute kidney injury (AKI) is a common complication in critically ill patients with COVID-19. Initial studies have reported an incidence from 20 to almost 90% among patients admitted to the

*Correspondence: marten.renberg@sll.se

[1] Department of Perioperative Medicine and Intensive Care, Karolinska University Hospital, Solna, 171 76 Stockholm, Sweden

Full list of author information is available at the end of the article

intensive care unit (ICU) or in need of mechanical ventilation [1–4], of which up to one-third have been treated with renal replacement therapy (RRT) [5, 6]. COVID-19 patients who develop AKI may have a 13-fold increased risk of death compared to those who do not develop AKI [4, 7, 8].

Renal resistive index (RRI) is an ultrasonographic Doppler measurement of flow velocities in intraparenchymal renal arteries. Normal values are around 0.60 [9, 10] with 0.70 considered the upper normal threshold in adults [11]. Elevated RRI has shown promise in early detection and prognostication of AKI in mixed ICU populations [12–16], and the method seems feasible within the scope of point-of-care ultrasonography (POCUS) [17].

As thromboembolism and renal microangiopathy have gained interest as possible mechanisms giving rise to AKI in COVID-19 [18, 19], RRI may show to be an especially helpful tool to guide diagnosis and treatment of AKI in these patients. In a recent case–control study, reduced renal perfusion and substantially elevated RRI were described in ten COVID-19 patients with severe AKI [20]. However, RRI has not been described in larger populations of COVID-19 patients and its role in these patients remains unclear. The aim of this study was to describe the pattern of RRI in relation to AKI in patients with COVID-19 treated in the ICU. We specifically investigated if there was an association between RRI and AKI diagnosis, different AKI stages and urine output.

Methods

Study population

This was an observational cohort study conducted in six ICUs designated for COVID-19 patients (COVID-ICUs) at the Karolinska University Hospital, Stockholm, Sweden. Four ICUs were at one of two sites, and two at the other site. On specific dates, patients in each COVID-ICU were screened for participation. Inclusion criteria were infection with Severe Acute Respiratory Syndrome Coronavirus 2 (SARS-CoV-2) detected by a positive reverse transcriptase-polymerase chain reaction taken from upper or lower airways, admission to a COVID-ICU, and age ≥ 18 years. Exclusion criteria were end-stage renal disease (ESRD) before ICU admission, palliative phase of intensive care, ongoing irregular cardiac rhythm or treatment with extracorporeal membrane oxygenation (ECMO).

The study complied with the Declaration of Helsinki and was approved by the Swedish Ethical Review Authority. Requirement for signed informed consent was waived. A printed information sheet was sent to each patient or next of kin with the opportunity to retrospectively withdraw participation.

Definitions

AKI was defined according to the Kidney Disease Improving Global Outcomes (KDIGO) classification as an increase in serum creatinine concentration (sCr) and categorized into three stages [21]. The highest sCr from ICU admission to the day of RRI measurement was compared to baseline sCr. Baseline sCr was defined as the last known value measured in a disease-free phase before admission. When no previous sCr value existed, hospital admission sCr was used. The AKI stages were defined as the following: stage 1, $\geq$ 1.5- to 1.9-fold increase or an absolute increase $\geq$ 26 µmol/l; stage 2, $\geq$ 2.0- to 2.9-fold increase; stage 3, $\geq$ 3.0-fold increase or an absolute increase > 354 µmol/l or initiation of RRT. The KDIGO urine output criteria were not used since hourly urine output was not always registered in the medical records. If the sCr elevation occurred more than 7 days before the RRI measurement and its value had returned to < 1.5-fold or < 26 µmol/l higher than from baseline, the patient was evaluated as having recovered from an AKI episode and was classified into the no AKI group. Oliguria at the time of RRI measurement was defined as urine output < 0.5 ml/kg ideal body weight/hour for 24 h regardless of diuretic drug administration [22]. Ideal body weight was calculated using the gender-specific Acute Respiratory Distress Syndrome Network formula [23]. Chronic kidney disease (CKD) was defined as estimated glomerular filtration rate (eGFR) < 60 mL/min/1.73 m^2, ESRD was defined as eGFR < 15 mL/min/1.73 m^2, and eGFR was calculated using the Chronic Kidney Disease Epidemiology Collaboration (CKD-EPI) equation [24]. For this, baseline sCr was used when classifying patients as having CKD or ESRD, and a combination of sCr and cystatin C was used when calculating eGFR at the time of RRI measurement. Comorbidities were considered present if documented in the patient's medical record or if the patient was prescribed medication for the current state. The cardiovascular disease group included patients with cardiac failure, atrial arrhythmia, prior myocardial infarction or prior cardiac surgery.

RRI measurements

All RRI measurements were performed by one of two operators (MR and OJ). Both operators had more than one year's clinical experience of the RRI method. For each site a designated ultrasound device with a curvilinear probe of 1.0–6.0 MHz was used (GE Vivid S70N, US and GE Logiq E10, US at the two sites, respectively). The patients were examined in their ICU bed in supine or prone position depending on their respiratory requirements. Both kidneys were examined, and measurements were made on both or the most accessible side since the difference in RRI values between the right and left kidney has been shown to be negligible both in healthy and critically ill patients [9, 12, 17]. After obtaining a complete view of the kidney, color-Doppler was applied to visualize the global organization of intrarenal blood vessels. Pulse waved Doppler at the smallest possible width between 2 and 5 mm was used to measure flow velocities in an interlobular or arcuate artery in the upper, middle and lower kidney pole. The Doppler gain was set to obtain a clear outline of flow waves with minimal background noise. The pulse waved Doppler spectrum was considered optimal when at least three consecutive similar-looking waveforms for each pole were visualized. RRI was calculated for each pole as [(peak systolic velocity–end-diastolic velocity)/peak systolic velocity]. From the pole RRI values, a mean RRI was computed.

Data collection

The following clinical data were collected for each patient at the time of RRI measurement: hemodynamic parameters, vasopressor requirements, sedatives dose and ventilator settings if mechanically ventilated. Severity of illness was graded on the day of measurement using the Sequential Organ Failure Assessment (SOFA) (originally the Sepsis-related Organ Failure Assessment) score [25]. Information on comorbidities, regular and current medication and laboratory data were collected from medical records.

Statistical analysis

Patient characteristics and variables are presented using frequencies and percentages for categorical data, and medians with interquartile range (IQR) and minimum/maximum (min/max) values for continuous data. Clinical characteristics of patients with or without AKI were compared using Fisher's exact test for dichotomous variables and Wilcoxon rank-sum test for continuous variables. Median RRI between different groups were compared using the Wilcoxon rank-sum test. To elucidate potential confounding of the association between RRI and AKI, a multivariable logistic regression model was performed including RRI as a continuous and AKI as a dichotomous variable. Variables in our dataset that were associated with AKI with a p-value < 0.2 in bivariate logistic regression were selected for a manual forward selection procedure. Variables with the strongest association with AKI were included first, and variables that no longer were associated with AKI (p-value > 0.2) during forward selection were excluded. Remaining variables constituted the final model. Odds ratios (OR) and 95% confidence intervals (CI) were calculated. Goodness-of-fit of the model was assessed using the Hosmer–Lemeshow test. For all analyses a p-value < 0.05 was considered significant. The following variables had missing data: hospital admission sCr ($n = 7$ [14%]) and urine output at the day of RRI measurement ($n = 2$ [4%]). Missing data on height ($n = 1$ [2%]) were substituted with the median value according to sex. Statistical analyses were performed using Stata version 15.1 (StataCorp, College Station, US).

Results

Between April 15 and May 15 in 2020, the six COVID-ICUs were screened on specific dates for each ICU when at least one of the operators was available and able to perform measurements. Out of 71 screened patients, 20 were excluded, and a total of 51 patients were analyzed (Fig. 1).

Patient characteristics of the study population are presented in Table 1. Median age was 63 (IQR 57–67, min/max 29/74) and 88% were male. At the time of RRI measurement 23 patients (45%) had AKI (stage 1, $n = 4$ (8%); stage 2, $n = 2$ (4%); stage 3, $n = 17$ (33%) with $n = 13$ (25%) treated with continuous RRT [CRRT]). Among the 28 patients (55%) who did not have AKI, 11 patients (22%) previously during the ICU course had an AKI episode but had recovered (recovered from stage 1, $n = 7$ (14%); from stage 2, $n = 2$ (4%); from stage 3, $n = 2$ [4%]) and 17 patients (33%) never had AKI. Compared to patients without AKI, the AKI patients had a higher body mass index (BMI) and a lower incidence of cardiovascular disease. At the time of RRI measurement, AKI patients had a higher SOFA score, a higher incidence of mechanical ventilation and vasopressor use, lower eGFR and were more often oliguric compared to patients without AKI.

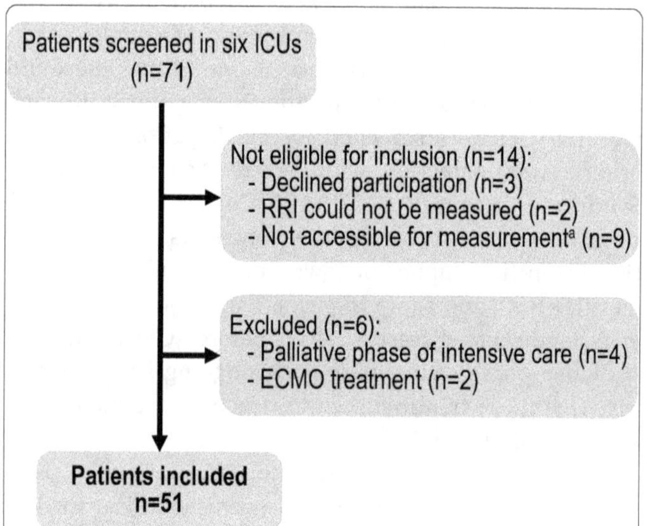

Fig. 1 Selection of the study population. ICU, intensive care unit; ECMO, extracorporeal membrane oxygenation. [a] Not accessible due to ongoing resuscitation, delirium/agitation, ongoing long period of mobilization/physiotherapy or unknown reason

Table 1 Patient characteristics of all patients and those with and without AKI

	All patients ($n=51$)	No AKI ($n=28$)	AKI ($n=23$)	p-value no AKI vs AKI
Age, median (IQR)	63 (57–67)	63 (58–68)	64 (53–65)	0.48
Sex, n (%)				0.027
Male	45 (88)	22 (79)	23 (100)	
Female	6 (12)	6 (21)	0 (0)	
BMI, median (IQR)	28.7 (25.2–31.2)	26.8 (24.6–29.9)	30.9 (27.0–34.7)	0.012
Risk factors for AKI, n (%)				
Hypertension	29 (57)	15 (54)	14 (61)	0.78
Diabetes	10 (20)	5 (18)	5 (22)	0.74
Chronic lung disease	11 (22)	7 (25)	4 (17)	0.73
Cardiovascular disease	6 (12)	6 (21)	0 (0)	0.027
Chronic kidney disease[a, c]	6 (12)	1 (4)	5 (22)	0.079
End-stage renal disease[b, c]	0 (0)			
No risk factor[d]	15 (29)	7 (25)	8 (35)	0.54
Data at RRI measurement				
ICU day, median (IQR)	18 (6–29)	16 (6–26)	19 (10–31)	0.19
SOFA score, median (IQR)	5 (4–8)	4 (3–7)	7 (5–10)	0.003
Mechanical ventilation, n (%)	38 (75)	17 (61)	21 (91)	0.022
Prone position, n (%)	9 (18)	5 (18)	4 (17)	1.00
Vasopressors, n (%)	26 (51)	10 (36)	16 (70)	0.025
eGFR[c], median (IQR)	58 (41–75)	70 (52–80)	26 (13–41)	<0.001
Oliguria[e], n (%)	5 (24)	0 (0)	5 (24)	0.011
RRT, n (%)				
Continuous RRT	13 (25)	0 (0)	13 (57)	<0.001
Intermittent HD	0 (0)			
Treatment in ICU[f], n (%)				
Mechanical ventilation	49 (96)	26 (93)	23 (100)	0.49
Vasopressors	49 (96)	26 (93)	23 (100)	0.49
RRT				
Continuous RRT	13 (25)	0 (0)	13 (57)	<0.001
Intermittent HD	1 (2)	0 (0)	1 (4)	0.45
Diuretics	48 (94)	25 (89)	23 (100)	0.24
Anti-inflammatory drugs				
Corticosteroids	37 (73)	21 (75)	16 (70)	0.76
Tocilizumab	3 (6)	3 (11)	0 (0)	0.24
Antiviral drugs				
Chloroquine phosphate	1 (2)	0 (0)	1 (4)	0.45
Remdesivir	2 (4)	2 (7)	0 (0)	0.49
Anticoagulation drugs				
LMWH	51 (100)	28 (100)	23 (100)	
Antiplatelets	33 (65)	21 (75)	12 (52)	0.14
Episode of thrombolysis	4 (8)	1 (4)	3 (13)	0.32

AKI acute kidney injury, *BMI* body mass index (kg/m^2), *RRI* renal resistive index, *ICU* intensive care unit, *SOFA score* Sequential Organ Failure Assessment score, *eGFR* estimated glomerular filtration rate (ml/min/1.73 m^2), *RRT* renal replacement therapy, *HD* hemodialysis, *LMWH* low-molecular-weight heparin

[a] Chronic kidney disease was defined as eGFR before ICU admission < 60 ml/min/1.73 m^2

[b] End-stage renal disease was defined as eGFR before ICU admission < 15 ml/min/1.73 m^2

[c] eGFR was calculated using the CKD-EPI equation using serum creatinine for classification of chronic kidney disease and end-stage renal disease, and a combination of serum creatinine and cystatin C at the time of RRI measurement

[d] Patients without history of smoking, chronic diagnoses or regular medications at hospital admission

[e] Oliguria was defined as urine output < 0.5 ml/kg ideal body weight/hour for 24 h

[f] Treatment from ICU admission to RRI measurement

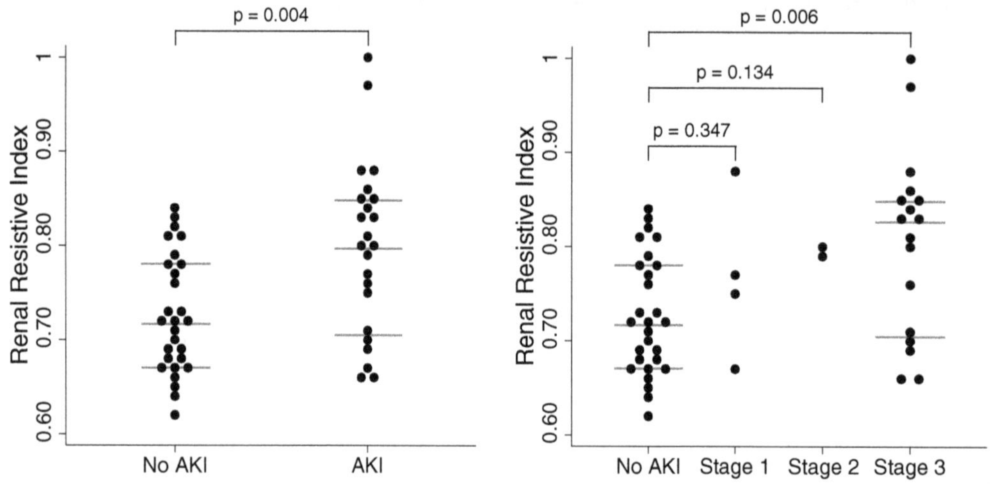

Fig. 2 Dot plot illustrating the association between renal resistive index and acute kidney injury (AKI) in patients with or without AKI (left) and patients with different stages of AKI (right). Each dot represents a patient. The horizontal lines represent the median, upper and lower quartiles

RRI was measured most often in the third week of the ICU and hospital course (median ICU day 18, IQR 6–29, min/max 0/37; median hospital day 20, IQR 10–30, min/max 2/37) and 4 weeks from symptom debut of COVID-19 (median 28, IQR 22–40, min/max 7/72). In 27 patients (53%) RRI was calculated from measurements in the right kidney, in 12 patients (23,5%) from measurements in the left kidney and in 12 patients (23,5%) from measurements in both kidneys. Forty-two patients (82%) were examined in supine and nine patients (18%) in prone position.

RRI in relation to AKI and AKI stage

Median RRI in the study population was 0.76 (IQR 0.69–0.82, min/max 0.62/1.0). One patient had completely diminished end-diastolic blood flow resulting in an RRI of 1.0. Median RRI in patients with AKI was 0.80 (IQR 0.71–0.85, min/max 0.66/1.0) compared to 0.72 (IQR 0.67–0.78, min/max 0.62/0.84) in patients without AKI ($p=0.004$) (Fig. 2). There was no difference in RRI between AKI stage 1 (median 0.76, IQR 0.71–0.83, min/max 0.67/0.88) or AKI stage 2 (median 0.79, min/max 0.79/0.80, $n=2$) compared to no AKI ($p=0.347$ and 0.134, respectively), but RRI was higher in patients with AKI stage 3 (median 0.83, IQR 0.71–0.85, min/max 0.66/1.0) compared to patients without AKI ($p=0.006$) (Fig. 2).

RRI in relation to non-AKI, recovered AKI and ongoing AKI

RRI did not differ within the no AKI group when comparing patients who never had AKI (median 0.72, IQR 0.69–0.78, min/max 0.62/0.83) to patients with recovered AKI (median 0.68, IQR 0.67–0.81, min/max 0.65/0.84) ($p=0.621$), but RRI was higher in the AKI group compared to both these groups ($p=0.015$ and 0.021, respectively) (Fig. 3).

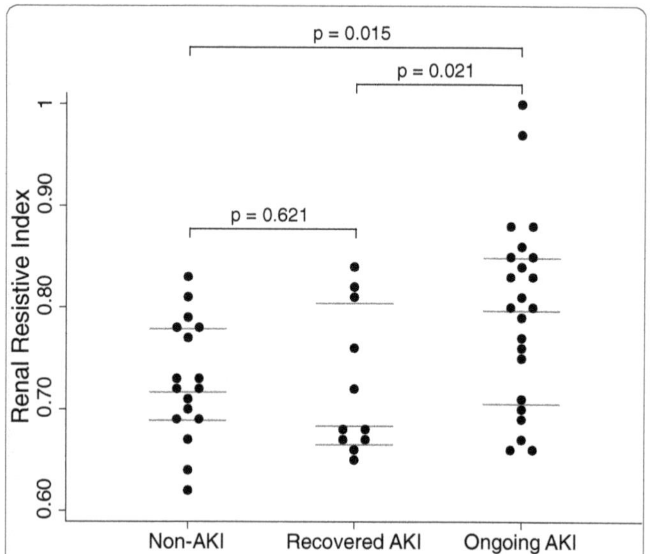

Fig. 3 Dot plot illustrating the association between renal resistive index and acute kidney injury (AKI) in patients who did not develop AKI, developed AKI but recovered, and had an ongoing AKI episode at the time of measurement. Each dot represents a patient. The horizontal lines represent the median, upper and lower quartiles

RRI in relation to oliguria

RRI was higher in oliguric patients (median 0.84, IQR 0.83–0.85, min/max 0.80/0.97) compared to non-oliguric patients (median 0.74, IQR 0.69–0.81, min/max 0.62/1.0) ($p=0.009$) (Fig. 4).

Multivariable analysis

Bivariate and multivariable logistic regression analysis is presented in Table 2. Possible confounders eligible for inclusion in the multivariable model are all variables presented in Table 1 except those that could be influenced by

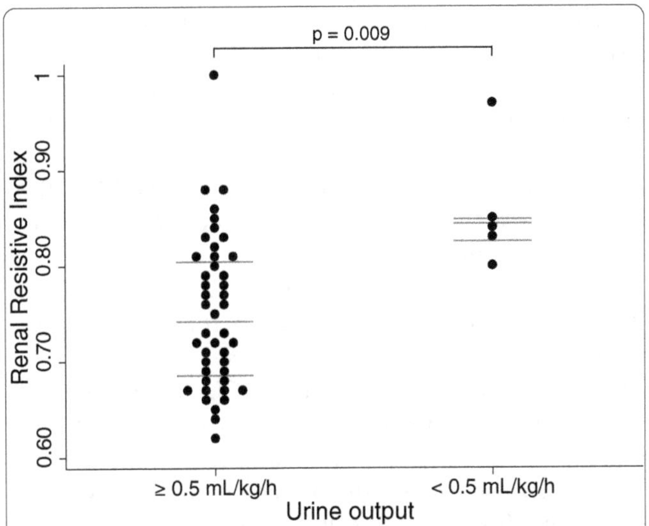

Fig. 4 Dot plot illustrating the association between renal resistive index and oliguria defined as urine output < 0.5 ml/kg ideal body weight/hour for 24 h. Each dot represents a patient. The horizontal lines represent the median, upper and lower quartiles

AKI and hence be part of a causal chain (ICU day, SOFA score, eGFR, oliguria, RRT, administration of diuretics). The following variables were omitted due to perfect prediction in the AKI groups (sex, cardiovascular disease, mechanical ventilation during ICU course, vasopressors during ICU course, tocilizumab, chloroquine phosphate, remdesivir, low-molecular-weight heparin). Variables included in the final model were RRI, BMI, CKD, vasopressors at measurement and administration of antiplatelet drugs. After multivariable adjustment, RRI was independently associated with AKI (OR for 0.01 increments of RRI 1.22, 95% CI 1.07–1.41). Goodness-of-fit had $p = 0.705$.

Discussion

This study presents novel findings of the pattern of RRI in critically ill patients with COVID-19. RRI was higher in patients with AKI compared to patients without AKI, and the difference was significant in patients with AKI stage 3 but not in patients with AKI stage 1 or 2. RRI was higher in patients with an ongoing AKI episode compared to

Table 2 Bivariate and multivariable analysis showing the association with AKI

	Bivariate analysis		Multivariable analysis[a]	
	OR (95% CI)	*p*-value	OR (95% CI)	*p*-value
RRI (0.01 unit step)	1.13 (1.04–1.23)	0.005	1.22[b] (1.07–1.41)	0.004
Age	0.97 (0.91–1.03)	0.296		
BMI	1.11 (0.99–1.23)	0.067	1.23 (1.02–1.48)	0.031
Risk factors for AKI				
Hypertension	1.35 (0.44–4.13)	0.601		
Diabetes	1.28 (0.32–5.10)	0.729		
Chronic lung disease	0.63 (0.16–2.50)	0.513		
Chronic kidney disease[c]	7.50 (0.81–70)	0.076	175 (3.72–8281)	0.009
No risk factor[d]	1.60 (0.48–5.37)	0.447		
Data at RRI measurement				
Mechanical ventilation	6.79 (1.32–35)	0.022	[f]	
Prone position	0.97 (0.23–4.12)	0.965		
Vasopressors	4.11 (1.27–13)	0.019	27 (2.68–268)	0.005
Treatment in ICU[e]				
Anti-inflammatory drugs				
Corticosteroids	0.76 (0.22–2.61)	0.666		
Anticoagulation drugs				
Antiplatelets	0.36 (0.11–1.19)	0.094	0.18 (0.03–1.17)	0.073
Episode of thrombolysis	4.05 (0.39–42)	0.241		

AKI acute kidney injury, *OR* odds ratio, *CI* confidence interval, *RRI* renal resistive index, *BMI* body mass index (kg/m^2), *ICU* intensive care unit

[a] Goodness-of-fit $p = 0.705$

[b] An increase of 0.01 in RRI increased the risk of having AKI at measurement by 22%

[c] Chronic kidney disease was defined as eGFR before ICU admission < 60 ml/min/1.73 m^2

[d] Patients without history of smoking, chronic diagnoses or regular medications at hospital admission

[e] Treatment from ICU admission to RRI measurement

[f] Variable excluded from multivariable logistic regression model during forward selection

patients who had recovered from AKI earlier during the ICU course. Oliguric patients had higher RRI compared to non-oliguric patients. The association between RRI and AKI remained significant after adjustment for possible confounding.

Our results are in line with previous studies on mixed or septic ICU patients instead designed to investigate the role of RRI to predict and prognosticate AKI [12, 13, 16, 26, 27]. These studies have suggested RRI to be able to distinguish severe or persistent AKI from no or transient AKI, with optimal cut-off values for this discrimination varying from 0.69 to 0.80. The median RRI of 0.80 in patients with AKI in our population must be considered high in comparison, but may partly be due to the large proportion of patients with AKI stage 3. This is in line with the results of a recent case–control study which presented higher RRI in ten COVID-19 patients with AKI stage 3 compared to ten patients with AKI from septic shock [20]. Notably, also patients without AKI in our study had higher RRI (median 0.72) compared to non-AKI patients in ICU populations without COVID-19 where reported values typically are lower than 0.65 [12, 14, 28]. It is not clear if elevated RRI in patients without AKI but infected with SARS-CoV-2 is specifically related to the infection itself, or if it reflects severity of illness as indicated by the long length of ICU stay as well as the high incidence of mechanical ventilation and vasopressor use in our population.

There is growing evidence of reduced renal microperfusion in patients with COVID-19-related AKI, both from contrast enhanced ultrasonographic measurements in patients with severe AKI [20] as well as from post-mortem findings of microvascular obstruction [29]. In addition, numerous studies have reported high rates of thrombotic complications in hospitalized COVID-19 patients in general [30–32], and thrombi in the renal microcirculation has been mentioned as a possible mechanism contributing to AKI in these patients [2]. Even if several renal and extrarenal factors influence the final profile of the RRI flow wave and value [33], it is conceivable that renal microcirculatory disturbances further contributed to the generally high RRI values observed in our population.

Previous studies on critically ill patients without COVID-19 have in general focused on prediction of AKI from RRI measurements performed within the first day of ICU admission [12, 14–16, 26]. However, the ability of early RRI measurements to predict short-term AKI reversibility within 3 days recently has been challenged [34, 35]. Our finding of higher RRI in COVID-19 patients with an ongoing AKI episode compared to patients who had recovered from an AKI episode earlier during the ICU course suggests that RRI values decrease with recovered renal function. This indicates that RRI also might have a role later in the ICU or hospital course, but its exact role for prediction of renal recovery or progression towards CKD while the patient still is in hospital needs to be investigated in properly designed studies. In outpatients with already established CKD, RRI $\geq$ 0.70 notably has shown to be predictive of both CKD progression [36, 37] and mortality [38].

Our finding of elevated RRI in COVID-19-related AKI indicates that RRI may have a role in the assessment of this new and unique disease. Further, RRI has shown potential as a precocious ICU monitoring tool for detecting progression of shock states [39, 40], and together with Doppler assessments of other splanchnic organs RRI can expand the bedside monitoring window for hypoperfusion in critically ill patients in general [41]. As a non-invasive and repeatable method that has been demonstrated to be fast to learn also for non-experienced sonographers [17, 42], RRI should be applicable within POCUS protocols for ICU clinicians and thereby contributing as a valuable tool in the present resource scarce times of a pandemic.

Our study has several limitations. First, our study population was small and although we were still able to adjust our analysis for a number of possible confounders, the results should therefore be interpreted with caution. The small number of patients with AKI stage 1 and 2 further makes it difficult to draw conclusions on the association between RRI and AKI in these specific subgroups. Second, due to the challenges of conducting clinical research during a pandemic, RRI measurements were performed at different time points in different patients and most of the measurements were made late in the ICU course. The Karolinska University Hospital is a tertiary referral hospital, and many patients were transferred to its ICUs from other hospitals when they had already received several days of intensive care. This meant there was a delay from ICU admission to accessibility in some of the patients, and we were therefore not able to perform early measurements to investigate the ability of RRI as an early predictor of subsequent AKI development. Third, intra- and inter-observer variability for the operators were not investigated. Our group has previously shown that RRI measurements by inexperienced sonographers were reliable, accurate and precise compared to an expert after only a brief training session [17], and both operators in our study were experienced with the RRI method. Lastly, our study was affected by some of the well-known pitfalls in AKI research. The use of hospital admission sCr as baseline level in patients in whom pre-admission sCr was missing might have resulted in an underestimation of the AKI incidence. Further, using sCr decline to define recovery from an AKI episode could in patients with muscle wasting during a prolonged ICU course lead to overestimation of renal function recovery [43]. However, we used eGFR calculations based on a combination of sCr and cystatin C at the time of RRI measurement and still observed a difference in estimated renal function between patients classified with or without AKI, suggesting any such misclassification was negligible.

Conclusion

Critically ill COVID-19 patients with AKI have higher RRI compared to those without AKI, and elevated RRI may have a role in identifying severe and oliguric AKI at the bedside in these patients. The exact role of RRI as a POCUS application for AKI assessment and monitoring of ICU patients with COVID-19 should be established in further studies.

Abbreviations

COVID-19: Coronavirus disease 2019; AKI: Acute kidney injury; ICU: Intensive care unit; RRT: Renal replacement therapy; RRI: Renal resistive index; POCUS: Point-of-care ultrasonography; COVID-ICU: Intensive care unit designated for care of COVID-19 patients; SARS-CoV-2: Severe acute respiratory syndrome coronavirus 2; ESRD: End-stage renal disease; ECMO: Extracorporeal membrane oxygenation; KDIGO: Kidney Disease Improving Global Outcomes; sCr: Serum creatinine concentration; eGFR: Estimated glomerular filtration rate; CKD-EPI: Chronic Kidney Disease Epidemiology Collaboration; CKD: Chronic kidney disease; SOFA: Sequential Organ Failure Assessment; IQR: Interquartile range; min/max: Minimum/maximum; OR: Odds ratio; CI: Confidence interval; CRRT: Continuous renal replacement therapy; BMI: Body mass index.

Acknowledgements

We would like to thank all ICU health care workers that made measurements and data collection possible with their flexibility during a stressful time.

Authors' contributions

MR, DH, MB, and CRS conceived the study. MR, OJ and NK performed the data collection. MR and DH conducted the analyses and interpretation of the data. MR drafted the manuscript. DH, MB, CRS, OJ and NK substantially revised the manuscript. DH and MB supervised the process. All authors read and approved the final manuscript.

Author details

[1] Department of Perioperative Medicine and Intensive Care, Karolinska University Hospital, Solna, 171 76 Stockholm, Sweden. [2] Department of Physiology and Pharmacology, Karolinska Institutet, Stockholm, Sweden. [3] Department of Radiology, Karolinska University Hospital, Huddinge, Stockholm, Sweden.

References

1. Yang X, Jin Y, Li R, Zhang Z, Sun R, Chen D (2020) Prevalence and impact of acute renal impairment on COVID-19: a systematic review and meta-analysis. Crit Care 24:356. https://doi.org/10.1186/s13054-020-03065-4
2. Gabarre P, Dumas G, Dupont T, Darmon M, Azoulay E, Zafrani L (2020) Acute kidney injury in critically ill patients with COVID-19. Intensive Care Med 46:1339–1348. https://doi.org/10.1007/s00134-020-06153-9
3. Hirsch JS, Ng JH, Ross DW, Sharma P, Shah HH, Barnett RL, Hazzan AD, Fishbane S, Jhaveri KD (2020) Acute kidney injury in patients hospitalized with COVID-19. Kidney Int 98:209–218. https://doi.org/10.1016/j.kint.2020.05.006
4. Hansrivijit P, Qian C, Boonpheng B, Thongprayoon C, Vallabhajosyula S, Cheungpasitporn W, Ghahramani N (2020) Incidence of acute kidney injury and its association with mortality in patients with COVID-19: a meta analysis. J Investig Med. https://doi.org/10.1136/jim 2020 001407
5. Karagiannidis C, Mostert C, Hentschker C, Voshaar T, Malzahn J, Schillinger G, Klauber J, Janssens U, Marx G, Weber-Carstens S, Kluge S, Pfeifer M, Grabenhenrich L, Welte T, Busse R (2020) Case characteristics, resource use, and outcomes of 10 021 patients with COVID-19 admitted to 920 German hospitals: an observational study. Lancet Respir Med. https://doi.org/10.1016/s2213-2600(20)30316-7
6. Cummings MJ, Baldwin MR, Abrams D, Jacobson SD, Meyer BJ, Balough EM, Aaron JG, Claassen J, Rabbani LE, Hastie J, Hochman BR, Salazar-Schicchi J, Yip NH, Brodie D, O'Donnell MR (2020) Epidemiology, clinical course, and outcomes of critically ill adults with COVID-19 in New York City: a prospective cohort study. Lancet 395:1763–1770. https://doi.org/10.1016/s0140-6736(20)31189-2
7. Cheng Y, Luo R, Wang K, Zhang M, Wang Z, Dong L, Li J, Yao Y, Ge S, Xu G (2020) Kidney disease is associated with in-hospital death of patients with COVID-19. Kidney Int 97:829–838. https://doi.org/10.1016/j.kint.2020.03.005
8. Lim MA, Pranata R, Huang I, Yonas E, Soeroto AY, Supriyadi R (2020) Multiorgan failure with emphasis on acute kidney injury and severity of COVID-19: systematic review and meta-analysis. Can J Kidney Health Dis 7:2054358120938573. https://doi.org/10.1177/2054358120938573
9. Ponte B, Pruijm M, Ackermann D, Vuistiner P, Eisenberger U, Guessous I, Rousson V, Mohaupt MG, Alwan H, Ehret G, Pechere-Bertschi A, Paccaud F, Staessen JA, Vogt B, Burnier M, Martin PY, Bochud M (2014) Reference values and factors associated with renal resistive index in a family-based population study. Hypertension 63:136–142. https://doi.org/10.1161/hypertensionaha.113.02321
10. Keogan MT, Kliewer MA, Hertzberg BS, DeLong DM, Tupler RH, Carroll BA (1996) Renal resistive indexes: variability in Doppler US measurement in a healthy population. Radiology 199:165–169. https://doi.org/10.1148/radiology.199.1.8633141
11. Tublin ME, Bude RO, Platt JF (2003) Review. the resistive index in renal doppler sonography: where do we stand? AJR Am J Roentgenol 180:885–892. https://doi.org/10.2214/ajr.180.4.1800885
12. Haitsma Mulier JLG, Rozemeijer S, Rottgering JG, Spoelstra-de Man AME, Elbers PWG, Tuinman PR, de Waard MC, Oudemans-van Straaten HM (2018) Renal resistive index as an early predictor and discriminator of acute kidney injury in critically ill patients; a prospective observational cohort study. PLoS ONE 13:e0197967. https://doi.org/10.1371/journal.pone.0197967
13. Boddi M, Bonizzoli M, Chiostri M, Begliomini D, Molinaro A, Tadini Buoninsegni L, Gensini GF, Peris A (2016) Renal Resistive Index and mortality in critical patients with acute kidney injury. Eur J Clin Invest 46:242–251. https://doi.org/10.1111/eci.12590
14. Song J, Wu W, He Y, Lin S, Zhu D, Zhong M (2018) Value of the combination of renal resistance index and central venous pressure in the early prediction of sepsis-induced acute kidney injury. J Crit Care 45:204–208. https://doi.org/10.1016/j.jcrc.2018.03.016
15. Lerolle N, Guerot E, Faisy C, Bornstain C, Diehl JL, Fagon JY (2006) Renal failure in septic shock: predictive value of Doppler-based renal arterial resistive index. Intensive Care Med 32:1553–1559. https://doi.org/10.1007/s00134-006-0360-x
16. Garnier F, Daubin D, Larcher R, Bargnoux AS, Platon L, Brunot V, Aarab Y, Besnard N, Dupuy AM, Jung B, Cristol JP, Klouche K (2020) Reversibility of acute kidney injury in medical icu patients: predictability performance of urinary tissue inhibitor of metalloproteinase-2 x Insulin-like growth factor-binding protein 7 and renal resistive index. Crit Care Med. https://doi.org/10.1097/ccm.0000000000004218
17. Renberg M, Kilhamn N, Lund K, Hertzberg D, Rimes-Stigare C, Bell M (2020) Feasibility of renal resistive index measurements performed by an intermediate and novice sonographer in a volunteer population. Ultrasound J 12:28. https://doi.org/10.1186/s13089-020-00175-6
18. Ostermann M, Lumlertgul N, Forni LG, Hoste E (2020) What every Intensivist should know about COVID-19 associated acute kidney injury. J Crit Care 60:91–95. https://doi.org/10.1016/j.jcrc.2020.07.023
19. Batlle D, Soler MJ, Sparks MA, Hiremath S, South AM, Welling PA, Swaminathan S (2020) Acute kidney injury in COVID-19: emerging Evidence of a distinct pathophysiology. J Am Soc Nephrol 31:1380–1383. https://doi.org/10.1681/asn.2020040419
20. Watchorn J, Huang DY, Joslin J, Bramham K, Hutchings SD (2020) Critically ILL COVID-19 patients with acute kidney injury have reduced renal blood

flow and perfusion despite preserved cardiac function. Shock, A Case-Control Study Using Contrast Enhanced Ultrasound. https://doi.org/10.1097/shk.0000000000001659
21. Kidney Disease: Improving Global Outcomes (KDIGO) Acute Kidney Injury Work Group. KDIGO Clinical Practice Guideline for Acute Kidney Injury (2012). Kidney inter, Suppl:1–138
22. Fliser D, Laville M, Covic A, Fouque D, Vanholder R, Juillard L, Van Biesen W (2012) A european renal best practice (ERBP) position statement on the Kidney Disease Improving Global Outcomes (KDIGO) clinical practice guidelines on acute kidney injury: part 1: definitions, conservative management and contrast-induced nephropathy. Nephrol Dial Transplant 27:4263–4272. https://doi.org/10.1093/ndt/gfs375
23. Brower RG, Matthay MA, Morris A, Schoenfeld D, Thompson BT, Wheeler A (2000) Ventilation with lower tidal volumes as compared with traditional tidal volumes for acute lung injury and the acute respiratory distress syndrome. N Engl J Med 342:1301–1308. https://doi.org/10.1056/nejm200005043421801
24. Levey AS, Stevens LA, Schmid CH, Zhang YL, Castro AF 3rd, Feldman HI, Kusek JW, Eggers P, Van Lente F, Greene T, Coresh J (2009) A new equation to estimate glomerular filtration rate. Ann Intern Med 150:604–612. https://doi.org/10.7326/0003-4819-150-9-200905050-00006
25. Vincent JL, Moreno R, Takala J, Willatts S, De Mendonça A, Bruining H, Reinhart CK, Suter PM, Thijs LG (1996) The SOFA (Sepsis-related Organ Failure Assessment) score to describe organ dysfunction/failure. On behalf of the working group on sepsis-related problems of the european society of intensive care medicine. Intensive Care Med 22:707–710. https://doi.org/10.1007/bf01709751
26. Schnell D, Deruddre S, Harrois A, Pottecher J, Cosson C, Adoui N, Benhamou D, Vicaut E, Azoulay E, Duranteau J (2012) Renal resistive index better predicts the occurrence of acute kidney injury than cystatin C. Shock 38:592–597. https://doi.org/10.1097/SHK.0b013e318271a39c
27. Darmon M, Schortgen F, Vargas F, Liazydi A, Schlemmer B, Brun-Buisson C, Brochard L (2011) Diagnostic accuracy of Doppler renal resistive index for reversibility of acute kidney injury in critically ill patients. Intensive Care Med 37:68–76. https://doi.org/10.1007/s00134-010-2050-y
28. Oliveira RAG, Mendes PV, Park M, Taniguchi LU (2019) Factors associated with renal Doppler resistive index in critically ill patients: a prospective cohort study. Ann Intensive Care 9:23. https://doi.org/10.1186/s13613-019-0500-4
29. Su H, Yang M, Wan C, Yi LX, Tang F, Zhu HY, Yi F, Yang HC, Fogo AB, Nie X, Zhang C (2020) Renal histopathological analysis of 26 postmortem findings of patients with COVID-19 in China. Kidney Int 98:219–227. https://doi.org/10.1016/j.kint.2020.04.003
30. Helms J, Tacquard C, Severac F, Leonard-Lorant I, Ohana M, Delabranche X, Merdji H, Clere-Jehl R, Schenck M, Fagot Gandet F, Fafi-Kremer S, Castelain V, Schneider F, Grunebaum L, Anglés-Cano E, Sattler L, Mertes PM, Meziani F (2020) High risk of thrombosis in patients with severe SARS-CoV-2 infection: a multicenter prospective cohort study. Intensive Care Med 46:1089–1098. https://doi.org/10.1007/s00134-020-06062-x
31. Klok FA, Kruip M, van der Meer NJM, Arbous MS, Gommers D, Kant KM, Kaptein FHJ, van Paassen J, Stals MAM, Huisman MV, Endeman H (2020) Confirmation of the high cumulative incidence of thrombotic complications in critically ill ICU patients with COVID-19: An updated analysis. Thromb Res 191:148–150. https://doi.org/10.1016/j.thromres.2020.04.041
32. Bilaloglu S, Aphinyanaphongs Y, Jones S, Iturrate E, Hochman J, Berger JS (2020) Thrombosis in hospitalized patients with COVID-19 in a New York City health system. JAMA. https://doi.org/10.1001/jama.2020.13372
33. Di Nicolo P, Granata A (2019) Renal intraparenchymal resistive index: the ultrasonographic answer to many clinical questions. J Nephrol 32:527–538. https://doi.org/10.1007/s40620-018-00567-x
34. Darmon M, Bourmaud A, Reynaud M, Rouleau S, Meziani F, Boivin A, Benyamina M, Vincent F, Lautrette A, Leroy C, Cohen Y, Legrand M, Morel J, Terreaux J, Schnell D (2018) Performance of Doppler-based resistive index and semi-quantitative renal perfusion in predicting persistent AKI: results of a prospective multicenter study. Intensive Care Med 44:1904–1913. https://doi.org/10.1007/s00134-018-5386-3
35. Wiersema R, Kaufmann T, van der Veen HN, de Haas RJ, Franssen CFM, Koeze J, van der Horst ICC, Keus F (2020) Diagnostic accuracy of arterial and venous renal Doppler assessment for acute kidney injury in critically ill patients: a prospective study. J Crit Care 59:57–62. https://doi.org/10.1016/j.jcrc.2020.05.012
36. Sugiura T, Wada A (2011) Resistive index predicts renal prognosis in chronic kidney disease: results of a 4-year follow-up. Clin Exp Nephrol 15:114–120. https://doi.org/10.1007/s10157-010-0371-3
37. Parolini C, Noce A, Staffolani E, Giarrizzo GF, Costanzi S, Splendiani G (2009) Renal resistive index and long-term outcome in chronic nephropathies. Radiology 252:888–896. https://doi.org/10.1148/radiol.2523080351
38. Toledo C, Thomas G, Schold JD, Arrigain S, Gornik HL, Nally JV, Navaneethan SD (2015) Renal resistive index and mortality in chronic kidney disease. Hypertension 66:382–388. https://doi.org/10.1161/hypertensionaha.115.05536
39. Corradi F, Brusasco C, Vezzani A, Palermo S, Altomonte F, Moscatelli P, Pelosi P (2011) Hemorrhagic shock in polytrauma patients: early detection with renal Doppler resistive index measurements. Radiology 260:112–118. https://doi.org/10.1148/radiol.11102338
40. Anile A, Ferrario S, Campanello L, Orban MA, Castiglione G (2019) Renal resistive index: a new reversible tool for the early diagnosis and evaluation of organ perfusion in critically ill patients: a case report. Ultrasound J 11:23. https://doi.org/10.1186/s13089-019-0138-3
41. Corradi F, Via G, Tavazzi G (2020) What's new in ultrasound-based assessment of organ perfusion in the critically ill: expanding the bedside clinical monitoring window for hypoperfusion in shock. Intensive Care Med 46:775–779. https://doi.org/10.1007/s00134-019-05791-y
42. Schnell D, Reynaud M, Venot M, Le Maho AL, Dinic M, Baulieu M, Ducos G, Terreaux J, Zeni F, Azoulay E, Meziani F, Duranteau J, Darmon M (2014) Resistive Index or color-Doppler semi-quantitative evaluation of renal perfusion by inexperienced physicians: results of a pilot study. Minerva Anestesiol 80:1273–1281
43. Ravn B, Rimes-Stigare C, Bell M, Hansson M, Hansson LO, Martling CR, Larsson A, Mårtensson J (2019) Creatinine versus cystatin C based glomerular filtration rate in critically ill patients. J Crit Care 52:136–140. https://doi.org/10.1016/j.jcrc.2019.04.007

24

Novel role of focused airway ultrasound in early airway assessment of suspected laryngeal trauma

Osman Adi[1*], Kok Meng Sum[2], Azma Haryaty Ahmad[1], Mahathar Abd. Wahab[3], Luca Neri[4] and Nova Panebianco[5]

Abstract

Background: Upper airway injury secondary to blunt neck trauma can lead to upper airway obstruction and potentially cause a life-threatening condition. The most important aspect in the care of laryngeal trauma is to establish a secure airway. Focused airway ultrasound enables recognition of important upper airway structures, offers early opportunity to identify life-threatening upper airway injury, and allows assessment of the extent of injury. This information that can be obtained rapidly at the bedside has the potential to facilitate rapid intervention.

Case presentation: We report a case series that illustrate the diagnostic value of focused airway ultrasound in the diagnosis of laryngeal trauma in patients presenting with blunt neck injury.

Conclusion: Early recognition, appropriate triaging, accurate airway evaluation, and prompt management of such injuries are essential. In this case series, we introduce the potential role of focused airway ultrasound in suspected laryngeal trauma, and the correlation of these exam findings with that of computed tomography (CT) scanning, based on the Schaefer classification of laryngeal injury.

Keywords: Ultrasound, Airway management, Point-of-care ultrasound, Focused airway ultrasound, Laryngeal trauma

Background

Laryngeal injuries are often undiagnosed in the initial evaluation of the trauma patient. They are rare, with an estimated incidence of one in every 30,000 emergency department admissions [1]. Delayed recognition and intervention may prove fatal in the presence of upper airway obstruction [2].

Blunt laryngeal trauma may present with varying degrees of severity, from mild to life-threatening extremes. A tracheostomy may be required to gain airway access distal to the site of injury. A systematic classification and management approach of blunt laryngeal trauma is crucial to guide early decision-making and improve patient outcome in the emergency department.

Current standard of care for laryngeal trauma is determined according to the Schaefer classification of laryngeal injury. Schaefer group 1 and group 2 with minor endolaryngeal injuries can be managed conservatively with observation, antibiotics, steroids, voice rest and anti-reflux medications. However, for more severe Schaefer type 3–5 injuries, open surgical repair will be required to secure a definitive airway [1, 2].

Good history taking, detailed clinical examination and a high index of suspicion are critical in the diagnosis of laryngeal trauma. The diagnosis can be aided using flexible nasendoscopy by direct visualization of the airway. CT scanning of the neck is still considered the gold standard to grade the severity of the injury and to direct appropriate management. Obtaining a timely CT scan may often be challenging due to logistical problems,

*Correspondence: osman.adi@gmail.com
[1] Department of Emergency and Trauma, Raja Permaisuri Bainun Hospital, Jalan Raja Ashman (Jalan Hospital), Jalan Raja Ashman, 30400 Ipoh, Perak, Malaysia
Full list of author information is available at the end of the article

primarily availability of radiology service support especially in resource-limited area, and stability for patient transfer.

Of late, studies have integrated the use of upper airway ultrasound into point-of-care ultrasound examination, a paradigm shift in upper airway assessment [3–5]. The incorporation of ultrasound into the diagnostic arm may expedite the intervention process by removing some logistics problem and provide rapid information to guide timely management.

We discuss the role of focused airway ultrasound in upper airway trauma performed by point-of-care ultrasound trained emergency physician and propose a focused airway ultrasound classification in relation to Schaefer classification of laryngeal injury.

Case presentation

Case 1—endolaryngeal hematoma without detectable fracture (Schaefer group 1)

A 24-year-old male presented with neck swelling without signs of respiratory distress after a traumatic blunt neck injury. There was swelling of the anterior neck without palpable crepitus. Airway ultrasound showed disruption of the air–mucosal interface suggesting endolaryngeal disruption (Fig. 1b). CT scan confirmed the diagnosis of endolaryngeal disruption without cartilaginous fracture. The patient was conservatively managed and discharged well on the third day.

Case 2—undisplaced thyroid cartilage fracture (Schaefer group 2)

A 66-year-old motorcyclist, was injured in a collision with a van. He presented with mild neck pain, difficulty in breathing, hoarseness, dysphagia and odynophagia. He had stridor, and his neck was swollen and tender with subcutaneous emphysema.

Airway ultrasound using a 15-MHz linear transducer found discontinuity of the anterior cortex of thyroid cartilage with minimal surrounding tissue edema, consistent with Schaefer group 2 (Fig. 2c). CT scan confirmed the ultrasound findings, showing a defect in the posterolateral wall of the trachea and the esophagus, with fracture of the right anterior lamina of the thyroid cartilage and superior cornu of the left thyroid cartilage (Fig. 2d).

He was immediately intubated and was started on intravenous dexamethasone to reduce inflammation and edema, a proton pump inhibitor to prevent reflux and laryngeal irritation, nebulized adrenaline and a prophylactic antibiotic in the emergency department. The patient was managed conservatively and was discharged well from intensive care unit on the fifth day post trauma.

Case 3—displaced thyroid cartilage fracture (Schaefer group 3)

A 28-year-old male martial art athlete was kicked by his opponent and sustained a blow to the anterior part of the neck. He complained of pain, dysphagia and hoarseness. There was an abrasion to the anterior part of his neck, which was tender to palpation with localized crepitus.

Bedside airway ultrasound revealed a displaced fracture of the thyroid cartilage, disruption of anterior cortex of thyroid cartilage with surrounding mixed echogenicity denoting endolaryngeal edema (Fig. 3a and Additional file 1: Video S1) and paralyzed right vocal cord (Fig. 3e), consistent with Schaefer group 3.

Direct visualization using a flexible fibreoptic scope revealed an edematous and medially deviated right arytenoid with paralyzed and erythematous right vocal cord. He was intubated and intravenous dexamethasone,

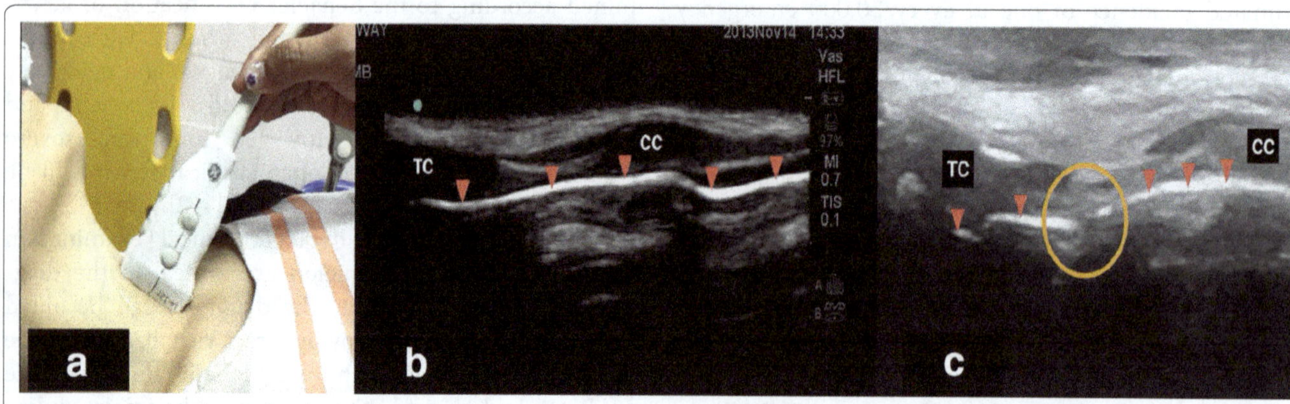

Fig. 1 **a** Surface landmark of probe position (in longitudinal view) in relation to scanning the area for **b** and **c**. **b** Normal sonoanatomy of upper airway showing the relationship between thyroid cartilage, cricoid cartilage, air–mucosal interface and surrounding soft tissues. A continuous and undisrupted line of air–mucosal interface seen as hyperechoic line (arrowhead) **c** Airway ultrasound showed disruption air–mucosal interface without obvious detectable laryngeal fracture (circle). SM: sternocleidomastoid muscle; TC: thyroid cartilage; CC: cricoid cartilage

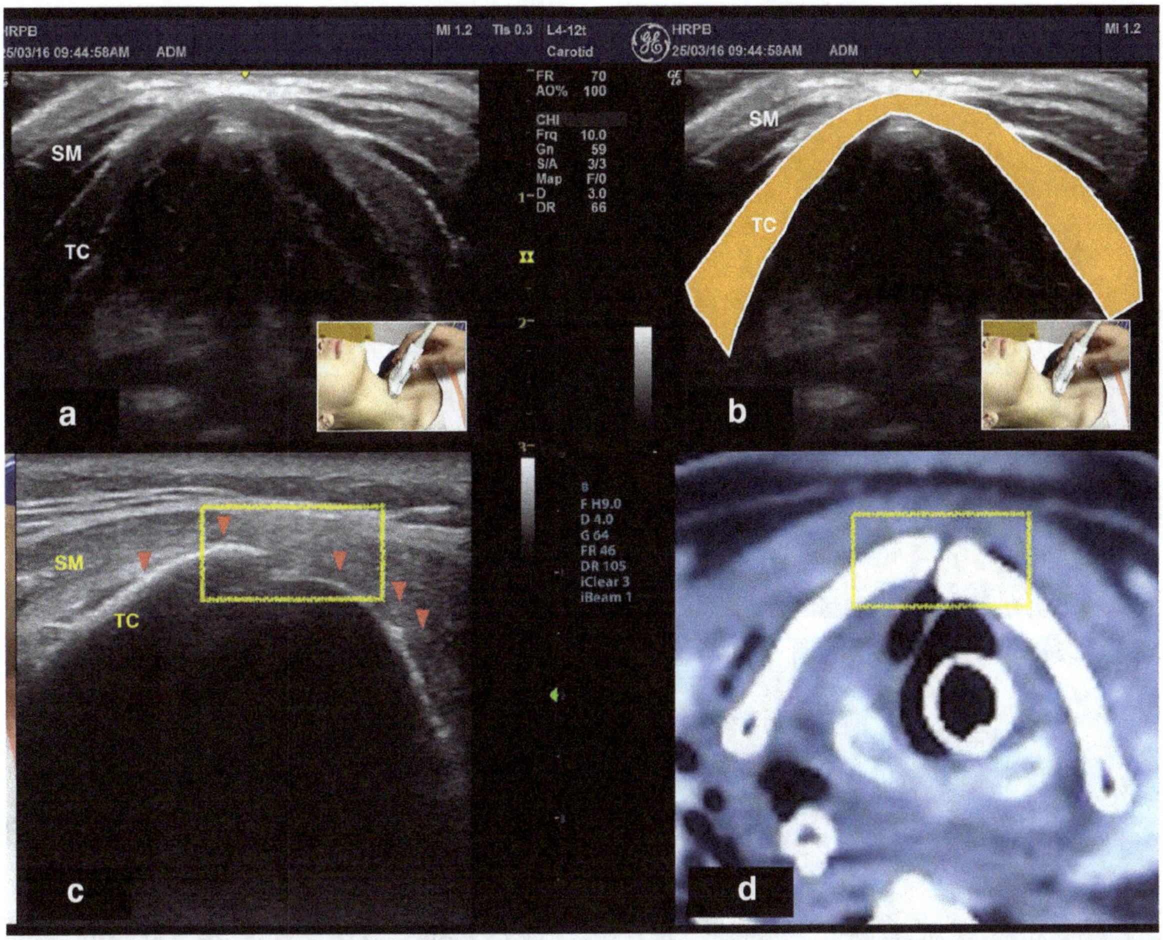

Fig. 2 **a**, **b** Surface landmark of the probe position and ultrasound image of the normal thyroid cartilage (in transverse view). **c** Airway ultrasound showing undisplaced fracture of the thyroid cartilage (box) and disruption of the anterior cortex of the thyroid cartilage (arrowhead). **d** A Computerized tomography (CT) scan image shown right thyroid lamina fracture with surrounding prevertebral edema and hematoma. SM: sternocleidomastoid muscle; TC: thyroid cartilage

proton pump inhibitor, nebulized adrenaline and prophylactic antibiotic were initiated early in the emergency department. The patient was sent for CT neck after stabilization, which showed a defect in the posterolateral wall of the trachea with a displaced fracture of right anterior lamina of thyroid cartilage and superior cornu of left thyroid cartilage, consistent with Schaefer group 3 (Fig. 3b), and that found on bedside ultrasound. The patient was stable throughout his entire hospitalization after open surgical repair and was allowed home on day nine with outpatient follow up.

Case 4—displaced thyroid cartilage fracture (Schaefer group 3)

A 35-year-old male lorry driver hit his neck against the steering wheel when he thrown forwards during a head-on collision. He presented with neck pain, severe swelling over the whole anterior region of the neck, stridor, hypoxia and a compromised airway. The patient was immediately intubated and ventilated.

Focused airway ultrasound showed disruption of the air–mucosal interface, a displaced thyroid cartilage fracture with formation of endolaryngeal hematoma and a cricoid cartilage fracture (Fig. 4b). He was treated as Schaefer group 3 and was started on intravenous dexamethasone, proton pump inhibitor, nebulized adrenaline, prophylactic antibiotic and open surgical repair was planned.

CT scan revealed a defect in the posterolateral wall of the trachea with a displaced fracture of the left anterior lamina of thyroid cartilage and hematoma surrounding the thyroid and cricoid cartilages. This confirmed the classification and injury details categorized under Schaefer group 3, which correlated with that of ultrasound assessment. Hospital stay was uneventful, and he went home after 2 weeks, to be reviewed in the outpatient department.

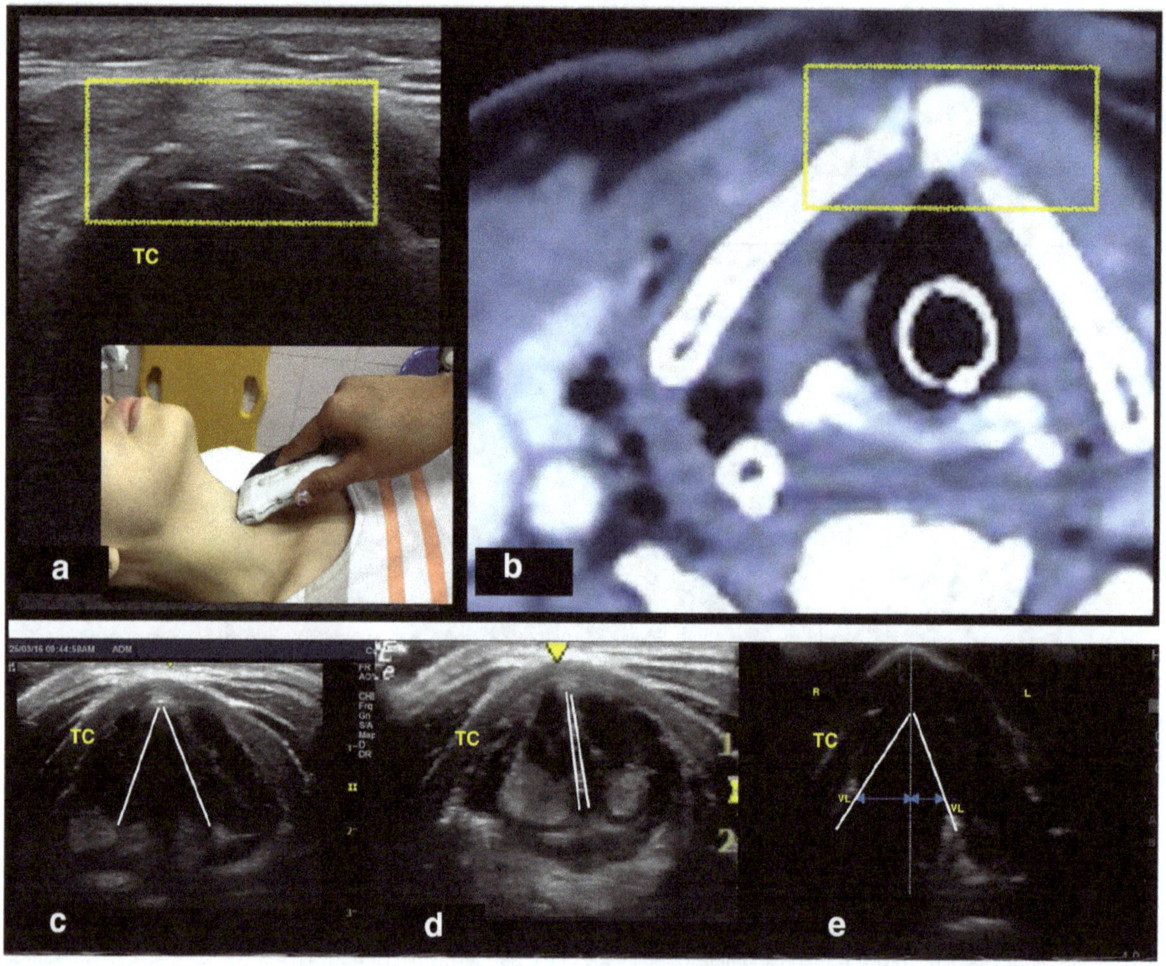

Fig. 3 **a** Image of focused airway of displaced thyroid cartilage fracture and disruption of anterior cortex of the thyroid cartilage (box). **b** A computerized tomography (CT) scan image showing defect in posterolateral wall of trachea with fracture of right anterior lamina of thyroid cartilage and superior cornu of left thyroid cartilage. **c**, **d** Assessment of vocal cord mobility can be done by looking at the movement of vocal ligament (white line) during abduction and adduction. **e** Blue arrow indicates reduced movement of the right vocal ligament (white line) to the midline during adduction compare to the left vocal ligament. R: right; L: left; VL: vocal ligament, TC: thyroid cartilage

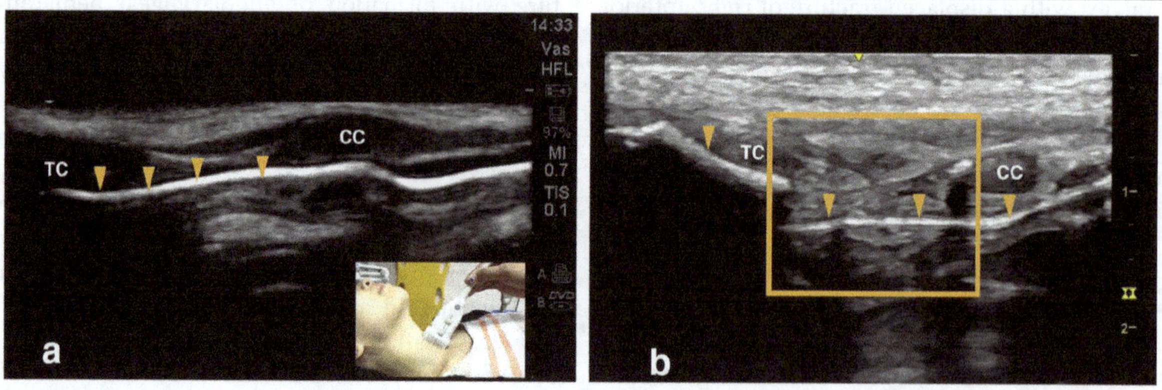

Fig. 4 **a** Normal sonoanatomy in longitudinal scan showing continuous and intact air–mucosal interface (arrowhead) in relation to thyroid and cricoid cartilage. **b** Airway ultrasound image in longitudinal scan showing disruption of the air–mucosal interface (arrowhead) and formation of endolaryngeal hematoma and fracture cricoid cartilage (box). TC: thyroid cartilage; CC: cricoid cartilage

Discussion

The ABCs of trauma, a mantra that prioritizes the primary survey starts, with "A" for airway. In this case series, we describe four encounters in which ultrasound of the upper airway was performed for suspected laryngeal trauma and correlated with CT scan assessment of severity based on the Schaefer classification of laryngeal injury.

Upper airway obstruction as a consequence of laryngeal injury may be catastrophic. Apart from blunt force trauma, iatrogenic injuries can occur after percutaneous dilatational tracheostomy, fiberoptic bronchoscopy, airway manipulations and procedures, even tracheal intubation [6, 7, 8]. The lack of correlation between symptoms, physical findings and severity of laryngeal injury may result in delayed recognition of such injuries. Additionally, patients with laryngeal injury are at risk of false passages, transforming an incomplete fracture to total separation of the upper airway, converting mild upper airway obstruction to complete obstruction especially in undiagnosed laryngeal trauma [9–11]. For these reasons upper airway ultrasound may play an important role in the early assessment for laryngeal injury.

For the past three decades the internationally accepted Schaefer classification of laryngeal injury stratification system has been used to categorize laryngeal injury. This classification not only categorizes, but it also guides management. It divides the management plan into 2 categories; non-invasive or conservative airway management for group 1 and group 2 injuries, and invasive airway management for higher grade injuries (group 3 to group 5). Further study is needed to determine if focused upper airway ultrasound can reliably be used to determine injury grade [1].

While the authors could not find previous publication of ultrasound assessment for upper airway injury in trauma, prior research by Osman et al. and You-Ten et al. briefly illustrated the usage of airway ultrasound in a step-by step manner to delineate the normal sonoanatomy of the upper airway such as thyroid cartilage, epiglottis, cricoid cartilage, cricothyroid membrane, tracheal cartilages, esophagus and the surrounding soft tissues [3–5]. Schick et al. published promising evidence on the use of airway ultrasound in the emergency setting to identify airway edema and impending threats to the airway [12]. Airway ultrasound can also be used to assess laryngeal edema in the post-extubation period. [13–15]. Kameda et al. [16] identified airway edema as hypoechoic thickening of the tracheal wall on airway ultrasound in a patient with inhalational burns. The findings on the sonogram were later confirmed by CT scan, demonstrating good correlation between focused ultrasound and CT Scan.

Cheng et al. [17] found good correlation between sonographic visualization of abnormal vocal cords movement and laryngoscopic examination. They demonstrated that clinician-performed airway ultrasound is an accurate screening tool for preoperative assessment of vocal cord movement.

Upper airway ultrasound findings that correlate with the Schaefer Classification System may be especially relevant in hemodynamically unstable patients where CT imaging is not feasible. While larger trials are needed, we propose that focused airway ultrasound can be used to correlate with the Schaefer Classification System (Table 1) and therefore propose it be assimilated into the work-up of laryngeal trauma.

Possible advantages of focused upper airway ultrasound in the diagnostic classification of blunt laryngeal trauma are:

- In centers without CT scan capabilities—focused airway ultrasound can complement emergency department triage protocol to enable early airway management planning in blunt laryngeal injury.
- In centers with CT scan facility—focused airway ultrasound can hasten airway management planning prior to airway catastrophe during an emergency situation when transfer to the radiology suite is deemed unsuitable.
- In resource-limited situation such as—scarce resources, remote area, and humanitarian medical mission in environmental disasters and war-torn regions—focused airway ultrasound can supplement disaster and transfer protocol facilitating decision for early airway intervention while preparing for emergency transfer.
- It has the added advantage of real-time visualization of dynamic vocal cords function.

Limitations

Ultrasound evaluation of the airway may not be practical in every case. Subcutaneous emphysema, posterior laryngeal injury, cartilage calcification and foreign bodies may result in artifacts interfering with ultrasound images and interpretation. Furthermore, ultrasound techniques and interpretation are operator-dependent, and have a steep learning curve. Adequate competency training and reproducibility is important to standardize findings.

Future directions

Further studies to identify optimal management strategies for patients with laryngeal injury are required. Areas of interest include:

Table 1 Proposed focused airway ultrasound findings in correlation to the Schaefer Classification System and standard management of laryngeal injury

Group -Based on Schaefer classification [1]	CT scan findings -Based on Schaefer classification [1]	Focused airway ultrasound findings	Standard management and intervention [1, 2]
Group 1	Minor endolaryngeal hematoma or laceration without detectable fracture	Endolaryngeal hematoma without detectable fracture	Supportive care including observation, antibiotics, humidified air, supplemental oxygen, anti-reflux medications, voice rest and early steroid administration.
Group 2	Edema, hematoma, minor mucosal disruption without exposed cartilage, nondisplaced fracture noted on CT	Edema, endolaryngeal hematoma, minor mucosal disruption without exposed cartilage, nondisplaced fracture Mucosal hematoma/edema Nondisplaced fracture of cartilage framework	*Patients with Group 2 injuries should be serially examined, since the injuries may worsen or progress with time. Occasionally group 2 injuries may require a tracheotomy
Group 3	Massive edema, mucosal tear, exposed cartilage, cord immobility, displaced fracture	Edema, cord immobility, displaced fracture Vocal fold immobility Obvious displaced fracture	Direct laryngoscopy, esophagoscopy and immediate open surgical repair is deemed necessary due to extension of injuries
Group 4	Addition of more than two fracture lines or massive trauma to laryngeal mucosa	Addition of more than two fracture lines Comminuted fracture of laryngeal cartilage framework	
Group 5	Complete laryngeal separation		

- Validation studies comparing accuracy of focused airway ultrasound to CT scan findings across a range of injury types.
- Management outcome, cost effectiveness, accuracy and time of diagnosis of focused airway ultrasound compared to existing radiological modalities.
- Reproducibility of results by different operators at different stages of seniority and proficiency level, their abilities to accurately detect pathology and studies on learning curve of this procedure.

Conclusion

Ultrasound assessment of the upper airway is a promising adjunct in the rapid evaluation of patients with suspected laryngeal trauma. Early diagnosis and injury classification stratification with point-of-care ultrasound may play an important role in trauma patient care, particularly those too unstable for CT imaging or when advanced imaging is unavailable.

Supplementary information

Additional file 1: Video S1. Bedside airway ultrasound revealed a displaced fracture of the thyroid cartilage, disruption of anterior cortex of thyroid cartilage with surrounding mixed echogenicity denoting endolaryngeal edema.

Abbreviations

POCUS: Point-of-care ultrasound; CT: Computed tomography; Sm: Sternocleidomastoid muscle; Tc: Thyroid cartilage; Vm: Vocalis muscle; VL: Vocalis ligament; AC: Arytenoid cartilage.

Acknowledgements

We would like to thank Ms. Anusha Bala, Cheong Chee Keong, Tan Wan Chuan, Lai Si Qi and World Integrated Network for Focused Ultrasound (WINFOCUS) Malaysia, and Society of Critical Ipoh Emergency Medicine Society (IEMS) and Emergency Sonography (SUCCES) for their assistance.

Declaration

I declare that this manuscript which depicts the clinical management of patient with laryngeal trauma. Contributions from respective authors have been explicitly mentioned in the respective segment. This work has not been submitted to any other publication for publishing.

Authors' contributions

OA and KMS: primary author, involved in the management of case, and drafting, reviewing, editing, preparing, and final approval of the manuscript. AHA, MAW and LN: involved in the management of case, reviewing, editing, preparing, and final approval of the manuscript. NP: involved indirectly in reviewing, editing, and preparing the manuscript. All authors read and approved the final manuscript.

Author details

[1] Department of Emergency and Trauma, Raja Permaisuri Bainun Hospital, Jalan Raja Ashman (Jalan Hospital), Jalan Raja Ashman, 30400 Ipoh, Perak, Malaysia. [2] Department of Anesthesiology & Intensive Care, Beacon Hospital, No. 1, Jalan 215, Off Jalan Templer, Section 51, 46050 Petaling Jaya, Selangor, Malaysia. [3] Department of Emergency and Trauma, Kuala Lumpur Hospital, Jalan Pahang, 50586 Kuala Lumpur, Wilayah Persekutuan Kuala Lumpur, Malaysia. [4] A.O Niguarda Ca' Granda' Hospital, Piazza dell'Ospedale Maggiore, 3, 20162 Milan, MI, Italy. [5] Division of Emergency Ultrasound, Department of Emergency Medicine, Hospital of the University of Pennsylvania, 3400 Spruce St, Philadelphia, PA 19104, USA.

References

1. Schaefer SD (1992) The acute management of external laryngeal trauma. A 27-year experience. Arch Otolaryngol Head Neck Surg 118(6):598–604

2. Atkins BZ, Abbate S, Fisher SR, Vaslef SN (2004) Current management of laryngotracheal trauma: case report and literature review. J Trauma 56:185Y190
3. Osman A, Sum KM (2016) Role of upper airway ultrasound in airway management. J Intensive Care 4:52
4. Osman A, Sum KM, Farid S, Wahab A (2019) Focused airway ultrasound: an armamentarium in future airway management. J Emerg Crit Care Med 3:31
5. You-Ten KE, Siddiqui N, Teoh WH, Kristensen MS (2018) Point-of-care ultrasound (POCUS) of the upper airway. Can J Anaesth. https://doi.org/10.1007/s12630-018-1064-8
6. Bent JP 3rd, Silver JR, Porubsky ES (1993) Acute laryngeal trauma: a review of 77 patients. Otolaryngol Head Neck Surg 109(3 Pt 1):441–449
7. Hotchkiss KS, McCaffrey JC (2003) Laryngotracheal injury after percutaneous dilational tracheostomy in cadaver specimens. Laryngoscope. 113:16–20
8. Maktabi MA, Hoffman H, Funk G, From RP (2002) Laryngeal trauma during awake fiberoptic intubation. Anesth Analg 95:1112–1114
9. Chen FH, Fetzer JD (1993) Complete cricotracheal separation and third cervical spinal cord transection following blunt neck trauma: a case report of one survivor. J Trauma 35:140–142
10. Minard G, Kudsk KA, Croce MA, Butts JA, Cicala RS, Fabian TC (1992) Laryngotracheal trauma. Am Surg 58:181–187
11. O'Connor PJ, Russell JD, Moriart DC (1998) Anesthetic implication of laryngeal trauma. Anesth Analg 87:1283–1284
12. Schick M, Grether-Jones K (2016) Point-of-care sonographic findings in acute upper airway edema. West J Emerg Med 17(6):822–826 **(Epub 2016 Oct 4)**
13. Pluijms WA, van Mook WN, Wittekamp BH et al (2015) Postextubation laryngeal edema and stridor resulting in respiratory failure in critically ill adult patients: updated review. Crit Care 19:295
14. Tikotekar A, Jagpal S, Nagella N (2014) A clinical prediction tool for prognosis in patients with cystic fibrosis, short-term glucocorticoid therapy for chronic obstructive pulmonary disease, and laryngeal ultrasound for prediction of postextubation laryngeal edema. Am J Respir Crit Care Med 189:482–483
15. Sutherasan Y, Teerawit P, Hongphanut T et al (2013) Predicting laryngeal edema in intubated patients by portable intensive care unit ultrasound. J Crit Care 28(5):675–680
16. Kameda T, Fujita M (2014) Point-of-care ultrasound detection of tracheal wall thickening caused by smoke inhalation. Ultrasound J. 6(1):11. https://doi.org/10.1186/2036-7902-6-11
17. Cheng SP, Lee JJ, Liu TP, Lee KS, Liu CL (2012) Preoperative ultrasonography assessment of vocal cord movement during thyroid and parathyroid surgery. World J Surg 36:2509–2515

Cardiac ultrasound in resource-limited settings (CURLS): towards a wider use of basic echo applications in Africa

Michaëla A. M. Huson[1], Dan Kaminstein[2], Daniel Kahn[3], Sabine Belard[4,5], Prakash Ganesh[6,7], Vanessa Kandoole-Kabwere[8], Claudia Wallrauch[9], Sam Phiri[6,10,11,12], Benno Kreuels[8,13] and Tom Heller[6*]

Abstract

Background: Point-of-care ultrasound is increasingly being used as a diagnostic tool in resource-limited settings. The majority of existing ultrasound protocols have been developed and implemented in high-resource settings. In sub-Saharan Africa (SSA), patients with heart failure of various etiologies commonly present late in the disease process, with a similar syndrome of dyspnea, edema and cardiomegaly on chest X-ray. The causes of heart failure in SSA differ from those in high-resource settings. Point-of-care ultrasound has the potential to identify the underlying etiology of heart failure, and lead to targeted therapy. Based on a literature review and weighted score of disease prevalence, diagnostic impact and difficulty in performing the ultrasound, we propose a context-specific cardiac ultrasound protocol to help differentiate patients presenting with heart failure in SSA.

Results: Pericardial effusion, dilated cardiomyopathy, cor pulmonale, mitral valve disease, and left ventricular hypertrophy were identified as target conditions for a focused ultrasound protocol in patients with cardiac failure and cardiomegaly in SSA. By utilizing a simplified 5-question approach with all images obtained from the subxiphoid view, the protocol is suitable for use by health care professionals with limited ultrasound experience.

Conclusions: The "Cardiac ultrasound for resource-limited settings (CURLS)" protocol is a context-specific algorithm designed to aid the clinician in diagnosing the five most clinically relevant etiologies of heart failure and cardiomegaly in SSA. The protocol has the potential to influence treatment decisions in patients who present with clinical signs of heart failure in resource-limited settings outside of the traditional referral institutions.

Keywords: Cardiac ultrasound, Protocol, POCUS, Resource-limited setting, Africa

Background

Point-of-care ultrasound is increasingly being used as a diagnostic tool in resource-limited settings. With more portable and affordable machines, providers from small clinics to large hospitals have increasing access to this technology. The majority of ultrasound protocols aimed at cardiac pathology have been developed and implemented in high-resource settings where more advanced imaging technology is usually available to help the clinician confirm their ultrasound diagnosis. As cardiovascular disease is an increasing cause of morbidity and mortality in sub-Saharan Africa (SSA) [1], there is a need for context-specific ultrasound protocols suited to the needs and available resources in this setting.

In SSA, patients with heart disease often present late in their clinical course with signs and symptoms of heart failure [2]. The etiology of heart disease in this context falls into several categories which are difficult to distinguish at the end stages, including hypertension and coronary artery disease [3], as well as communicable diseases such as tuberculosis (TB) and rheumatic fever [3]. There are striking differences in

*Correspondence: echnatom@web.de
[6] Lighthouse Clinic, Kamuzu Central Hospital, Lilongwe, Malawi
Full list of author information is available at the end of the article

the epidemiology of heart diseases when comparing SSA with the United States or Europe [4]. Based on a number of studies comparing patients from SSA with patients from Europe, the Americas and Asia, African patients with heart failure are younger, more likely to be female and less likely to suffer from ischemic heart disease [4–6].

Patients with heart failure of various etiologies commonly present with a similar syndrome of dyspnea, edema and cardiomegaly on chest X-ray. In tropical settings common cardiac causes of dyspnea and edema are dilated cardiomyopathy (e.g., peripartum or HIV-associated cardiomyopathy), hypertensive cardiomyopathy, pericardial effusion with tamponade (most commonly due to TB), post-rheumatic heart disease (RHD) and cor pulmonale [7, 8]. Point-of-care ultrasound may be the only tool available to clinicians to help them make definitive diagnoses allowing for targeted treatment.

A large body of evidence has demonstrated the feasibility and clinical utility of point-of-care cardiac ultrasound performed by non-cardiologists [9–13]. In SSA, studies on handheld echocardiography showed promising results in screening children for RHD by both cardiologists and non-experts, trained in a simplified screening protocol [9–11, 14, 15]. In addition, focused cardiopulmonary ultrasound was demonstrated to improve diagnostic accuracy in emergency care in Ghana, particularly in patients with cardiac disease such as cardiogenic shock, congestive heart failure or acute valvular disease [16]. More widespread use of echocardiography in low- and middle-income countries beyond referral centers has great potential. A recent study performed in a district hospital in South Africa demonstrated that patient management was influenced by echocardiography in 83.8% of patients, who predominantly suffered from valvular heart disease [17]. A study in Rwanda demonstrated that trained nurses were able to accurately diagnose different causes of heart failure and provide care for heart failure patients using a simplified echocardiography protocol [18]. Similarly clinical officers in Kenya were able to improve their diagnosis of cardiac conditions using a focused protocol after an 8-h training [12]. These studies demonstrate the numerous applications and practical possibilities to expand the use of echocardiography in SSA.

As ultrasound becomes more ubiquitous, there is a need for context-specific training protocols. In the following pages, we outline a cardiac ultrasound protocol specifically for providers working in sub-Saharan Africa (SSA). This protocol is based on a literature review of locally prevalent conditions, and created for ease of use both in regards to performing ultrasound with basic B mode software capabilities and for teaching cardiac ultrasound in a way that is most relevant for healthcare professionals in SSA.

Methods

Literature review on prevalence of cardiac conditions

We searched PubMed with the following search string: "Africa" [MeSH Terms] AND "heart diseases" [MeSH Terms] and extracted information on the frequency of causes of heart failure. Our search was conducted on 1 August 2018, and an additional search on 11 October 2019. We limited our search to papers published in the last 5 years and relevant references cited herein published within the last 10 years. We excluded papers focusing on pediatric populations, ECG findings, surgery, cardiovascular risk or stroke, studies outside SSA, case reports and studies focusing on clinical characteristics of specific groups, such as HIV patients or patients with congenital heart disease. Review papers were included to search for additional relevant references. Geographic area, number of assessed patients and relative frequencies of underlying conditions were extracted. These data were subsequently used to identify the most relevant conditions that need to be assessed in a cardiac ultrasound protocol.

Weighting of cardiac ultrasound application

Given that our goal is to create a protocol that is most relevant for clinicians in resource-limited settings, epidemiology was combined with ease of use and predicted clinical relevance to create a scoring system that would identify the high-yield ultrasound applications. Each application was assessed on three components: disease prevalence, diagnostic impact, and ultrasound difficulty (Table 1). The weight of disease prevalence was based on data from our literature review. We considered approximate average frequencies above 15% as frequent (weight = 3) and below 5% as rare (weight = 1). As the populations under study varied in age and sex distribution, and may thus not be comparable, no overall average prevalence was calculated. Prevalence was weighted as 3 if the prevalence was > 15% in the majority of studies. Weighting ultrasound difficulty was based on expert consensus between co-authors with experience in ultrasound teaching in resource-limited settings (TH, DKam, MH, VK, BK); weight of therapeutic impact by consensus of co-authors experienced in treating cardiac patients in clinical practice in these settings (DKah, PG, CW). Although the multifactorial weighting model has not been formally validated and the weights are partially subjective, the method first proposed by Van Hoving et al. [19] is transparent and easy to apply. Therefore, we consider it currently the best option to inform decisions about relevant curriculum content in various settings. The weighting of cardiac ultrasound applications allowed

Table 1 Weighting of prevalence, diagnostic impact and difficulty of POCUS applications

Weight	Disease prevalence	Diagnostic impact of US	US difficulty and technical requirements
1	Rare (< 5%)	Minor or no management change	Technically advanced, often requiring special equipment like TEE probe, cw-Doppler, cardiac software
2	Relatively common (5–15%)	Management change	Moderate, may require color-Doppler
3	Very common (> 15%)	Urgent management change (possibly life threatening)	Technically easy, only basic b/w US

For prevalence and impact the numbers indicate the following levels: 1 = low, 2 = medium, 3 = high. For difficulty, scoring is reversed with numbers indicating the following levels: 1 = high, 2 = medium, and 3 = low. This allows for a composite score where the higher numbers correspond to increasing relevance and applicability of POCUS

US ultrasound, *TEE* transesophageal echocardiography, *cw* continuous wave, *b/w* black and white

us to generate a protocol for focused cardiac ultrasound in resource-limited settings (CURLS) that is based on the most relevant applications and prioritizes practicality and ease of use for non-expert sonographers.

Results

Epidemiology of heart disease in sub-Saharan Africa

878 titles and abstracts were screened; nine papers provided relevant information on etiologies of cardiac failure in SSA [20–28], nine additional papers were identified by reviewing references [18, 29–36]. Geographic distribution of the study areas of included studies is presented in Fig. 1, showing the wide geographic range. The literature review flowchart and baseline characteristics of included studies are given in Additional file 1: Figure S1 and Table S1. Relative frequencies of the etiologies of heart failure are summarized in Table 2. Hypertension was the most common cause of heart failure in all studies, except in one study from Djibouti where ischemic heart disease was the most common cause [32]. Cardiomyopathy was the second most common cause in most studies. Ischemic

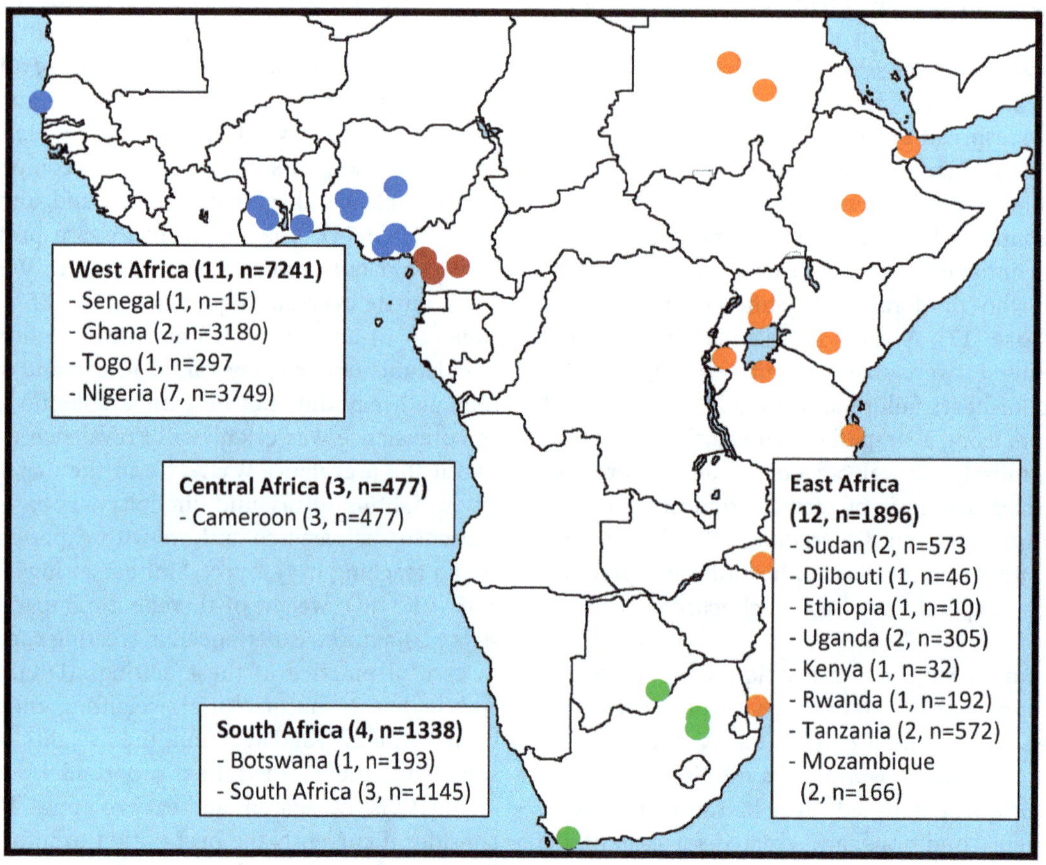

Fig. 1 Geographic area of the 18 included studies on frequency of causes of cardiac failure. Note that some studies included multiple sites. Therefore, there are more study sites in the figure than included studies

Table 2 Etiology of heart failure in sub-Saharan Africa

First author, year	Patients with HF (*n*)	Hypertension (%)	Dilated cardiomyopathy (%)[a]	Ischemic (%)	Valvular (%)	Right-sided HF/cor pulmonale (%)	Effusion (%)	Endomyocardial fibrosis (%)	Congenital (%)
Ansa, 2016	339	48.6	35.4		1.4				
Appiah, 2017	1916	52.3	19.8	4	7.6				0.4
Bonsu, 2017	1488	61.2	19.9	12.9					
Boombhi, 2017	148	30.2	28.6	6.4	11.9	8.7	4		
Damasceno, 2012	1006	45.4	18.8	7.7	14.3		6.8	1.3	
Dokainish, 2017	1294	35	14.2	20	11				0.1
Kingery, 2017	588	42.8	19.3	6.2	16.6	7.6			
Kwan, 2013	192	8	54		25		1.4	0.7	5
Makubi, 2014	427	45	22.4	9	12				
Massoure, 2013	45	13	7	62					
Mwita, 2017	193	40.4	19.6	5.7	9.3		6.2		
Nkoke, 2017	529	43.2	17.6	9.6	11.7	8.8	3.8		2.1
Ogah, 2013	452	78.5	7.5	0.4	2.4	4.4	3.3	0.9	0.4
Ojji, 2013	1515	60.6	12	0.4	9.4				
Onwuchekwa, 2009	423	56.3	7.3	0.2	4.3	2.1			
Pio, 2014	297	43.1	5.9	19.2	11.8	2.7	1.7		2.7
Stewart, 2008	844	33	28	9	8	27			

HF heart failure

[a] The majority of this group consists of idiopathic dilated cardiomyopathy. Peripartum cardiomyopathy and HIV-related cardiomyopathy were mentioned in several studies, while thyrotoxicosis, alcohol and diabetes were mentioned incidentally as causes for dilated cardiomyopathy

Table 3 Ranking of cardiac ultrasound applications according to prevalence, impact and difficulty

Echocardiographic finding	Prevalence (P)	Impact (I)	Difficulty (D)	PxIxD	Rank
LV hypertrophy	3	2	2	12	1
Rheumatic mitral disease (stenosis suggested by large LA)	2	2	3	12	1
Cardiomyopathy, severe	3	2	2	12	1
Cor pulmonale	2	2	3	12	1
Pericardial effusion	1	3	3	9	2
Regurgitation (MV, AV, TV by color Doppler)	2	2	2	8	3
Rheumatic mitral stenosis (valve morphology only)	2	2	1	4	4
Rheumatic aortic stenosis (valve morphology only)	2	2	1	2	4
Endocarditis (large vegetations seen on TTE)	1	2	2	4	4
RV function grading (e.g., TAPSE)	2	2	1	4	4
Mitral stenosis grading (PHT)	2	2	1	4	4
Aortic stenosis grading (continuation equation)	2	2	1	4	4
Regional hypokinesia	2	2	1	4	4
LV function grading (e.g., ejection fraction)	3	1	1	3	5
Endocarditis (TEE)	1	2	1	2	6
Endomyocardial fibrosis	1	1	2	2	6
Congenital heart diseases	1	2	1	2	6
Pulmonary artery pressure (dTR)	2	1	1	2	6

For prevalence and impact the numbers indicate the following levels: 1 = low, 2 = medium, 3 = high. For difficulty, scoring is reversed with numbers indicating the following levels: 1 = high, 2 = medium, and 3 = low. For prevalence and impact the numbers indicate the following levels: 1 = low, 2 = medium, 3 = high. For difficulty scoring is reversed with numbers indicating the following levels: 1 = high, 2 = medium, and 3 = low. This allows for a composite score where the higher numbers correspond to increasing relevance and applicability of POCUS

LV left ventricular, *LA* left atrium, *MV* mitral valve, *AV* aortic valve, *TV* tricuspid valve, *TEE* transesophageal echocardiogram, *RV* right ventricle, *TAPSE* tricuspid annular plane systolic excursion, *PHT* pressure half-time, *dTR* pressure gradient measured in tricuspid regurgitation

and valvular causes were less common, but reported by most studies. Endomyocardial fibrosis, pericardial effusion, cor pulmonale and congenital causes were only reported by a selected number of publications and their frequency was low.

The cardiac ultrasound in resource-limited settings (CURLS) protocol

Based on the 5 highest ranking conditions (Table 3), we propose a protocol that focuses on the identification of pericardial effusion, dilated cardiomyopathy, cor pulmonale, rheumatic mitral disease, and left ventricular hypertrophy. The proposed protocol answers 5 key questions summarized in Box 1. All 5 questions can be answered using a single subxiphoid view in B mode. More advanced sonographers have the option of additional views as outlined in Table 4 (Additional files 2, 3, 4, 5, 6, 7).

Box 1: Cardiac ultrasound in resource-limited settings (CURLS) protocol—5 questions

CURLS protocol: 5 questions	Interpretation
1. Is a pericardial effusion present?	Yes: consider cardiac tamponade No: consider alternative cause of heart failure
2. Is the left ventricular function reduced?	Yes: consider cardiomyopathy of various causes No: consider alternative cause of heart failure
3. Is the right ventricle larger than the left ventricle?	Yes: consider pulmonary artery hypertension or pulmonary embolism No: consider alternative cause of heart failure
4. Is the left atrium larger than the left ventricle?	Yes: consider mitral stenosis or regurgitation, possibly caused by rheumatic heart disease No: Consider alternative cause of heart failure
5. Is the left ventricle wall (septum) thicker than 12 mm?	Yes: consider hypertension, or aortic stenosis/regurgitation No: consider alternative cause of heart failure

1. Is a pericardial effusion present?

Pericardial effusion is easily identified in a subxiphoid view and usually presents as an anechoic rim around the heart. If a significant pericardial effusion is present, the heart should be evaluated for signs of tamponade. If jugular veins are distended, the patient has tachycardia and low blood pressure, obstructive shock and tamponade may be present. Right atrial systolic collapse and right ventricle (RV) diastolic collapse suggest tamponade physiology. It is important to be aware that if the rate of fluid accumulation is rapid, even a small effusion can cause hemodynamic compromise. In a patient with cardiac tamponade emergency pericardiocentesis can be life-saving. In resource-limited settings an ultrasound-guided intercostal approach with a simple cannula can be used [37].

2. Is the left ventricular function reduced?

Dilated cardiomyopathy can have multiple causes, but sonographically, the end stage is similar with global enlargement of both atria and ventricles with reduced left ventricular systolic function. Unfortunately, most symptomatic patients present in a late stage of the disease. Formal measurement of the ejection fraction and assessment of regional wall motion abnormalities is mostly confined to referral centers as it requires dedicated echocardiographic software and substantial experience. However, a broad classification of left ventricular contractility as hyperdynamic, normal, moderately impaired and severely impaired, can be made by estimating whether contraction is symmetrical towards the center, whether the myocardium thickens as it contracts, and whether the mitral valve opens normally during diastole. In an enlarged heart, this can usually be achieved in a subxiphoid view.

3. Is the right ventricle larger than the left ventricle?

An enlarged RV can indicate cor pulmonale. Cardiac ultrasound can demonstrate sonographic features of cor pulmonale by evaluating shape, size and pressure of the right side of the heart. In the subxiphoid view, in the presence of a normal-sized left ventricle (LV), the RV is typically 2/3 the size of the LV, any larger suggests RV enlargement. If the RV is equal in size to the LV, it is considered moderately enlarged. Pronounced dilatation of the RV such that it is larger than the LV is considered severe RV enlargement and cor pulmonale may be considered. In addition, movement of the intraventricular septum away from the RV indicates increased right ventricular pressure or volume, resulting in a D-shaped LV in the parasternal short axis view (optional view). The measurement of RV contractility and the calculation of the pressure gradient in the setting of tricuspid regurgitation can be helpful. However, this is technically more difficult and requires Doppler software, so it is best reserved for referral sites.

4. Is the left atrium larger than the left ventricle?

An enlarged left atrium (LA) is a feature of mitral stenosis and/or regurgitation, which may serve as a surrogate marker for RHD. The LA often becomes larger than the normal-sized LV by the time the patient presents. Additional findings include a thickened mitral valve with a diastolic hockey stick appearance or "doming" of the

Table 4 Clinical signs of heart failure or cardiomegaly on chest X-ray: narrowing differential diagnoses by cardiac ultrasound to guide management/and respective management (video clips of a normal heart and for each pattern are available as Additional file 2)

Ultrasound image	**Effusion**	**Dilated CMP**	**Right-sided heart failure**	**Valvular (mitral)**	**LV Hypertrophy**
	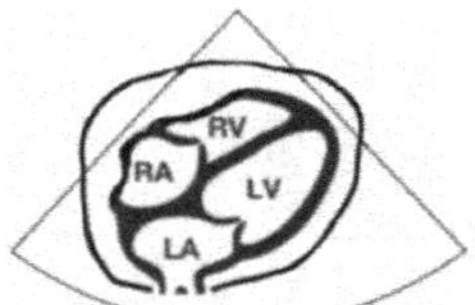 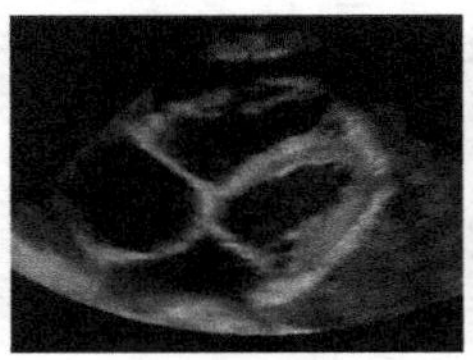	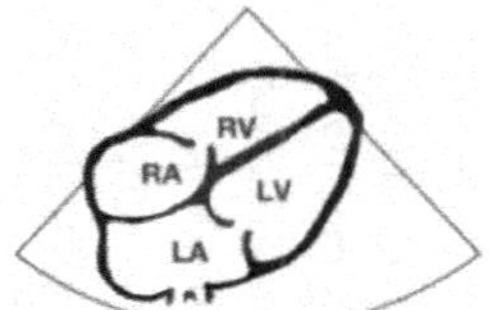 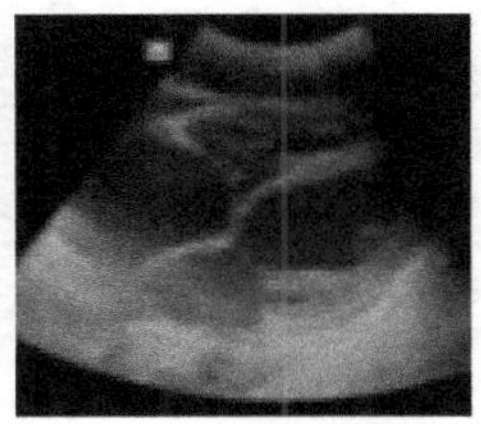	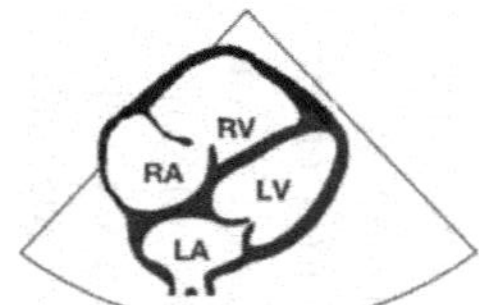 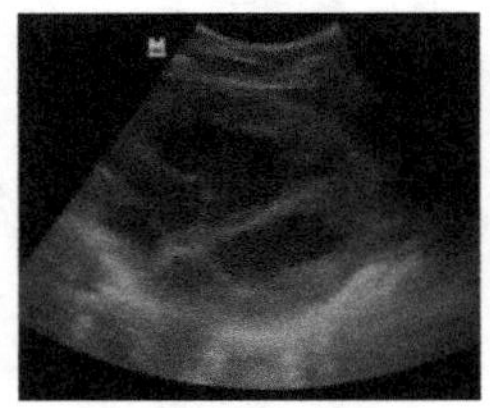	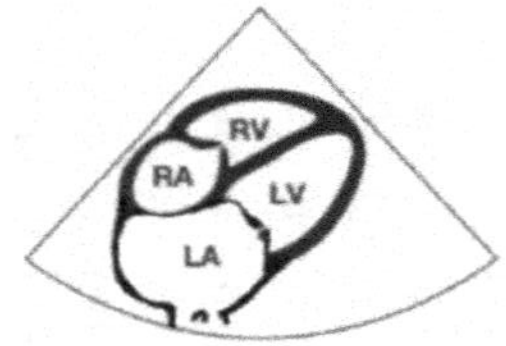 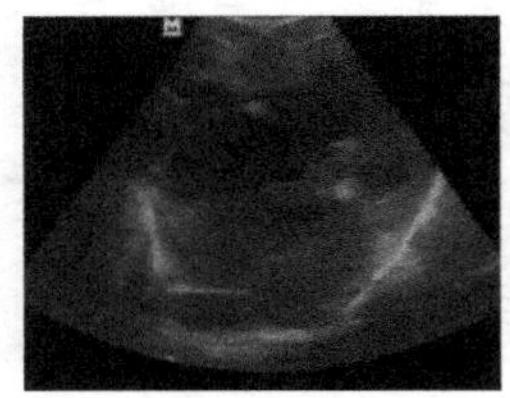	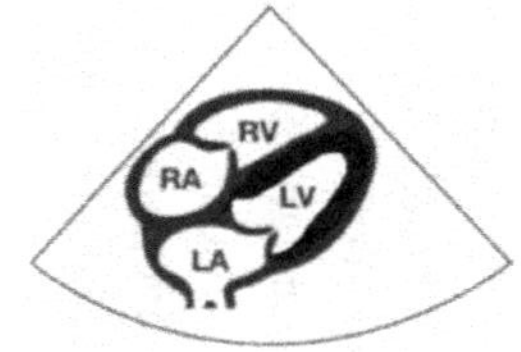 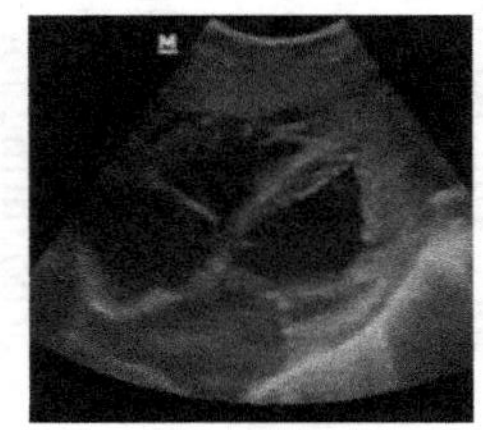
Scanning method	Subxiphoid view Optional: 4-chamber view	Subxiphoid view Optional: 4-chamber view	Subxiphoid view Optional: 4-chamber view, parasternal short	Subxiphoid view Optional: 4-chamber view, parasternal long	Subxiphoid view Optional: parasternal long
Key US features	Anechoic fluid surrounding the heart[a] In severe cases collapse of RV (tamponade)	Reduced inward movement of the LV wall Generalized dilatation of both atria and ventricles	Dilated RV in comparison to the left (ratio > 0.7) D-shaped LV in the parasternal short axis	Dilated LA Thickened mitral valve Mitral regurgitation on Doppler	Thickened LV (septum > 12 mm) Dilated LA Possibly secondary dilated right heart
Differential diagnosis	TB Malignancy Uremia Massive fluid overload Viral Auto-immune	HIV CMP Idiopathic dilated CMP (post-infectious) Peripartum CMP Alcoholic CMP Ischemic heart disease (severe)	Pulmonary embolism Pulmonary hypertension of other cause	Rheumatic heart disease	Hypertension Aortic stenosis Genetic hypertrophic CMP

RV right ventricle, *LV* left ventricle, *LA* left atrium, *CMP* cardiomyopathy, *TB* tuberculosis, *HIV* human immunodeficiency virus

[a] Use the parasternal long axis to differentiate between pleural and pericardial effusions. Pericardial effusions continue anterior to the descending aorta, whereas pleural effusions are found posterior to the descending aorta

valve leaflets. The right heart may also be enlarged due to the subsequent increase in pulmonary pressures. Post-rheumatic changes of the aortic valve are slightly more difficult to detect as they initially lead to left ventricular hypertrophy only and the aortic valve is more difficult to visualize on ultrasound from a subxiphoid view. The morphological assessment of the aortic valve is possible at referral centers, as is the detection of mitral and aortic regurgitation if color-Doppler is available. For the basic CURLS exam, these questions were not included.

5. Is the left ventricle wall (septum) thicker than 12 mm?

Left ventricular hypertrophy can be determined by measuring the intra-ventricular septum (IVS) at end diastole. The standard measurement of the IVS is performed in the parasternal long axis view and should be less than 12 mm. Nevertheless, the septum is generally visible in the subxiphoid view. The clinician should freeze the screen and scroll back to end diastole where the IVS is measured at the level of the mitral valve leaflet tips.

Discussion

The clinical syndrome of heart failure is prevalent around the world. However, the underlying pathology differs significantly between resource-limited and resource-affluent settings. Ischemic heart disease is the main underlying cause in high-resource settings, but is only observed in a minority of patients in SSA. On the other hand, dilated cardiomyopathy, RHD and pericarditis (mostly TB-related) are important causes of heart failure in resource-limited settings, which are less prevalent in high-resource settings. Limited cardiac ultrasound can play a significant role in differentiating between underlying causes. Based on our analysis of the frequency of cardiac conditions, the impact on treatment decisions and the ease of use, we identified five cardiac conditions relevant to SSA for the CURLS protocol. The protocol should serve in emergency departments or acute patient settings and is not intended for screening asymptomatic patients.

Our literature search identified hypertension as the most common cause of heart failure followed by dilated cardiomyopathy and valvular causes. Pericardial effusion and cor pulmonale were less frequently reported, but play a significant role in sub-populations such as HIV-infected patients. Our suggested "cardiac ultrasound for the resource-limited setting" (CURLS) protocol aims to identify these conditions in the "5-question" approach summarized in Box 1 and Table 4. The first question addresses pericardial effusion. Although less common then the other cardiac conditions, it is very easy to recognize and can have life-threatening implications when present. In African patients effusions that mimic congestive heart failure are a common presenting sign of TB [38]. Tuberculosis is the most common cause of pericarditis in Africa. In a South African study, TB pericarditis was responsible for 70% of all cases referred for diagnostic pericardiocentesis and 96% of those who were HIV infected [39]. The second question assesses LV function as dilated cardiomyopathy was the second most common cause of heart failure in SSA in our literature review, accounting for approximately 20% of cases in most studies. Causative factors include myocarditis, HIV-associated cardiomyopathy, alcohol, nutritional deficiency, thyrotoxicosis and pregnancy. In some areas, iron overload and other metabolic factors may play a role [40]. HIV-associated cardiomyopathy is reported in 9–57% of patients who are HIV-positive in Africa [41]. The third question focuses on RV size to detect cor pulmonale. While chronic obstructive pulmonary disease and pulmonary hypertension secondary to left-sided heart failure are seen in all settings, chronic fibrocavitary TB is a frequent underlying cause in Africa [42]. In addition, HIV, schistosomiasis, and pulmonary embolism can lead to chronic pulmonary hypertension eventually resulting in cor pulmonale [43, 44]. Moreover, patients with HIV may suffer from HIV-associated pulmonary artery hypertension. The fourth question considers left atrial size to assess for sequelae of mitral stenosis or mitral regurgitation. In contrast to high-resource settings, where valvular disease is largely degenerative in origin, in Africa valvular disease is almost invariably the result of infectious disease, either directly in infective endocarditis, or indirectly, following acute rheumatic disease [45]. Whereas degenerative valvular disease afflicts mainly the elderly, RHD is encountered in young, school-age children or young females of childbearing age. The course of RHD is more rapid than in degenerative disease and predisposes to cardiac failure, secondary endocarditis, atrial fibrillation and stroke [46]. Most patients with RHD have mixed mitral valve stenosis and regurgitation [47]. Aortic regurgitation is seen in less than 50% of the patients and it is found almost always in combination with mitral valve disease; aortic stenosis is rare [48]. Finally, the protocol addresses left ventricular hypertrophy, generally the result of uncontrolled hypertension. The prevalence of hypertension is high in many African settings, and remains frequently undiagnosed and inadequately treated [49]. It is therefore a frequently identified etiology for cardiac failure in SSA [50].

Ultrasound protocols designed specifically for resource-limited settings have proven effective in SSA. Heller et al. demonstrated that the FASH (focused assessment with sonography for HIV-associated tuberculosis) exam could be efficiently taught to ultrasound-naïve clinicians over a 2-day training period [51]. The FASH exam has now become widely established as an important ultrasound exam for clinicians working in African settings with a high burden of HIV [52]. Similar success in ultrasound training has been demonstrated with the application of the 10-point yes/no checklist for various point-of-care ultrasound applications in a tertiary referral hospital in Tanzania [53]. Recently, a study in Kenya demonstrated the utility of a focused cardiac protocol applied in patient care by clinical officers [54]. Henwood et al. also demonstrated that a longitudinal ultrasound training program could detect basic cardiac abnormalities with high sensitivity and specificity when compared to experienced sonographer interpretation [55]. These studies suggest that implementation of a focused CURLS protocol is feasible.

Some limitations of the protocol should be highlighted. The protocol has not been validated in clinical practice, so its sensitivity and specificity still need to be determined. While the use of only the subxiphoid view simplifies the protocol for non-expert sonographers, it is possible that the image quality is insufficient in some patients. Furthermore, as with any focused protocol, it is not a replacement of an expert cardiology ultrasound and difficult cases should be referred for more extensive workup. Finally, no evidence is available that the protocol enhances diagnosis of cardiac pathologies in resource-limited settings. Hence, the protocol we outline here is set forward as a research agenda and discussion point to encourage all providers to think about how the incredible potential of ultrasound can become more context specific for both patients and providers. Future studies need to assess if the CURLS protocol is trainable and whether significant cardiac findings are missed in comparison to "full specialist" echo exam even though this is not widely available.

Conclusions

Based on the epidemiology of heart disease in sub-Saharan Africa and expert consensus on difficulty and impact of cardiac sonographic examinations, we propose a protocol for screening symptomatic patients with signs of heart failure and/or cardiomegaly on chest X-ray in resource-limited settings. This protocol is unique in that uses primarily the subxiphoid view and is designed to have high clinical relevance whilst being easy to use for providers at the front line of patient care in these settings. The protocol assesses pericardial effusion, dilated cardiomyopathy, cor pulmonale, mitral valve disease, and left ventricular hypertrophy. The protocol has great potential to influence treatment of patients with heart failure in resource-limited settings. Future studies are needed to evaluate whether the protocol can easily be taught and implemented by clinicians, and if ultrasound findings have a positive influence on treatment decisions without missing important findings that would be observed by a specialist echocardiogram.

Supplementary information

Additional file 1: Figure S1. Literature search flowchart. **Table S1.** Baseline characteristics of included studies on etiologies of cardiac disease in SSA (2008–2018).

Additional file 2. Normal heart.

Additional file 3. Pericardial effusion.

Additional file 4. Dilated cardiomyopathy.

Additional file 5. Right sided heart failure.

Additional file 6. Rheumatic heart disease with mitral valve dysfunction.

Additional file 7. Left ventricular hypertrophy.

Abbreviations

AV: aortic valve; CMP: cardiomyopathy; CURLS: cardiac ultrasound for resource-limited settings; cw: continuous wave; dTR: pressure gradient measured in tricuspid regurgitation; FASH: focused assessment with sonography for HIV-associated tuberculosis; HF: heart failure; HIV: human immunodeficiency virus; LA: left atrium; LV: left ventricle; MV: mitral valve; PHT: pressure half-time; POCUS: point-of-care ultrasound; RHD: rheumatic heart disease; RV: right ventricle; SSA: sub-Saharan Africa; TAPSE: tricuspid annular plane systolic excursion; TB: tuberculosis; TEE: transesophageal echocardiography; TV: tricuspid valve; US: ultrasound.

Acknowledgements

Not applicable.

Authors' contributions

TH, DKam conceived the idea of cardiac protocol while teaching ultrasound in various geographic settings, MH conducted the literature review for prevalence, TH, DKam, MH, VK and BK assessed the difficulty of teaching, CW, PG and DKah assessed the relevance with respect to treatment, MH and TH drafted the first manuscript, SB, DKah, Dkam, PG, VK, BK and SP commented extensively on the drafts. All authors read and approved the final manuscript.

Author details

[1] Department of Microbiology and Infectious Diseases, Erasmus Medical Centre, Rotterdam, The Netherlands. [2] Department of Emergency Medicine, Medical College of Georgia, Augusta University, Augusta, GA, USA. [3] Department of Internal Medicine, University of California, Los Angeles, CA, USA. [4] Department of Paediatric Pulmonology, Immunology and Intensive Care Medicine, Charité–Universitätsmedizin Berlin, Berlin, Germany. [5] Berlin Institute of Health, Berlin, Germany. [6] Lighthouse Clinic, Kamuzu Central Hospital, Lilongwe, Malawi. [7] International Training and Education Centre for Health, University of Washington, Seattle, WA, USA. [8] Department of Internal Medicine, College of Medicine, University of Malawi, Blantyre, Malawi. [9] Division of Infectious Diseases and Tropical Medicine, University Hospital, LMU, Munich, Germany. [10] Department of Global Health, University of Washington, Seattle, USA. [11] Department of Medicine, University of North Carolina School of Medicine, Chapel Hill, NC, USA. [12] Department of Public Health, College of Medicine, School of Public Health and Family Medicine, University of Malawi, Lilongwe, Malawi. [13] Department of Tropical Medicine, Bernhard Nocht Institute for Tropical Medicine, I. Department of Medicine, University Medical Center Hamburg-Eppendorf, Hamburg, Germany.

References

1. Mensah GA, Roth GA, Sampson UK, Moran AE, Feigin VL, Forouzanfar MH et al (2015) Mortality from cardiovascular diseases in sub-Saharan Africa, 1990–2013: a systematic analysis of data from the Global Burden of Disease Study 2013. Cardiovasc J Afr. 26(2 Suppl 1):S6–S10

2. Sliwa K, Wilkinson D, Hansen C, Ntyintyane L, Tibazarwa K, Becker A et al (2008) Spectrum of heart disease and risk factors in a black urban population in South Africa (the Heart of Soweto Study): a cohort study. Lancet 371(9616):915–922
3. Sliwa K (2016) The heart of Africa: succeeding against the odds. Lancet 388(10063):e28–e36
4. Sliwa K (2013) Is all heart failure the same around the globe? Eur Heart J 34(40):3091–3092
5. Dokainish H, Teo K, Zhu J, Roy A, AlHabib KF, ElSayed A et al (2017) Global mortality variations in patients with heart failure: results from the International Congestive Heart Failure (INTER-CHF) prospective cohort study. Lancet Glob Health. 5(7):e665–e672
6. Makubi A, Hage C, Sartipy U, Lwakatare J, Janabi M, Kisenge P et al (2016) Heart failure in Tanzania and Sweden: Comparative characterization and prognosis in the Tanzania Heart Failure (TaHeF) study and the Swedish Heart Failure Registry (SwedeHF). Int J Cardiol 220:750–758
7. Heller T, Mtemang'ombe EA, Huson MA, Heuvelings CC, Bélard S, Janssen S et al (2017) Ultrasound for patients in a high HIV/tuberculosis prevalence setting: a needs assessment and review of focused applications for Sub-Saharan Africa. Int J Infect Dis. 56:229–236
8. Mayosi BM (2007) Contemporary trends in the epidemiology and management of cardiomyopathy and pericarditis in sub-Saharan Africa. Heart 93(10):1176–1183
9. Beaton A, Lu JC, Aliku T, Dean P, Gaur L, Weinberg J et al (2015) The utility of handheld echocardiography for early rheumatic heart disease diagnosis: a field study. Eur Heart J Cardiovasc Imaging. 16(5):475–482
10. Ploutz M, Lu JC, Scheel J, Webb C, Ensing GJ, Aliku T et al (2016) Handheld echocardiographic screening for rheumatic heart disease by non-experts. Heart 102(1):35–39
11. Sims Sanyahumbi A, Sable CA, Karlsten M, Hosseinipour MC, Kazembe PN, Minard CG et al (2017) Task shifting to clinical officer-led echocardiography screening for detecting rheumatic heart disease in Malawi, Africa. Cardiol Young 27(6):1133–1139
12. Barasa E, Rogo K, Mwaura N, Chuma J (2018) Kenya National Hospital Insurance Fund Reforms: implications and lessons for universal health coverage. Health Syst Reform 4:346–361
13. Nelson BP, Sanghvi A (2013) Point-of-care cardiac ultrasound: feasibility of performance by noncardiologists. Glob Heart 8(4):293–297
14. Beaton A, Aliku T, Okello E, Lubega S, McCarter R, Lwabi P et al (2014) The utility of handheld echocardiography for early diagnosis of rheumatic heart disease. J Am Soc Echocardiogr 27(1):42–49
15. Lu JC, Sable C, Ensing GJ, Webb C, Scheel J, Aliku T et al (2015) Simplified rheumatic heart disease screening criteria for handheld echocardiography. J Am Soc Echocardiogr 28(4):463–469
16. Becker TK, Tafoya CA, Osei-Ampofo M, Tafoya MJ, Kessler RA, Theyyunni N et al (2017) Cardiopulmonary ultrasound for critically ill adults improves diagnostic accuracy in a resource-limited setting: the AFRICA trial. Trop Med Int Health 22(12):1599–1608
17. Bedeker WF, Lachman AS, Borkum M, Hellenberg D, Cupido CS (2015) Impact of transthoracic echocardiography at district hospital level. S Afr Med J 105(10):817–822
18. Kwan GF, Bukhman AK, Miller AC, Ngoga G, Mucumbitsi J, Bavuma C et al (2013) A simplified echocardiographic strategy for heart failure diagnosis and management within an integrated noncommunicable disease clinic at district hospital level for sub-Saharan Africa. JACC Heart Fail. 1(3):230–236
19. van Hoving DJ, Lamprecht HH, Stander M, Vallabh K, Fredericks D, Louw P et al (2013) Adequacy of the emergency point-of-care ultrasound core curriculum for the local burden of disease in South Africa. Emerg Med J. 30(4):312–315
20. Appiah LT, Sarfo FS, Agyemang C, Tweneboah HO, Appiah NABA, Bedu-Addo G et al (2017) Current trends in admissions and outcomes of cardiac diseases in Ghana. Clin Cardiol 40(10):783–788
21. Bonsu KO, Owusu IK, Buabeng KO, Reidpath DD, Kadirvelu A (2017) Clinical characteristics and prognosis of patients admitted for heart failure: a 5-year retrospective study of African patients. Int J Cardiol 238:128–135
22. Damasceno A, Mayosi BM, Sani M, Ogah OS, Mondo C, Ojji D et al (2012) The causes, treatment, and outcome of acute heart failure in 1006 Africans from 9 countries. Arch Intern Med 172(18):1386–1394
23. Dokainish H, Teo K, Zhu J, Roy A, AlHabib KF, ElSayed A et al (2016) Heart failure in Africa, Asia, the Middle East and South America: The INTER-CHF study. Int J Cardiol 204:133–141
24. Makubi A, Hage C, Lwakatare J, Kisenge P, Makani J, Ryden L et al (2014) Contemporary aetiology, clinical characteristics and prognosis of adults with heart failure observed in a tertiary hospital in Tanzania: the prospective Tanzania Heart Failure (TaHeF) study. Heart 100(16):1235–1241
25. Mwita JC, Dewhurst MJ, Magafu MG, Goepamang M, Omech B, Majuta KL et al (2017) Presentation and mortality of patients hospitalised with acute heart failure in Botswana. Cardiovasc J Afr 28(2):112–117
26. Nkoke C, Makoge C, Dzudie A, Mfeukeu LK, Luchuo EB, Menanga A et al (2017) A predominance of hypertensive heart disease among patients with cardiac disease in Buea, a semi-urban setting, South West Region of Cameroon. BMC Res Notes 10(1):684
27. Ojji D, Stewart S, Ajayi S, Manmak M, Sliwa K (2013) A predominance of hypertensive heart failure in the Abuja Heart Study cohort of urban Nigerians: a prospective clinical registry of 1515 de novo cases. Eur J Heart Fail 15(8):835–842
28. Pio M, Afassinou Y, Pessinaba S, Baragou S, N'Djao J, Atta B et al (2014) Epidemiology and etiology of heart failure in Lome. Pan Afr Med J 18:183
29. Ansa V, Otu A, Oku A, Njideoffor U, Nworah C, Odigwe C (2016) Patient outcomes following after-hours and weekend admissions for cardiovascular disease in a tertiary hospital in Calabar, Nigeria. Cardiovasc J Afr 27(5):328–332
30. Boombhi J, Moampea M, Kuate L, Menanga A, Hamadou B, Kingue S (2017) Clinical pattern and outcome of acute heart failure at the Yaounde Central Hospital. Open Access Lib J 4:1
31. Kingery JR, Yango M, Wajanga B, Kalokola F, Brejt J, Kataraihya J et al (2017) Heart failure, post-hospital mortality and renal function in Tanzania: a prospective cohort study. Int J Cardiol 243:311–317
32. Massoure PL, Roche NC, Lamblin G, Topin F, Dehan C, Kaiser E et al (2013) Heart failure patterns in Djibouti: epidemiologic transition. Med Sante Trop 23(2):211–216
33. Ogah OS, Stewart S, Falase AO, Akinyemi JO, Adegbite GD, Alabi AA et al (2014) Contemporary profile of acute heart failure in Southern Nigeria: data from the Abeokuta Heart Failure Clinical Registry. JACC Heart Fail 2(3):250–259
34. Ogah OS, Adegbite GD, Akinyemi RO, Adesina JO, Alabi AA, Udofia OI et al (2008) Spectrum of heart diseases in a new cardiac service in Nigeria: an echocardiographic study of 1441 subjects in Abeokuta. BMC Res Notes 1:98
35. Onwuchekwa AC, Asekomeh GE (2009) Pattern of heart failure in a Nigerian teaching hospital. Vasc Health Risk Manag 5:745–750
36. Stewart S, Wilkinson D, Hansen C, Vaghela V, Mvungi R, McMurray J et al (2008) Predominance of heart failure in the Heart of Soweto Study cohort: emerging challenges for urban African communities. Circulation 118(23):2360–2367
37. Heller T, Lessells RJ, Wallrauch C, Brunetti E (2010) Tuberculosis pericarditis with cardiac tamponade: management in the resource-limited setting. Am J Trop Med Hyg 83(6):1311–1314
38. Desai HN (1979) Tuberculous pericarditis. A review of 100 cases. S Afr Med J 55(22):877–880
39. Reuter H, Burgess LJ, Doubell AF (2005) Epidemiology of pericardial effusions at a large academic hospital in South Africa. Epidemiol Infect 133(3):393–399
40. Sliwa K, Damasceno A, Mayosi BM (2005) Epidemiology and etiology of cardiomyopathy in Africa. Circulation 112(23):3577–3583
41. Ntsekhe M, Hakim J (2005) Impact of human immunodeficiency virus infection on cardiovascular disease in Africa. Circulation 112(23):3602–3607
42. Aderaye G (2004) Causes and clinical characteristics of chronic corpulmonale in Ethiopia. East Afr Med J 81(4):202–206
43. Klein SK, Slim EJ, de Kruif MD, Keller TT, ten Cate H, van Gorp EC et al (2005) Is chronic HIV infection associated with venous thrombotic disease? A systematic review. Neth J Med 63(4):129–136
44. Ramlakhan R, Andronikou S, Rajkumar A (2017) The prevalence and radiological findings of pulmonary embolism in HIV-positive patients referred for computed tomography pulmonary angiography in the Western Cape of South Africa. Cardiovasc J Afr 28(4):221–228

45. Strasser T (1980) Community control of rheumatic heart disease in developing countries: 1 a major public health problem. WHO Chron 34(9):336–345
46. Essop M, Nkomo V (2005) Rheumatic and nonrheumatic valvular heart disease: epidemiology, management, and prevention in Africa. Circulation 112(23):3584–3591
47. Malla R, Thapaliya S, Gurung P, Bogati A, Khadka S, Shrestha S et al (2016) Patterns of Valvular Involvement in Rheumatic Heart Disease patients taking Benzathine Penicillin at Shahid Gangalal National Heart Centre, Kathmandu, Nepal. Nepal Heart J 13(2):25–27
48. Faheem M, Hafizullah M, Gul A, Ullah Jan H, Asghar Khan M. Pattern of valvular lesions in rheumatic heart disease. J Postgrad Med Inst. 2007;21(2):99–103
49. Addo J, Smeeth L, Leon DA (2007) Hypertension in sub-saharan Africa: a systematic review. Hypertension 50(6):1012–1018
50. Amoah AG, Kallen C (2000) Aetiology of heart failure as seen from a National Cardiac Referral Centre in Africa. Cardiology 93(1–2):11–18
51. Heller T, Wallrauch C, Lessells RJ, Goblirsch S, Brunetti E (2010) Short course for focused assessment with sonography for human immunodeficiency virus/tuberculosis: preliminary results in a rural setting in South Africa with high prevalence of human immunodeficiency virus and tuberculosis. Am J Trop Med Hyg 82(3):512–515
52. Salmon M, Landes M, Hunchak C, Paluku J, Malemo Kalisya L, Salmon C et al (2017) Getting it right the first time: defining regionally relevant training curricula and provider core competencies for point-of-care ultrasound education on the african continent. Ann Emerg Med 69(2):218–226
53. Stanley A, Wajanga BM, Jaka H, Purcell R, Byrne L, Williams F et al (2017) The impact of systematic point-of-care ultrasound on management of patients in a resource-limited setting. Am J Trop Med Hyg 96(2):488–492
54. Barasa FB, DeLong A, Kimaiyo S, Koech M, Binanay C, Foster M et al (2018) Diagnostic accuracy of focused cardiac ultrasound for common cardiac conditions in a Kenyan hospital. J Kenya Assoc Phys 1(1):5–13
55. Henwood PC, Mackenzie DC, Liteplo AS, Rempell JS, Murray AF, Leo MM et al (2017) Point-of-care ultrasound use, accuracy, and impact on clinical decision making in rwanda hospitals. J Ultrasound Med 36(6):1189–1194

26

Hepatic and portal vein Dopplers in the clinical management of patients with right-sided heart failure: two case reports

Matthew Jefkins and Barry Chan*

Abstract

Background: Patients with right heart failure pose significant volume management challenges for hemodynamic optimization. We present two cases in which point of care ultrasound (POCUS) of the hepatic and portal veins contributed to the venous hypertension assessment and decongestive strategy for patients with right-sided heart failure.

Case presentation: Patient A was 91 years old with known pulmonary hypertension and right ventricular systolic dysfunction who presented in septic shock requiring vasopressor support. Hepatic and portal vein Dopplers were consistent with right heart failure and significant venous congestion, therefore, diuresis was initiated which resulted in portal flow normalization, renal recovery, and cessation of vasopressor support. Patient B was 82 years old with severe idiopathic pulmonary fibrosis on home oxygen who presented in decompensated right heart failure. Despite aggressive diuresis, a negative fluid balance was not achieved. The patient continued to deteriorate and prior to their death portal vein, Doppler showed significant flow reversal.

Conclusion: Hepatic and portal vein Doppler ultrasounds are venous hypertension assessment tools that can be readily used at the bedside by clinicians trained in POCUS that may contribute holistically to the hemodynamic profiling for patients with right heart failure and direct therapeutic interventions.

Keywords: Congestive heart failure, Point of care ultrasound, Portal vein, Doppler

Introduction

Congestive heart failure is a complex condition with effects on other organ systems including liver and kidneys. Patients with right heart failure and concurrent illness such as sepsis pose significant challenges in managing volume status for hemodynamic optimization. Point of care ultrasound (POCUS) is a non-invasive, readily available tool with increasing numbers of clinical applications to assess and help guide management of patients.

In hepatic vein ultrasonography, the normal hepatic waveform is triphasic with 4 components including a retrograde A wave (atrial systole), anterograde S wave (ventricular systole), transitional V wave (atrial overfilling transition wave), and an anterograde D wave (ventricular diastole) [1]. Normally, the magnitude of the S wave is larger than the D wave because the anterograde venous return velocity from the liver to the heart during ventricular systole is higher than the velocity during passive ventricular filling [1]. However, in right heart failure, the hepatic waveform exhibits a S to D wave ratio reversal due to the relatively greater anterograde blood flow during diastole than systole. In addition, tricuspid regurgitation, often coexisting with significant right heart failure, can result in a retrograde S wave [1].

In patients with significant right heart failure, portal vein Doppler demonstrates increased portal vein pulsatility due to an interplay between elevated right atrial pressure and tricuspid regurgitation wave transmission [2]. Conversely, in healthy patients, the portal vein normally shows continuous flow with minimal phasic variation throughout the cardiac cycle [3]. Portal vein pulsatility

*Correspondence: barrytschan@gmail.com
Division of General Internal Medicine, Department of Medicine, Queen's University, Kingston, Ontario K7L 3N6, Canada

correlates with New York Heart Association classification, where class III and IV heart failure patients tend to demonstrate increased pulsatility or, at the extreme, flow reversal [2, 4].

The features and characteristics of portal vein Doppler ultrasonography in patients with heart failure have been described in the literature [2, 4, 5], and there have been case reports of clinical application in post-cardiac surgery patients [6] and critical care patients [7]. However, this technique is seldom known to most front-line clinicians. The aim of this report is to illustrate the clinical utility of portal vein Doppler in assessing venous hypertension, guiding the volume management, and the evolution of the waveforms through two patients with right-sided heart failure.

This study was approved by the Queen's University Health Sciences and Affiliated Teaching Hospitals Research Ethics Board.

Case presentation

Patient A who was 91 years old with moderate pulmonary hypertension and moderate right ventricular (RV) dysfunction was brought to the hospital for delirium who was found to have acute chronic kidney injury with a creatinine of 262 μmol/L (baseline 120 μmol/L) and in septic shock due to Staphylococcus *epidermidis* bacteremia of unknown source. The patient was initially aggressively volume expanded for hemodynamic resuscitation with no improvement in their mean arterial pressure (MAP), therefore, vasopressor support was started. Norepinephrine was started at 0.05 mcg/kg/min and titrated to a maximum of 0.13 mcg/kg/min to maintain a MAP of 65 mmHg.

Given the patient's predisposition to right heart failure, POCUS was deployed to assess for venous congestion on Day 1. Hepatic vein Doppler revealed D > S wave which suggested tricuspid regurgitation and/or right heart failure (Fig. 1a). Interrogation of the right portal vein, imaged longitudinally from the right mid-axillary line, revealed a pulsatile waveform characterized by intermittent anterograde and cessation of flow suggestive of significant venous congestion (Fig. 1b). Hence, to optimize end-organ perfusion pressure, volume expansion was terminated, and diuresis was pursued. Furosemide 80 mg intravenously once daily was administered on Days 1 and 2 which resulted in net negative fluid balance of 1.9 L and 4.9 L, respectively. Daily reassessment of portal flow demonstrated attenuation of pulsatile flow velocity by Day 2 (Fig. 1c), then a continuous and anterograde phasic flow was achieved by Day 3 (Fig. 1d). Of note, the portal flow velocity on Day 3 was reduced to approximately 10 cm/s (Fig. 1d). This was unlikely secondary to a technical factor as the angle of insonation of the pulse wave Doppler was virtually paralleled with the right portal vein. The cause was most likely secondary to portal hypertension from right heart failure given the clinical context.

The patient was off norepinephrine by Day 2; and signs of renal recovery began on Day 3 with a creatinine of 196 and trending down. The patient was discharged home on post-admission Day 11 with their creatinine recovered to 123 mmol/L.

Patient B was 82 years old with severe idiopathic pulmonary fibrosis (IPF) on 2 L/min home oxygen who was transferred to the hospital for being found hypoxic during a follow-up assessment. Of note, the patient noted increasing peripheral edema up to the proximal thighs that developed over the course of 2 months. CT chest demonstrated features indicative of an IPF flare and bilateral pleural effusions. On Day 1, cardiac POCUS (Fig. 2) revealed a small pericardial effusion, normal LV systolic function, dilated RV, reduced RV systolic function, severe tricuspid regurgitation, and interventricular septal flattening was observed only during diastole. The hepatic vein waveform demonstrated S wave retrograde flow (Fig. 3a) and a continuous yet phasic anterograde portal flow at a lower velocity of about 10 cm/s (Fig. 3b). Given these sonographic findings, right ventricular volume overload and portal venous hypertension were evident; therefore, a decongestive strategy was commenced with 40 mg of intravenous furosemide.

On Day 2, pulsatile flow within the portal vein was present which prompted diuresis escalation from furosemide 40 mg intravenously up to 160 mg. However, the patient failed to respond to high-dose furosemide 160 mg with the addition of metolazone 5 mg orally resulting in daily net volume retention with biochemical evidence of progressive acute kidney injury with creatinine of 111 mmol/L from a baseline of 60 mmol/L, congestive hepatopathy, and an increasing lactic acidosis. On Day 5, the patient developed overt shock whereby the portal vein was in retrograde flow for the majority of time (Fig. 3c). The patient died shortly thereafter.

Discussion

Volume optimization for patients with right heart failure is a ubiquitous challenge. High right-sided filling pressures and tricuspid regurgitation often confound the interpretation of the jugular venous pulse (JVP) rendering it of little clinical utility for volume management [8]. In addition, the JVP is either not readily visible, or there is substantial inter-examiner variability [9]. Increasing peripheral edema and serial weights are probably the most reliable bedside markers for a clinician. Nevertheless, when a history of change in edema cannot be elicited or reliable serial weights is not available, hepatic and portal vein Doppler are alternative

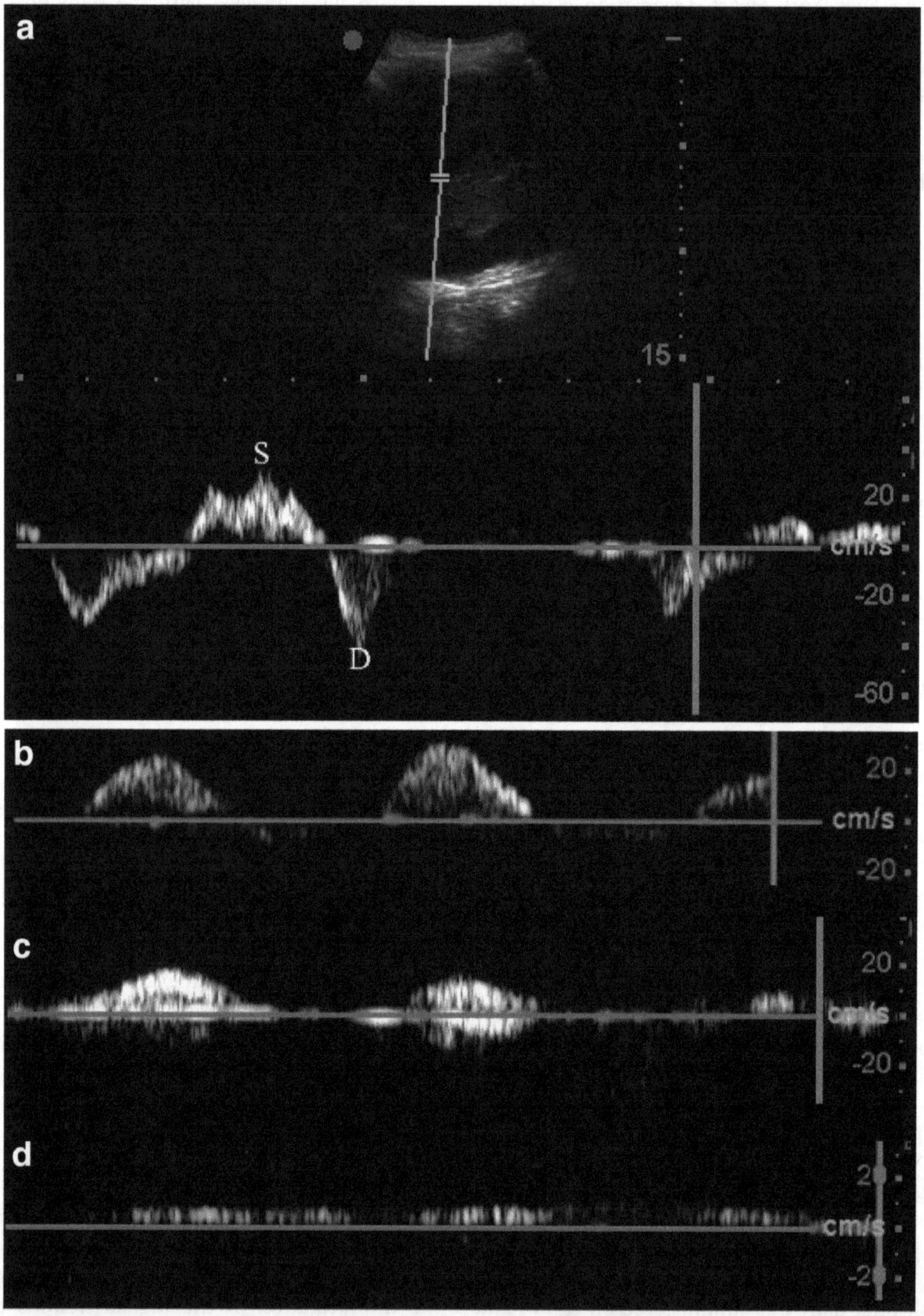

Fig. 1 **a** Doppler of the middle hepatic vein on Day 1 demonstrated S wave retrograde flow suggestive of tricuspid regurgitation and/or right heart failure. **b** Doppler of the right portal vein on Day 1 demonstrated pulsatile flow with intermittent flow cessation suggestive of venous congestion. **c** A net negative fluid balance of 1.9 L was achieved which resulted in on Day 2. **d** Then a net negative fluid balance of 4.9 L was achieved which resulted in the normalization to a continuous and anterograde phasic portal flow on Day 3

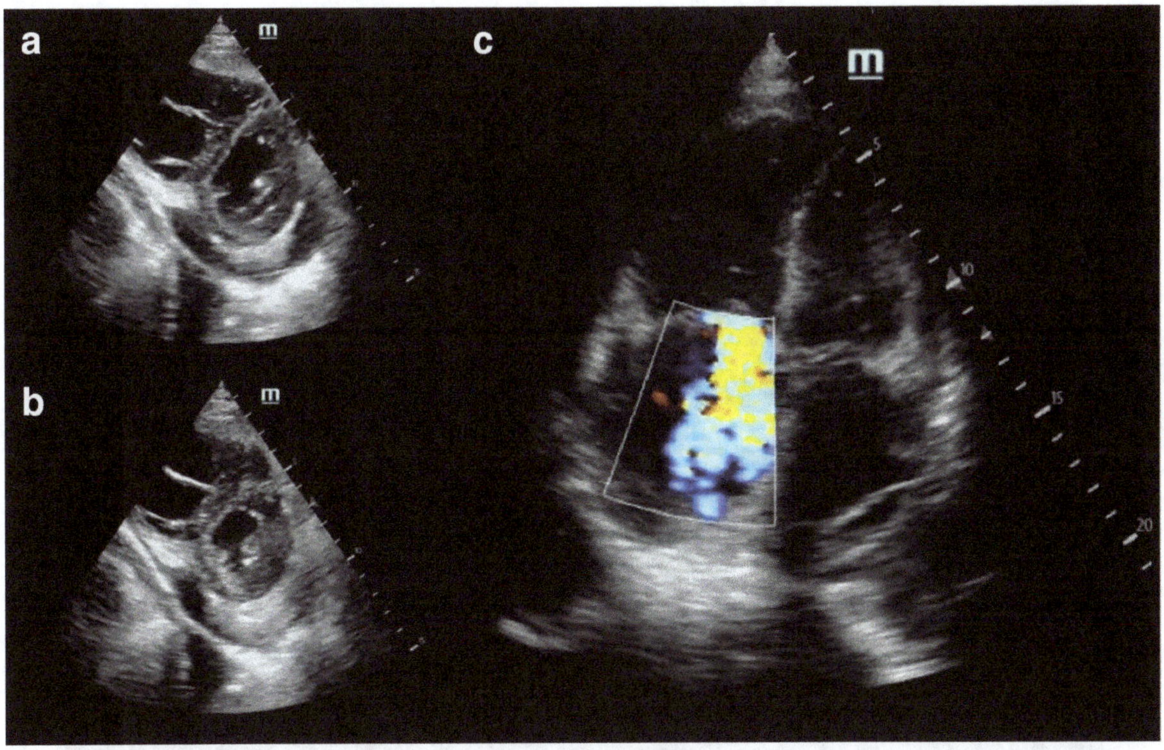

Fig. 2 Cardiac POCUS on Day 1, the parasternal short view demonstrated flattening of the interventricular septum only during diastole (**a**) and normalization during systole (**b**). The apical 4 view right ventricle was dilated with evidence of a tricuspid regurgitation jet (**c**)

evaluation tools that can be readily deployed. In both cases, the right portal vein was imaged with the same technique where the probe was positioned longitudinally at the level of the right mid-axillary line where the liver is situated.

In Case A, due to the patient's delirium and lack of collateral information, the aforementioned volume markers could not be obtained. Volume expansion was initiated but given the patient's right heart failure such an intervention can instead diminish end-organ perfusion due to reduction in cardiac output and venous hypertension. Hepatic and portal vein Dopplers were deployed to resolve this conundrum. The S wave is influenced by the state of compliance of the right atrium during systole and the presence of tricuspid regurgitation. Hence, the abnormal S wave does suggest abnormal right atrial compliance most commonly secondary to right heart dysfunction. The portal vein flow profile revealed a pulsatile flow with intermittent flow cessation suggestive of significantly high pressure downstream. As such, a net negative volume strategy was pursued which resulted in the normalization of the direction of portal flow. This was associated with the subsequent weaning of vasopressor support and renal recovery. The complex mechanisms of cardiointestinal and cardiorenal syndromes may explain these observed associations.

In cardiointestinal syndrome, intestinal hypoperfusion and gut edema are associated with systemic immune activation and increased levels of proinflammatory cytokines as a result of increased gut permeability secondary to gastrointestinal hypoperfusion and gut edema from venous congestion [10]. Hence, decongestive to relief venous hypertension may reduce proinflammatory cytokines and result in vasopressor cessation. In terms of the renal recovery, venous hypertension has been shown to result in increased renal resistance and, subsequently, reduction in renal blood flow. Hence, a net negative volume strategy can improve renal function [11].

Case B illustrated the natural history of decompensated right heart failure through the lens of portal venous flow profile. On presentation, despite having an anterograde and phasic portal venous flow, the reduced velocity indicated evidence of portal hypertension. To distinguish whether it is of cardiac or primary hepatic etiology, clinical context and corroborative investigation are needed [12, 13]. Sonographically, however, the former will be associated severe tricuspid regurgitation and concomitant S to D wave ratio reversal of the hepatic vein whereas the portal hypertension secondary to a primary liver disease should not have these associated findings. In this case, despite aggressive diuresis, daily net positive balance resulted. Eventually, the venous hypertension was

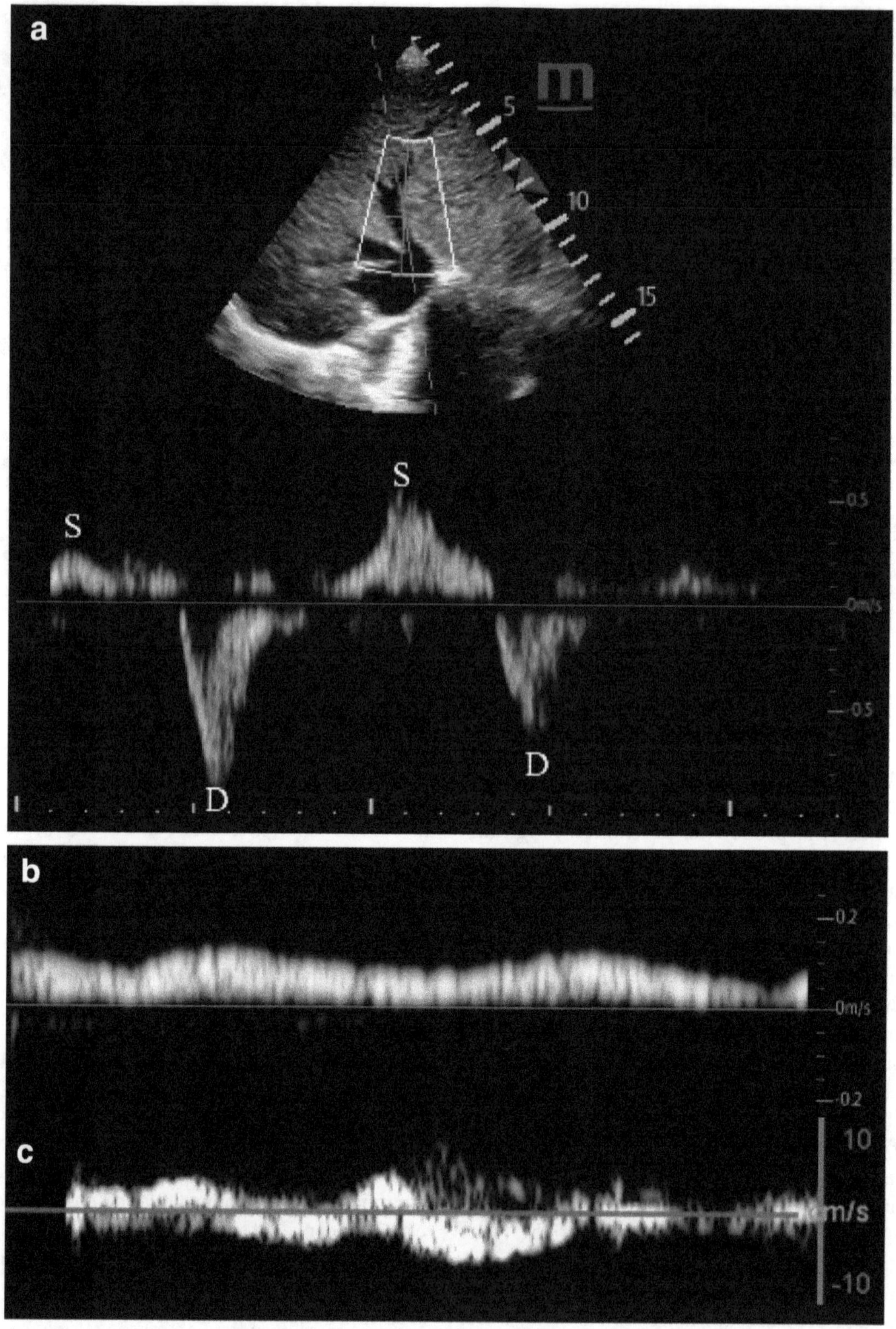

Fig. 3 Middle hepatic vein Doppler on Day 1 demonstrated S wave reversal suggestive of tricuspid regurgitation and/or right heart failure (**a**). Right portal vein Doppler on Day 1 demonstrating reduced portal venous flow suggestive of venous congestion (**b**). Right portal vein Doppler on Day 5 demonstrating portal venous flow reversal suggestive of severe heart failure and venous congestion

so severe such that the portal vein flow reversed which signified severely decompensated right-sided heart failure [4].

Both cases illustrate the utility of hepatic and portal venous Doppler to assess for venous hypertension for patients with right heart failure. Beaubien-Souligny et al. [6] demonstrated an association between portal vein pulsatility and the risk of acute kidney injury as manifested by venous congestion in a prospective cohort study in postoperative cardiac surgery patients. Similar to our cases, they found that portal vein pulsatility was associated with S to D wave ratio reversal of the hepatic vein waveform.

In terms of therapeutic intervention, for our two cases, a decongestive strategy was pursued to alleviate venous congestion to improve end-organ perfusion. Nevertheless, the added sonographic information from both hepatic and portal vein Doppler cannot be interpreted in isolation—they contribute to the assessment of a patient's hemodynamic profile holistically. Even if the portal flow demonstrates pulsatility or flow reversal, volume removal maybe deleterious should a high preload state is required to maintain cardiac output such as massive pulmonary embolism, or cardiac tamponade. The former requires afterload reduction and the latter necessitates relief from the intrapericardial pressure.

Conclusion

Hepatic and portal vein Doppler interrogations are venous hypertension assessment adjuncts for patients with right heart failure which may direct therapeutic interventions in conjunction with other hemodynamic parameters.

Abbreviations

IPF: idiopathic pulmonary fibrosis; JVP: jugular venous pulse; MAP: mean arterial pressure; NYHA: New York Heart Association; POCUS: point of care ultrasound; RV: right ventricle/right ventricular.

Acknowledgements

None.

Authors' contributions

MJ was a major contributor in writing of the manuscript. BC was responsible for acquiring the images and reviewing the manuscript. Both authors read and approved the final manuscript.

References

1. Scheinfeld MH, Bilali A, Koenigsberg M (2009) Understanding the spectral doppler waveform of the hepatic veins in health and disease. RadioGraphics 29(7):2081–2098
2. Catalano D, Caruso G, DiFazzio S, Carpinteri G, Scalisi N, Trovato GM (1998) Portal vein pulsatility ratio and heart failure. J Clin Ultrasound 26(1):5
3. Goncalvesova E, Lesny P, Luknar M, Solik P, Varga I (2010) Changes of portal flow in heart failure patients with liver congestion. Bratisl Lek Listy 111(12):635–639
4. Rengo C, Brevetti G, Sorrentino G, D'Amato T, Imparato M, Vitale DF et al (1998) Portal vein pulsatility ratio provides a measure of right heart function in chronic heart failure. Ultrasound Med Biol 24(3):327–332
5. Duerinckx AJ, Grant EG, Perrella RR, Szeto A, Tessler FN (1990) The pulsatile portal vein in cases of congestive heart failure: correlation of duplex Doppler findings with right atrial pressures. Radiology 176(3):655–658
6. Beaubien-Souligny W, Benkreira A, Robillard P, Bouabdallaoui N, Chassé M, Desjardins G et al (2018) Alterations in portal vein flow and intrarenal venous flow are associated with acute kidney injury after cardiac surgery: a prospective observational cohort study. J Am Heart Assoc 7:19
7. Beaubien-Souligny W, Elmi-Sarabi M, Desjardins G, Deanult AY (2017) Point-of-care ultrasonography to assess portal vein pulsatility and the effect of inhaled milrinone and epoprostenol in severe right ventricular failure: a report of 2 cases. A A Case Report 9(8):219–223
8. Konstam MA, Kiernan MS, Bernstein D et al (2018) Evaluation and management of right-sided heart failure: a scientific statement from the American Heart Association. Circulation 137:e578–e622
9. Cook DJ, Simel DL (1996) The Rational Clinical Examination. Does this patient have abnormal central venous pressure? JAMA 275:630–634
10. Sundaram V, Fang JC (2016) Gastrointestinal and liver issues in heart failure. Circulation 133(17):1696–1703
11. Rangaswami J, Bhalla V, Blair JEA, Chang TI, Costa S, Lentine KL et al (2019) Cardiorenal syndrome: classification, pathophysiology, diagnosis, and treatment strategies: a scientific statement from the American Heart Association. Circulation 139(16):e840–e878
12. Abu-Yousef MM, Milam SG, Farner RM (1990) Pulsatile portal vein flow: a sign of tricuspid regurgitation on duplex Doppler sonography. Am J Roentgenol 155(4):785–788
13. Iranpour P, Lall C, Houshyar R, Helmy M, Yang A, Choi J-I et al (2016) Altered Doppler flow patterns in cirrhosis patients: an overview. Ultrasonography 35(1):3–12

27

The effectiveness of a longitudinal ultrasound curriculum for general pediatricians working in a Puerto Rican emergency department

Veronica Sepulveda-Ortiz, Fred Warkentine, Rebecca Starr-Seal and Anna Rominger

Abstract

Background: The Hospital Pediatrico Universitario (HOPU) is the principal institution in Puerto Rico offering medical services to the children of the island and the Caribbean. There is limited use of point-of-care ultrasound (PoCUS) in their emergency department (ED) and obtaining an ultrasound through radiology is prohibitively time consuming. The objective of this study is to increase PoCUS knowledge and comfort by the ED physicians in the HOPU pediatric emergency department.

Results: Thirteen general pediatricians completed the entire PoCUS course, but only 10 completed both the pre- and post-tests and therefore included in the analysis ($N = 10$). Pretest scores ranged from 30 to 63.3% with a mean of 41.6% [standard deviation (SD) 9.95]. The posttest scores ranged from 55 to 96%, with a mean of 66.1% (SD 12.26). The mean difference in scores was 24.42% (95% confidence interval 17.9, 30.9) with a significance of $p < 0.05$ and range of 8.3–36.6%. Physician experience and confidence with each topic improved from baseline. After the course, the majority of the participants (> 70%) had at least some confidence in 5 of the 6 topics.

Conclusions: In EDs with limited resources, a longitudinal PoCUS educational curriculum is effective in improving the knowledge and comfort of physicians with limited PoCUS experience. The effectiveness of scheduled, repeated courses to refresh and refocus participants was highlighted following the unexpected challenges encountered during the course, including multiple natural disasters.

Keywords: Point-of-care ultrasound, POCUS, Pediatric emergency medicine, PoCUS education, Resource-limited settings

Background

PoCUS is an affordable, safe, and efficient imaging modality with a wide variety of uses in the medical field, particularly in the emergency setting. Medical providers in Europe have utilized ultrasound for decades and over the last 20 years; its use has exploded in the United States. A PoCUS examination is performed at bedside with immediate results, without radiation exposure to the patient or provider. In addition, ultrasonography is a fraction of the cost of other imaging modalities, including radiography, computed tomography (CT), and magnetic resonance imaging (MRI) which makes it a more accessible imaging option in financially strained circumstances.

Since 1985, the World Health Organization (WHO) has recommended ultrasonography for developing countries because it is portable, inexpensive, non-invasive, safe, and provides information immediately [6, 8]. Via et al. noted that point-of-care ultrasound (PoCUS) has a significant impact in undifferentiated shock, narrowing

*Correspondence: anna.rominger@louisville.edu
Division of Pediatric Emergency Medicine, Department of Pediatrics, University of Louisville, 571 S. Floyd Street, Suite 412, Louisville, KY 40202, USA

the differential diagnosis and improving the specificity of early recognition of hypovolemia and septic shock cardiovascular patterns [8]. Because of this, the authors suggest that PoCUS should have an integral role in management of unstable patients in developing countries [8]. In addition, lung PoCUS is very effective for the early diagnosis of various infectious respiratory conditions, which is a leading cause of childhood mortality in developing countries [8, 9]. Short-term medical mission trips to resource-limited regions have been using PoCUS for many years. However, the best strategy to make a lasting change in these areas is to equip local providers with ultrasound machines and the knowledge to use them so they can continuously provide a higher level of care to the local people.

Short-term PoCUS training programs are proven to deliver adequate knowledge and skills to novices [8]. Shah et al. conducted an educational intervention in Rwanda to create an effective PoCUS curriculum for inpatient providers at two of the local hospitals [6]. They concluded that PoCUS is a very teachable skill with an intensive training course and hands-on teaching [6]. They introduced a 9-week course with 1-h lectures three times per week for the first 3 weeks and then one time per week for the remaining 6 weeks with 1–2 h of guided scanning practice following each lecture [6, 7]. The most common clinical practice change noted after the course was a new plan to perform a surgical procedure following the results of the PoCUS [7]. The investigators found other types of changes in the patient care plan based on PoCUS results, including medication changes, referrals to a specialty clinic, cancellation of surgical procedures, and referrals for further radiologic evaluation with CT scanning [7].

More recently, Rominger et al. implemented a 12-month longitudinal PoCUS curriculum for primary care physicians working in rural outpatient clinics in Mexico [5]. They organized 4-day PoCUS teaching sessions each separated by approximately 3–4 months [5]. By having recurring short-term trips, the training did not interrupt the regular schedule of the local physicians and was more feasible for educators traveling to the area. The sessions included lectures and hands-on training focused on different topics at each session. They found that the use of PoCUS changed the patient diagnosis and clinical management in about 1/3 of cases [5]. They demonstrated that bedside PocUS education programs targeted to local physicians in outpatient settings is an effective strategy to equip them with a tool to improve the clinical management of their patients.

The effectiveness of a PoCUS curriculum is not limited to developing countries. A study by Clay et al. focused on United States (US) Internal Medicine residents, found that a single day of intensive PoCUS training at the beginning of the year yielded significant improvement in PoCUS interpretation skills [1, 2]. They used a 30-question assessment to measure bedside PoCUS knowledge prior to, immediately post, and 6 months post-training. Assessment performance increased by almost 25% and remained significantly better at 6 months [1, 2]. Noble et al. also performed an educational study directed towards United States (US) Emergency Medicine physicians and interns [4]. The participants of this study received an "introduction to PoCUS" course. An assessment before and 6 months after the introductory course was administered using a standardized image-based ultrasound test. There was a significant improvement in PoCUS knowledge for both faculty and interns, which also persisted for 6 months following the introductory course [4].

The Hospital Pediatrico Universitario (HOPU) is the principal institution in Puerto Rico offering medical services to the children of Puerto Rico and the Caribbean. HOPU is the pediatric academic institution for the University of Puerto Rico School of Medicine and the clinical center for the pediatric residency program. It is the only pediatric hospital to provide tertiary services to the island and guarantees that its services are accessible to children of all socio-economic levels, including the medically indigent. The Emergency Department (ED) at HOPU receives about 10,000 pediatric patients annually. It is generally a low-flow but high-acuity ED where general pediatricians and residents provide health care 24 h a day, 7 days a week. Prior to this study, there were no ultrasound machines in the Emergency Department and the physicians had no PoCUS training. Access to ultrasound was available through the Radiology Department but since the Radiology Department serves the entire Medical Center and not just the pediatric hospital, obtaining an official ultrasound report takes 24–48 h. Many of the conditions seen in the Emergency Department are easily identified and managed with the appropriate use of PoCUS. For example, the identification of cellulitis, abscess, free fluid in the abdomen (traumatic or nontraumatic), hydronephrosis, pericardial effusion, pleural effusion, appendicitis, intussusception, and global heart function. If the providers have basic PoCUS knowledge and skills, it would greatly aid in the local management of many medical conditions, reduce the number of referrals for imaging, and expedite the care of patients who do have a serious medical or surgical condition.

The objective of this study is to increase ultrasound knowledge and comfort by the ED physicians in the HOPU pediatric emergency department. Although Puerto Rico is a US territory, its pediatric health care model and funding can be likened to a resource-limited site with the closest additional pediatric resources located 1000 miles away in Miami, Florida. Therefore, it is a unique setting which cannot be simply grouped with US facilities or resource-limited ones, so many of the previous studies may not be easily generalizable to this particular institution. Therefore, the authors sought to identify an effective ultrasound curriculum for the HOPU ED providers.

Methods

This is a longitudinal educational curriculum conducted at the HOPU in San Juan, Puerto Rico. It is a pilot study to determine if a longitudinal approach would be an effective teaching strategy in this particular group of physicians. The instructors for the educational sessions included two pediatric emergency medicine (PEM) physicians, an emergency medicine (EM) physician and ultrasound fellow, and a PEM fellow from the University of Louisville. A PEM physician and ultrasound fellow from Indiana University joined the primary investigator on one of the trips. Both the University of Louisville and the University of Puerto Rico Institutional Review Boards reviewed this study and deemed it exempt.

Prior to initiation of the course work, the primary investigator conducted a needs assessment at HOPU with local physicians to determine the most relevant topics and commonly encountered regional pathologies. They designed the curriculum based on the findings in the needs assessment and desires of the local providers with a focus on trauma evaluation (FAST), bedsides cardiac evaluation for global function, identification of skin and soft tissue infections, and abdominal pathologies, specifically intussusception and appendicitis. To accommodate the schedules of the local physicians, the team taught the course in multiple sessions rather than one long conference, which the Puerto Rican providers preferred. In addition, the amount of information presented in one long conference can be overwhelming for novices and the investigators had concerns for adequate knowledge retention in a single course. The longitudinal approach allowed participants to master several PoCUS concepts before moving on to new ones. Lastly, this design put the educators at the site for multiple points in time to review previous concepts, answer additional questions, discuss images and cases, and review technique. The HOPU ED did not have an ultrasound machine in their department prior to the course; however, Norton Children's Hospital donated a Sonosite M-turbo ultrasound machine with low-frequency (curvilinear), phased-array, and high-frequency (linear) probes.

The curriculum was designed based on the previous work by Rominger et al. in Mexico. This structure was used due to the time constraints of the local providers and the fact that the providers were all general pediatricians without subspecialty training, similar to the general practitioners trained in Mexico. The curriculum consisted of three, 2-day sessions given over 12 months. The instructors taught the material in English and, as a US territory, all participants were fluent in English. The first day consisted of lectures with hands-on training on healthy volunteers. The class ratio was 5–7 learners per two instructors. The second day of the course focused on hands-on examination of patients with pathologic findings on ultrasound. Prior to the practice sessions, the instructors identified patients with relevant pathology throughout the hospital and obtained consent (and assents as applicable) to ultrasound for learning purposes.

The participants had all completed a 3-year general pediatrics residency and were working in the HOPU ED as independent providers and supervising physicians. The investigators tested the baseline ultrasound knowledge of each participant prior to the first session using a 25-question written test. The test was developed as part of the PEM PoCUS credentialing program at the University of Louisville used to demonstrate bedside PoCUS competency. The primary investigator distributed the same test to participants 3 months after the final session to assess ultrasound knowledge. The results of the test were withheld from participants until the completion of the post-curriculum evaluation. They each completed a questionnaire prior to each session and again 3 months following the last session, which assessed their subjective experience and confidence in the various PoCUS modalities. The first teaching course was in August 2017 and focused on care and use of the ultrasound machine, introduction to PoCUS, focused assessment with sonography in trauma (FAST), and basic bedside cardiac ultrasound. The next session was scheduled for November 2017, but the curriculum was adjusted following multiple natural disasters in Puerto Rico during the fall of 2017. The next session moved to February 2018 and it included a half-day review of the previous information plus the introduction of lung, skin and soft tissue, kidney, bladder, and ultrasound-guided procedures. The final session was May 2018 and focused on cardiovascular, abdominal, and ocular ultrasound. The instructors uploaded the presentations from each session onto a google drive that the participants had access to for their reference and review. The participants continued to order formal ultrasound examinations on patients through the HOPU radiology department throughout the study following their own bedside PoCUS and assessment. This was done for the safety of the patients until the providers could show competency with ultrasound by conducting at least 30 scans for each body area and completing a practical assessment of their skills.

There was a PoCUS log with the machine to document the type of study conducted, reason for the imaging, presumed diagnosis, and querying if the PoCUS findings confirmed or changed the presumed diagnosis for the patient. Information included the provider's initials, patient age, patient gender, and date of the study. This would allow the investigators to track the number of different PoCUS studies conducted and the number performed by each provider. This would allow the investigators to track the number of each type of study conducted by each participant. It would also allow investigators to determine if improved knowledge and experience with PoCUS was assisting diagnosis and treatment plans, specifically the clinical integration of the information. Participants downloaded de-identified images to a secure flash drive, which the senior investigator, who is a core instructor for the ultrasound curriculum at the University of Louisville and instructor at multiple national and international PoCUS courses, reviewed for technique, quality, and findings.

The investigators analyzed the basic demographic data for the participants and compared each one's change in confidence and experience from the beginning to the end of the yearlong curriculum. Investigators compared the pretest and posttest averages using a paired T test. They conducted all analyses in IBM SPSS statistics version 24.

Results

Ten physicians participated in all three PoCUS sessions and completed both the pretest and posttest. The posttest was distributed 3 months following the last PoCUS course. The pretest average score was 41.67% with a range of 30–63.3% and a standard deviation of 9.95 (Fig. 1). The posttest average was 66.1% with a range of 55–96% and a standard deviation of 12.26. The mean change in test score for the participants was 24.42% with a range of 8.3–36.6% and a standard deviation of 9.03 (p value < 0.01) (Fig. 1). Of note, this is meant to be a challenging test with a passing score of 75% for University of Louisville PEM physicians who are seeking bedside PoCUS credentialing.

Prior to the course, none of the participants expressed any confidence in their PoCUS examinations for FAST, lung, bedside cardiac, or nerve examination. "No confidence" was defined as no expectation of one's ability to obtain and interpret the appropriate PoCUS examination. "Little confidence" was defined as an expectation in one's abilities to obtain and correctly interpret the PoCUS image less than 50% of the time. "Moderate confidence" was defined as an expectation in one's abilities to obtain and correctly interpret the PoCUS image 50–90% of the time. Lastly, "very confident" was defined as an expectation in one's ability to obtain and correctly interpret the PoCUS image 90–100% of the time. There were nine of ten participants who had no confidence in their soft tissue and vascular access PoCUS examinations. Three months following the completion of the course, 80% were at least moderately confident with their FAST examinations and 50% were at least moderately confident with their cardiac and soft tissue examinations (Fig. 2). There were 70% of participants who had some confidence in their lung and 90% who had some confidence in their vascular access skills by the completion of the course (Fig. 2).

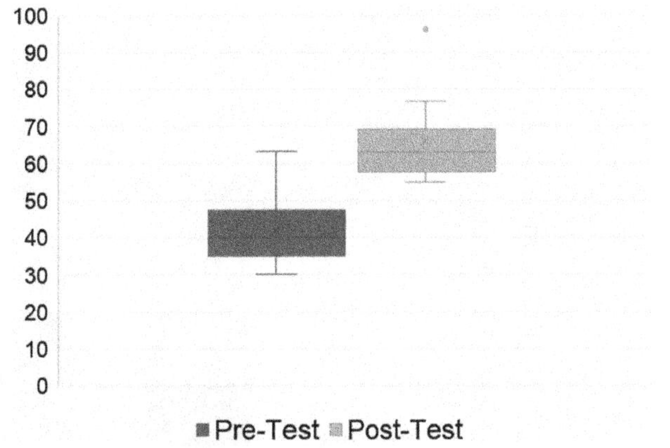

Fig. 1 Pre- and post-intervention scores of participants in the ultrasound course

Prior to the PoCUS course, 100% of participants had no experience with FAST, bedside cardiac, lung, and nerve blocks. There were 90% of participants who had no experience with soft tissue and 80% had no experience with vascular access PoCUS. With the exception of nerve blocks, the number of participants with experience in each of the studies increased following the course (Fig. 3).

There were 52 PoCUS studies saved on the ultrasound machine over the course of the curriculum (Fig. 4). The number of studies conducted had a sharp drop during the months of September, October, and November 2017 where there were only three recorded studies for all 3 months. This coincides with the devastation experienced on the island following multiple significant natural disasters. The providers recorded the most scans in August 2018, which is 12 months after the initiation of the educational curriculum and 3 months following the final session. The most commonly completed PoCUS studies were bedside cardiac (36.5%) and FAST (15.3%) (Table 1). The providers did not keep an accurate ultrasound log and for many months following the hurricane because the log was displaced from its position on the stand with the ultrasound machine. Therefore, it was impossible to determine the exact number of body

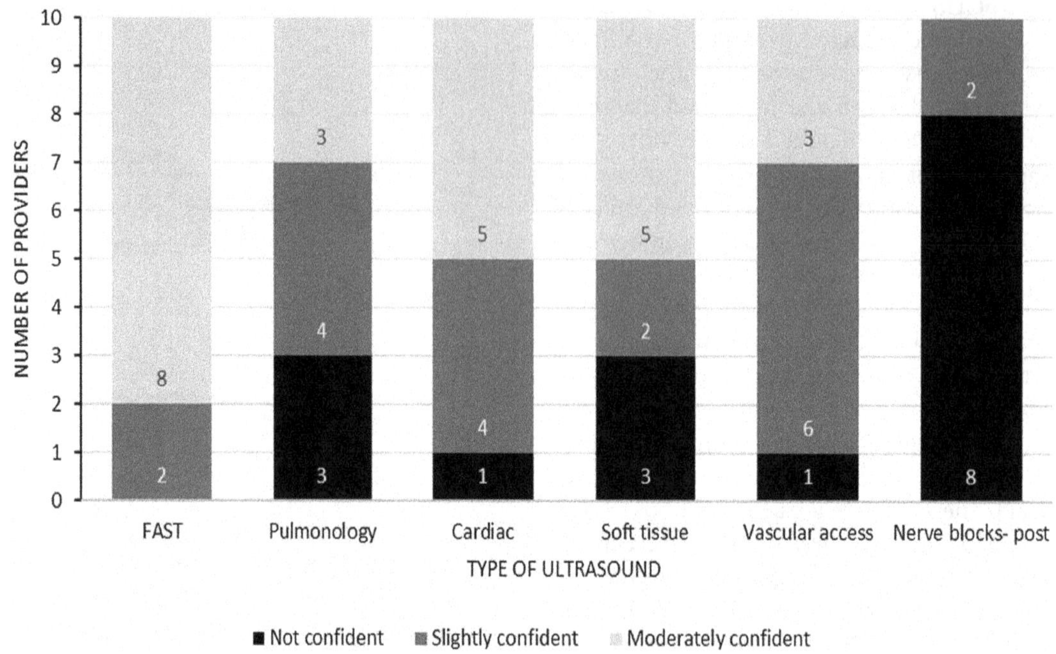

Fig. 2 Provider confidence in ultrasonography of the various types of studies

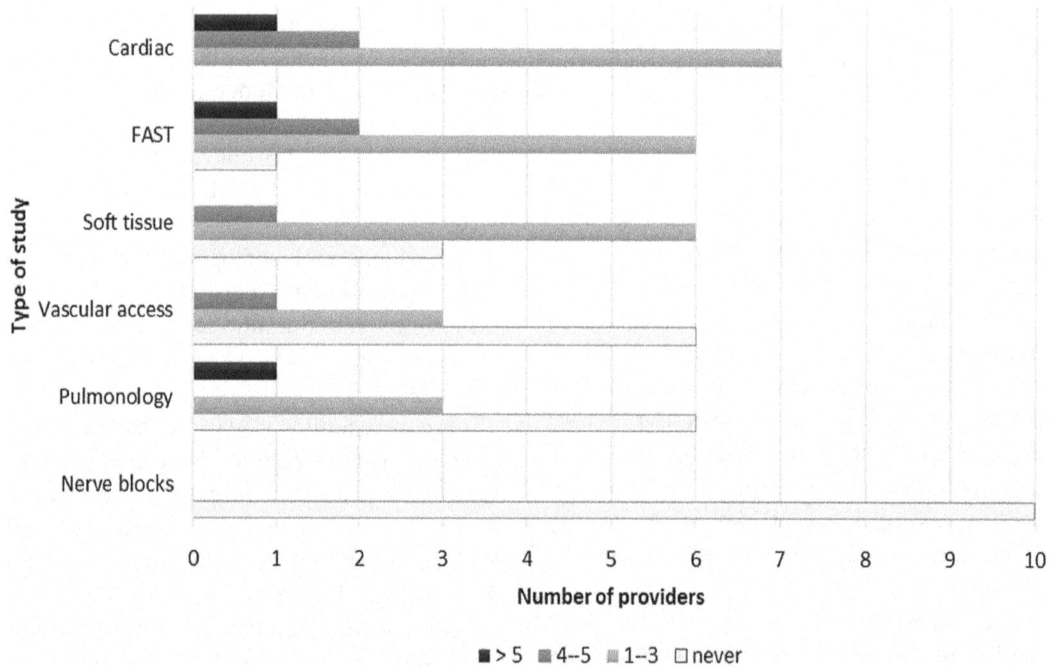

Fig. 3 The frequency of each type of ultrasound conducted throughout the ultrasound course

scans conducted by each provider to determine if anyone was eligible for a practical ultrasound assessment for independent scanning.

Ninety-four percent of the scans were reviewed for image quality. There were 3 scans that were not saved correctly and the images could not be reviewed. Of the images reviewed, 69% had good image quality and could be easily interpreted by the investigators. Good image quality was defined as an image that clearly identifies the organ or area of concern with appropriate scanning through its entirety. For example, a good-quality image of an abscess or cellulitis had a scan from the area of normal

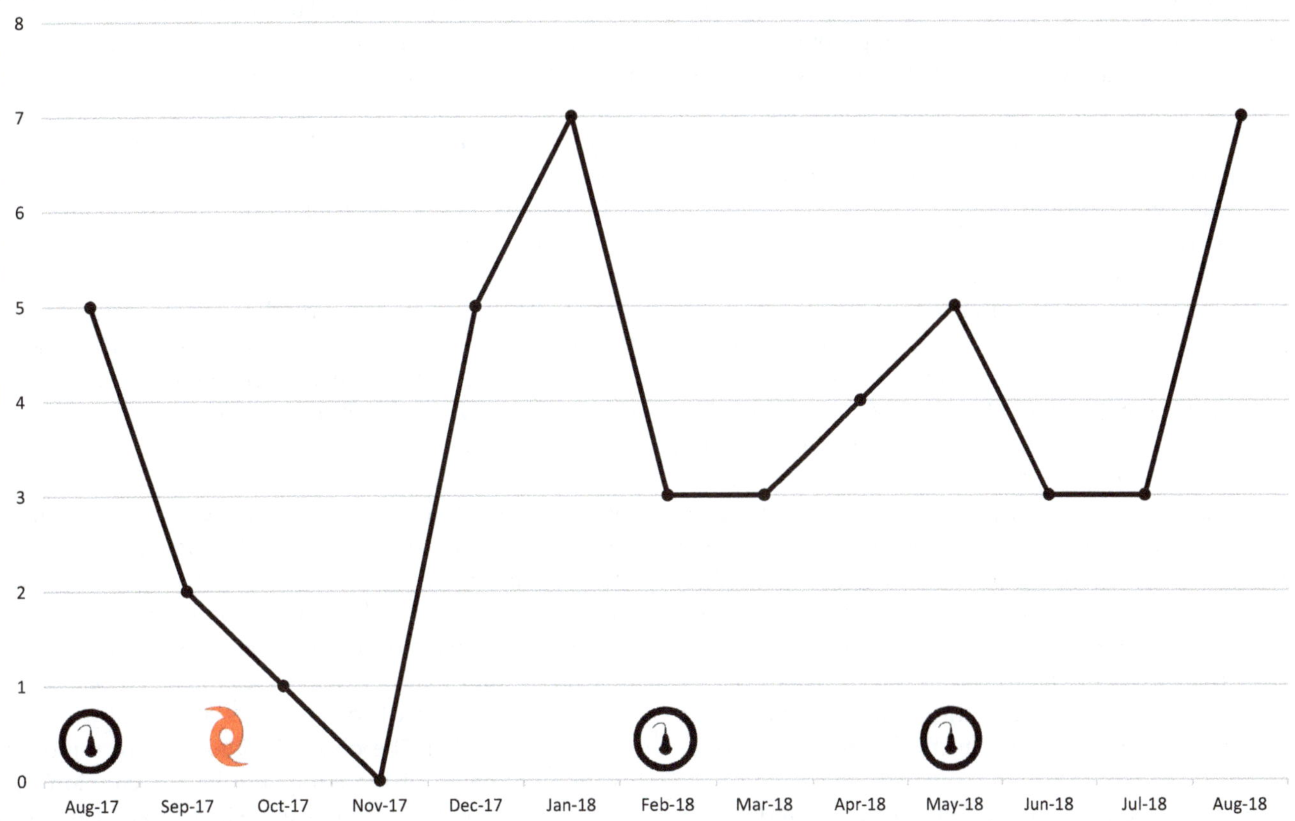

Fig. 4 The number of studies saved on the ultrasound machine over the 12-month curriculum. The images of the ultrasound probe correspond to each of the three teaching sessions. The hurricane symbol corresponds to the timing of the two hurricanes that devastated the island

Table 1 The number and type of PoCUS saved and recorded on the ultrasound machine

Type of study	Number of PoCUS	Percentage (%)
Cardiac	19	36.5
FAST	8	15.3
Renal/bladder	6	11.5
Lung	5	9.6
Skin/soft tissue	4	7.7
Eye	3	5.8
Aorta/IVC	2	3.8
Other	5	9.6

skin and soft tissue through the abnormal area back to the area of normal skin and soft tissue on the other side. It also had the appropriate amount of depth where the area of concern or question is in the center of the screen. A good-quality image would show the appropriate orientation of the probe based in the screen indicator and image (i.e., image is not backwards or upside down), have the appropriate probe and the appropriate windows. For example, an adequate bedside cardiac PoCUS would have the correct probe, orientation and windows for a parasternal long axis, parasternal short axis, subxiphoid, and/or apical 4 chamber views with at least 3 of the traditional cardiac windows.

Discussion

This study met the objective to increase the PoCUS knowledge of the physicians working in the HOPU pediatric ED. The participants' scores increased by an average of almost 25%. This is similar to the improvement in immediate posttest scores following a single day of intensive training demonstrated by Clay [1, 2]; however, their participants' average scores waned to an 18% increase 6 months following the initial intervention and may have decreased further if measured 12 months after the training. Noble showed a similar improvement of about 20% in ultrasound recognition scores after two back-to-back educational sessions and hands-on training [4]. Noble and Clay had the majority of the teaching sessions in a 1- or 2-day intense session with either no or optional teaching over the subsequent 6 months prior to repeat testing [1, 4]. Although both studies demonstrated improved PoCUS knowledge, Clay's study suggests that some of this knowledge wanes with time. The investigators obtained the Puerto Rican physicians' posttest scores 12 months after the initial intervention showing longer lasting knowledge retention of these initial concepts. This supports the notion that repeated short sessions has similar and somewhat improved long-term knowledge retention of basic ultrasound concepts compared to single, intense short-length interventions.

This curriculum consisted of 15 classroom/lecture hours, 15 required hands-on, and 10 optional extra hands-on hours over the course of the year, which is similar to the total training hours in the 9-week educational intervention in Rwanda [7]. The longitudinal approach is more feasible compared to Shah's study in settings where educators cannot be in one location for 9 weeks teaching PoCUS. Repeated short sessions are more practical for both presenters and participants who are balancing the course with their regular clinical responsibilities at their respective home sites. A recent educational curriculum conducted in Mexico shows the effectiveness of a longitudinal teaching design in an outpatient, resource-limited setting [5]. Although Puerto Rico is not considered a true "resource limited" site, the investigators demonstrate that this same design can be effectively applied to various settings.

The HOPU participants had little to no confidence in bedside PoCUS. Following the educational intervention, the majority of participants self-report at least some confidence and many had moderate confidence with five of the six imaging modalities presented over the course. The participants all conducted at least 5 of each type of body scan during the educational sessions and hands-on training. Keddis et al. also evaluated the confidence level in a similar 5-point Likert scale and showed a comparable improvement in confidence immediately following short-term PoCUS teaching sessions [3]. However, Keddis did not evaluate the long-term retention of confidence in POCUS, which the investigators demonstrate in this intervention with participant self-reporting 12 months following initial educational session [3].

The HOPU ED providers were novice ultrasonographers with little to no experience with PoCUS prior to the educational intervention. The initial design called for ultrasound logs to accurately document the total number, type, and intent of studies for each participant. However, due to multiple natural disasters, which occurred on the island shortly after the initiation of the curriculum, the logs were not accurately documented. Without accurate documentation of number of scans per provider, no providers were eligible for a practical ultrasound evaluation. The pilot phase of the study showed acquisition of knowledge and confidence with this type of training, so the next phase will focus on documentation and credentialing. The primary investigator will become the local ultrasound champion in the HOPU ED at the completion of her fellowship. With a local champion, the ultrasound logs will be more accurate and she can conduct practical ultrasound assessments of the local physicians when they have completed at least 30 scans of a particular body area.

There were 52 studies saved on the ultrasound machine which were used in the analysis. At the completion of the curriculum, the participants report conducting between 58 and 131 PoCUS studies. This discrepancy suggests that the HOPU physicians were not saving all of their images and using PoCUS more than documented. The number of overall PoCUS studies is lower than those documented in previous interventions by Rominger and Shah [5, 7]; however, there were 3 months during the 12-month intervention when PoCUS were unable to be obtained due to power outages and physical limitations following the natural disasters. In addition, the previous studies were not limited to pediatrics and between 1/3 and 1/2 of their studies were obstetric, which was not included in this curriculum [5, 7]. The most common PoCUS study was abdomen and cardiac which was consistent with previous studies when the obstetric studies were removed. In the next phase of the study, the local champion will encourage the providers to save the images and can cross check the ultrasound logs to the saved images weekly.

The intervention required curriculum modification following two major natural disasters (Hurricanes Irma and Maria), which affected the island in September 2017 after the first educational session. The hospital was with limited power and resources for 3 months following the hurricanes. The second session was originally scheduled for November 2017, but because power and communication had not been consistently restored, the session was moved to February 2018. Because there was a prolonged time between educational sessions, the educators gave a review of the August information before the scheduled February session. There was a significant drop in PoCUS use from September 2017 through November 2017, but once there was restoration of consistent power and communication, there was a dramatic increase in PoCUS use. It can be theorized that the providers utilized PoCUS as an effective diagnostic modality when there were still limited resources while the island was recovering from the hurricanes. This supports the usefulness of PoCUS training in this setting and the value of a longitudinal curriculum. Having a scheduled session following the disaster recovery period allowed the learners to review the previous information after a period of limited use. In addition, almost 25% of initial participants did not complete the full 12-month curriculum and their information was removed from the study. These providers left the island permanently following the natural disasters.

Limitations

The biggest limitation in this study was natural disasters, which resulted in loss of participants, decreased scanning months and adjustment of the originally scheduled curriculum. This also affected the documentation of images on the ultrasound logs which were used to track the number and type of study and the clinical applicability of the information. Upon discussion with the providers, it seemed that they were using the ultrasound machine much more frequently than they were documenting; however, only the documented studies could be used in analysis. This was beyond the control of the investigators; however, the remaining participants still showed increase in PoCUS knowledge, confidence and experience despite the circumstances. The total number of PoCUS studies and confidence level may have been affected by recall bias since each participant was asked to self-report this information at the completion of the course. The participants did not keep accurate ultrasound logs so the information was limited to subjective recall. In addition, the biggest limitation was no local ultrasound champion to oversee and answer real-time questions. This would have been helpful following the hurricanes when communication with providers on the island was limited.

Conclusions

The investigators show that a longitudinal PoCUS curriculum is an effective design to teach PoCUS to local physicians working in acute ED settings. Due to unforeseen circumstances, 6 months of the intervention occurred during a resource-limited time period for the HOPU, which further demonstrated its utility in this setting. This also highlighted the value of repeated, longitudinal sessions so the providers can refresh their knowledge following gap in ultrasound use due to challenging circumstances. At the completion of the course, all participants demonstrated a sustained increase in PoCUS knowledge, confidence and experience. A local champion, better documentation, and practical ultrasound assessments for independent scanning would be the next steps in continuing the PoCUS education program at HOPU.

Abbreviations

CT: Computed tomography; MRI: Magnetic resonance imaging; WHO: World Health Organization; PoCUS: Point-of-care ultrasound; US: United States; HOPU: Hospital Pediatrico Universitario; ED: Emergency department; PEM: Pediatric emergency medicine; EM: Emergency medicine; FAST: Focused assessment with sonography in trauma.

Acknowledgements

The authors acknowledge Kendra Sikes who assisted with the submission and maintenance of the IRB. Thank you to Corey Warf and Ben Nti who each went on one of the trips and assisted in the presentation of the educational material.

Authors' contributions

VS and AR conceptualized the study and did background research on the topic. VS conducted the needs assessment and initial planning meetings with the local physicians in Puerto Rico and was the primary liaison between HOPU and the University of Louisville. VS participated in all three of the teaching sessions and prepared the teaching materials. FW, BS, AR contributed to the design and development of the IRB. They also reviewed and revised the teaching materials prior to each trip. AR attended the first teaching trip and FW attended the second teaching trip. VS distributed and collected all the tests and questionnaires throughout the curriculum. AR analyzed the data. All authors read and approved the final manuscript.

References

1. Clay RD, Lee EC, Kurtzman MF, Dversdal RK (2016) Teaching the internist to see: effectiveness of a 1-day workshop in bedside ultrasound for internal medicine residents. Crit Ultrasound J 8(1):11. https://doi.org/10.1186/s13089-016-0047-7
2. Harris RD, Marks WM (2009) Compact ultrasound for improving maternal and perinatal care in low-resource settings: review of the potential benefits, implementation challenges, and public health issues. J Ultrasound Med 28(8):1067–1076
3. Keddis MT, Cullen MW, Reed DA, Halvorsen AJ, McDonald FS, Takahashi PY, Bhagra A (2011) Effectiveness of an ultrasound training module for internal medicine residents. BMC Med Educ 11:75. https://doi.org/10.1186/1472-6920-11-75
4. Noble VE, Nelson BP, Sutingco AN, Marill KA, Cranmer H (2007) Assessment of knowledge retention and the value of proctored ultrasound exams after the introduction of an emergency ultrasound curriculum. BMC Med Educ 7:40. https://doi.org/10.1186/1472-6920-7-40
5. Rominger AH, Gomez GAA, Elliott P (2018) The implementation of a longitudinal POCUS curriculum for physicians working at rural outpatient clinics in Chiapas. Mexico. Crit Ultrasound J 10(1):19. https://doi.org/10.1186/s13089-018-0101-8
6. Shah S, Noble VE, Umulisa I, Dushimiyimana JM, Bukhman G, Mukherjee J, Epino H (2008) Development of an ultrasound training curriculum in a limited resource international setting: successes and challenges of ultrasound training in rural Rwanda. Int J Emerg Med 1(3):193–196. https://doi.org/10.1007/s12245-008-0053-z
7. Shah SP, Epino H, Bukhman G, Umulisa I, Dushimiyimana JM, Reichman A, Noble VE (2009) Impact of the introduction of ultrasound services in a limited resource setting: rural Rwanda 2008. BMC Int Health Hum Rights 9:4. https://doi.org/10.1186/1472-698X-9-4
8. Via G, Storti E, Spreafico A, Melniker L, Neri L (2012) Point of care ultrasound for sepsis management in resource-limited settings: time for a new paradigm for global health care. Intensive Care Med 38(8):1405–1407. https://doi.org/10.1007/s00134-012-2606-0 **(author reply 1408-1409)**
9. Volpicelli G, Elbarbary M, Blaivas M, Lichtenstein DA, Mathis G, Kirkpatrick AW, International Liaison Committee on Lung Ultrasound for International Consensus Conference on Lung, U (2012) International evidence-based recommendations for point-of-care lung ultrasound. Intensive Care Med 38(4):577–591. https://doi.org/10.1007/s00134-012-2513-4

28

Giant rectus sheath hematoma

Gabriela Bello[1] and Pablo Blanco[2*]

Abstract

Background: Rectus sheath hematoma (RSH) is an uncommon entity associated with predisposing factors such as anticoagulation. It may mimic more frequent abdominal conditions and its accurate diagnosis is important to focus on the correct treatments and improve morbidity and mortality.

Case presentation: An elderly patient with shock, abdominal pain, palpable abdominal mass, and anemia was suspected of having a large RSH by point-of-care ultrasound (POCUS), which was then confirmed by computed tomography. Surgery was performed, markedly improving his clinical status.

Conclusions: POCUS has a good sensitivity for the diagnosis of RSH and it is also an excellent tool for patient follow-up.

Keywords: Rectus abdominis, Hematoma, Point of care, Ultrasound, Computed tomography, Critical care

Background

Rectus sheath hematoma (RSH) is an uncommon entity, accounting for less than 2% of patients complaining of acute abdominal pain [1]. It may mimic several more common conditions, such as intestinal obstruction, perforated peptic ulcer, pancreatitis, diverticulitis, tumors or a ruptured aortic aneurysm [2, 3]. Thus, a high index of suspicion and a careful diagnostic workup are mandatory to reach an accurate diagnosis, so as to focus on the correct treatment.

Known risk factors predisposing to RSH are anticoagulation (nearly invariably present); older age; female sex; pregnancy; trauma; iatrogenic/surgery; chronic medical conditions, such as hypertension, atherosclerosis or hematologic diseases; coughing and forceful rectus muscle contractions [2–4].

The overall mortality rate of RSH is around 4% and rises up to 25% in anticoagulated patients due to increased hemorrhage volume [2]; an early recognition of RSH may be associated with improved chances of survival [5].

We present the case of a patient with a large RSH suspected by the findings of point-of-care ultrasound (POCUS) and confirmed by computed tomography (CT) and discuss the importance of POCUS in the diagnosis and management of patients with this condition.

Case presentation

An 85 year-old-male patient with a history of congestive heart failure and atrial fibrillation under anticoagulation with enoxaparin was admitted to the intensive care unit (ICU) presenting with shock and abdominal pain. Extremely pale skin and mucous membranes were noted, along with an extensive ecchymosis occupying the left hemiabdomen (i.e., Grey Turner´s sign). The abdominal mass bulged on the left flank and was soft, painful and non-pulsating on palpation. Blood chemistry highlighted anemia (hemoglobin 5.7 g/dl), metabolic acidosis and elevation of creatinine and BUN; coagulation tests were normal. A POCUS abdominal ultrasound of the left flank (Fig. 1 and Additional file 1: Video 1) showed a large complex avascular cystic mass which extended to the pelvis, with echogenic particulate mobile contents in dependent areas, and multiple internal septations. Perisplenic free peritoneal fluid was also noted. No other anomalies were found. Given the described ultrasound features and in the context of this clinical presentation together with anemia, this mass was interpreted as a hematoma. However, because of its size, it could not be concluded with certainty whether it was an extra-abdominal (e.g., abdominal wall) or an intraabdominal structure. Thus,

*Correspondence: ohtusabes@gmail.com

[2] Intensive Care Unit, Clínica Cruz Azul, 2651, 60 St., Necochea 7630, Argentina

Full list of author information is available at the end of the article

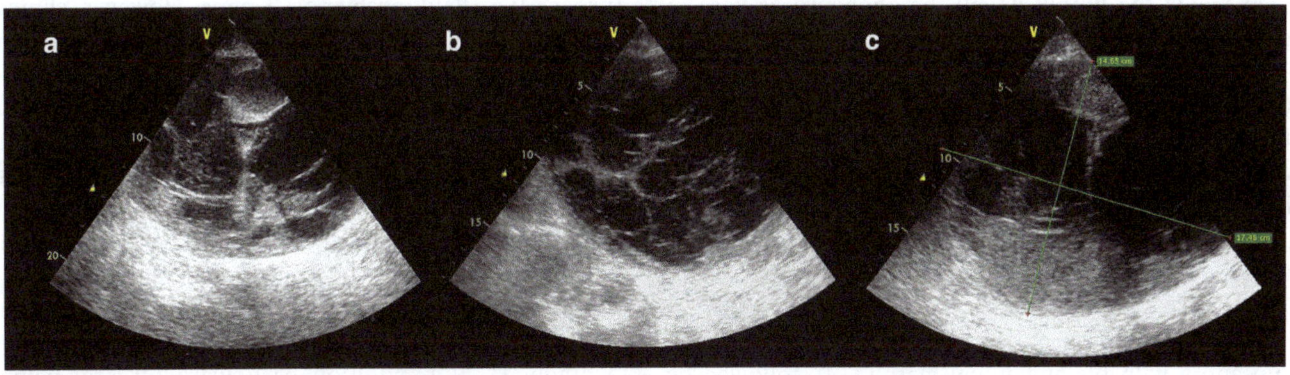

Fig. 1 Abdominal ultrasound from the left coronal view showing a complex cystic mass (**a** and **b**) with multiple internal septations, measuring approximately 18 cm × 15 mm (**c**), highly suggestive of a large rectus sheath hematoma (RSH)

an abdominopelvic CT with intravenous contrast was ordered. The CT showed a large heterogeneous fluid collection along the left rectus sheath which extended to the subperitoneal space (Fig. 2), showing signs of active contrast extravasation, suggestive of active bleeding (Fig. 2a). With the diagnosis of a large RSH complicated with hemodynamic instability, suspicion of abdominal compartment syndrome, and signs of active bleeding on the CT, the patient was immediately transferred to the operating room for surgical exploration. On laparotomy, 3 L of fresh blood mixed with clots was evacuated from the abdominal wall and subperitoneal space. The culprit vessel was identified as a branch of the left inferior epigastric artery, which was then successfully ligated. The patient´s hemodynamic parameters markedly improved after surgery and blood transfusions, and he was sent back to the ICU for further care, where he developed acute renal failure requiring hemodialysis. During the follow-up period, POCUS did not show signs of rebleeding within the rectus sheath. The patient died in the general ward after a prolonged length of stay in the ICU. The main complications observed were renal failure requiring hemodialysis as mentioned before, and nosocomial infections.

Discussion

Rectus sheath hematoma results from bleeding into the rectus sheath, after damage to the epigastric arteries or by direct muscle tear [2]. RSH is frequently localized below the umbilicus where the inferior epigastric artery (branch of the external iliac artery) penetrates the rectus muscles at the arcuate line and this vessel is relatively fixed, so branches are more prone to being injured [6]. Furthermore, below the arcuate line, which is approximately

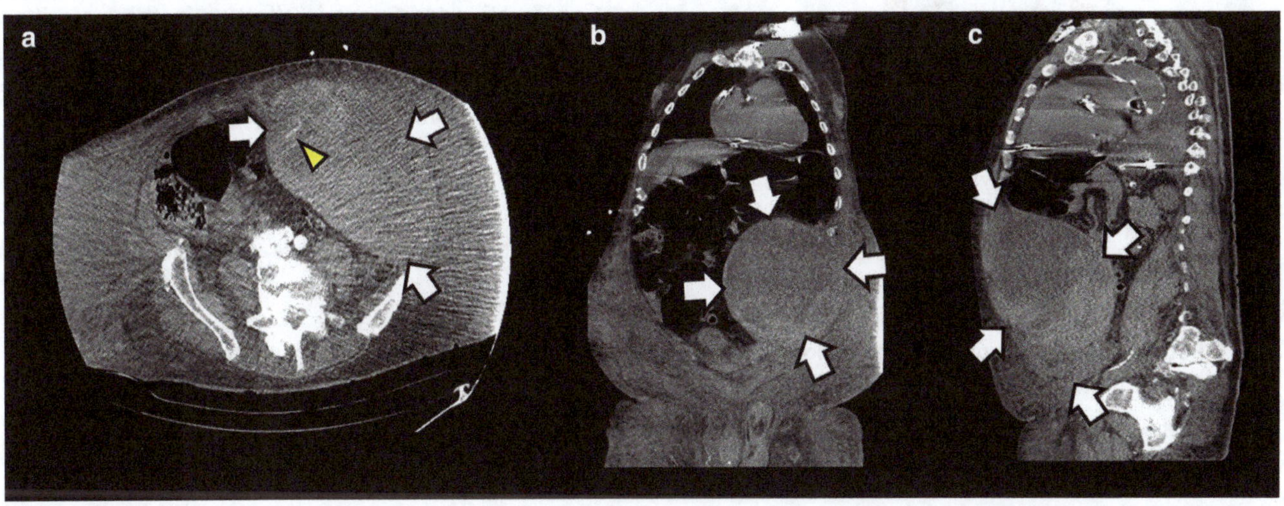

Fig. 2 Abdominopelvic computed tomography with intravenous contrast showing a large left RSH (arrows) extending to the pelvis. Signs of active contrast extravasation are shown in **a** (arrowhead), indicating active bleeding; **a** axial plane; **b** coronal plane; **c** sagittal plane

5 cm below the umbilicus, all the aponeuroses pass in front of the rectus abdominal muscle, thus creating a possibility for the hematoma to spread between the rectus muscle and fascia transversalis into the prevesical space, without other supporting planes (Fig. 3). Bleeding from the superior epigastric artery (terminal branch of the internal thoracic artery) is less common and minor, given the small caliber of this vessel as well as the effective supporting mechanism of the posterior rectus sheath [7].

The most common presentation of RSH is abdominal pain and a palpable abdominal mass [3, 4], followed by anemia [4]; very few patients may present with hemodynamic instability [3].

To reach a diagnosis, the clinical clues orienting toward an RSH are Carnett's sign (i.e., the abdominal pain worsens after voluntary contraction of the abdominal muscles), Fothergill's sign (i.e., the mass remains palpable after voluntary contraction of the abdominal muscles) and Cullen's (i.e., periumbilical ecchymosis) and Grey Turner's (i.e., flank ecchymosis) signs. However, clinical data are fairly unreliable, with a failure rate higher than 50% for the diagnosis of an RSH [1]. Conversely, diagnosis of RSH relies upon the use of imaging techniques. Given its widespread availability, bedside use, non-invasiveness, repeatability, lack of ionizing radiation and low costs, POCUS should be considered the first-line method, both to diagnose RSH and to rule in or out other common etiologies (e.g., ruptured abdominal aneurysm). Sensitivity of ultrasound for an RSH is around 90%, which indicates that some patients still remain undiagnosed using this technique [1, 2]. In addition, particularly for large hematomas, determining the exact origin of the mass is nearly impossible, and thus a CT is often required in these settings [2]. For abdominopelvic CT, the reported sensitivity and specificity for the diagnosis of an RSH reaches 100% and thus this method is often performed when the ultrasound is unreliable or a large hematoma is observed and active bleeding is suspected, proving that demonstrating signs of active bleeding, in addition to hemodynamic instability, points toward a non-conservative (embolization or surgery) treatment [2, 7]. Based on CT, a classification for RSH is well described [8] and this can be readily extrapolated to ultrasound (Table 1). Also, CT may even rule in or out other common diagnoses which could be missed by ultrasound. Common problems with CT are the need to transfer the patient to the radiology department and the use of ionizing radiation as well as iodinated contrast agents, which expose patients to allergic reactions as well as contrast-induced nephrotoxicity (CIN). Weighing the risks of CIN versus leaving an RSH undiagnosed should be assessed on an individual basis. In these cases, performing a CT without contrast media is a valid option, but demonstrating signs of active bleeding as well as eventually reaching an accurate diagnosis of other common pathologies will not be possible [9].

Conservative treatment is effective in the majority of patients with RSH. This group of patients is followed up by clinical and laboratory data, as well as serial ultrasound (US) examinations, measuring the size of the hematoma. US-guided drainage does not offer clear advantages compared to conservative treatment and may even prolong the length of hospital stay and predispose to a hematoma infection. Thus, this practice should not

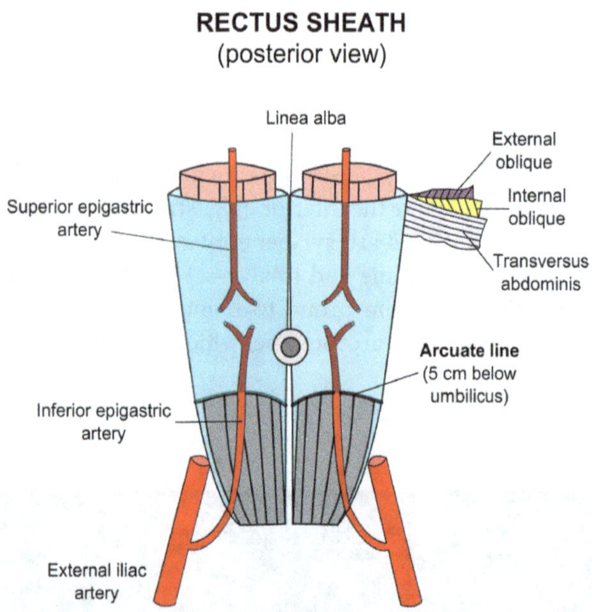

Fig. 3 Anatomy of the rectus sheath above and below the arcuate line observed from a posterior view. As noted, below the arcuate line, the posterior sheath is absent and thus the rectus muscle is in direct contact with the transversalis fascia

Table 1 Rectus sheath hematoma classification based on computed tomography. Modified from [8]

Type I	The hematoma is intramuscular and an increase in muscle size is observed, with an ovoid or fusiform aspect and hyperdense foci or diffusely increased density. The hematoma is unilateral and does not dissect along adjacent fascial planes
Type II	The hematoma is intramuscular (mimicking type I), but with blood between the muscle and the transversalis fascia. It may be uni- or bilateral, and no blood is seen occupying the prevesical space
Type III	The hematoma may or may not involve the muscle, and blood is seen between the transversalis fascia and the muscle, in the peritoneum, and in the prevesical space

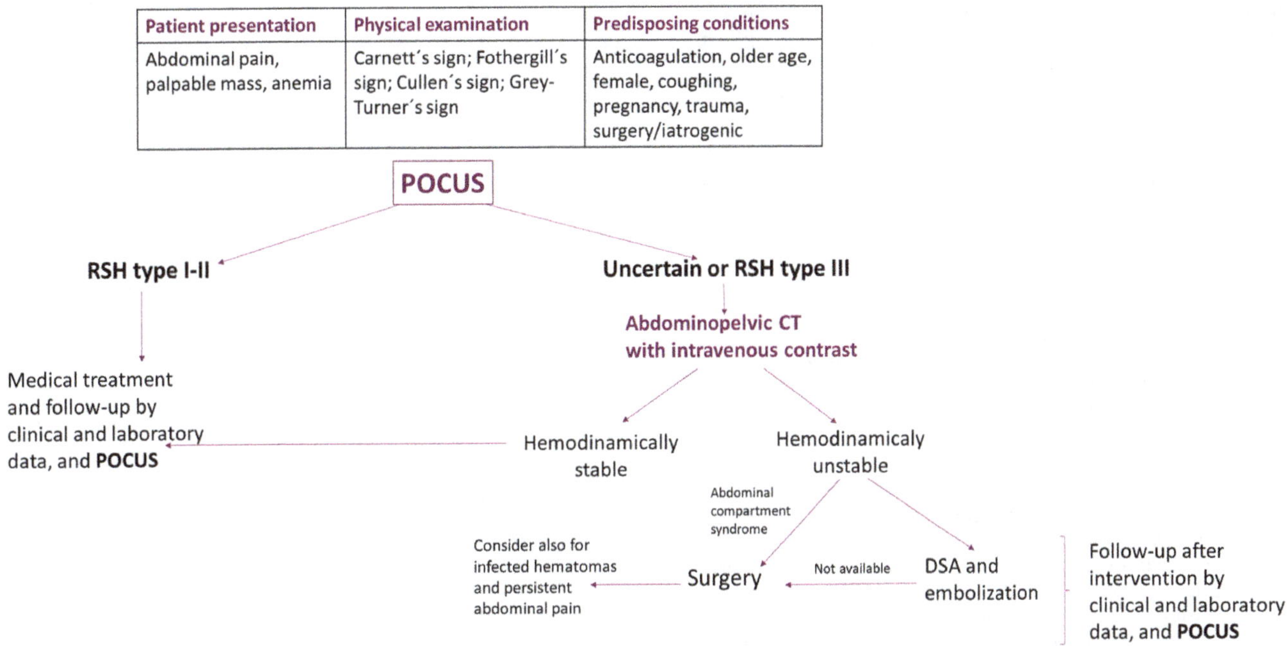

Fig. 4 Algorithm for diagnosing and managing a patient with an RSH. Modified from [2, 5]; RSH, rectus sheath hematoma; POCUS, point-of-care ultrasound; CT, computed tomography; DSA, digital subtraction angiography

be routinely recommended [6]. However, the use of US-guided diagnostic aspiration may be considered in those patients managed conservatively in whom an infected hematoma is suspected. On the other hand, patients with hemodynamic instability, persistent abdominal pain, those with suspicion of infected hematomas, as well as patients with elevated intraabdominal pressures developing an abdominal compartment syndrome (ACS) often need a more aggressive approach [2, 4, 7, 9]. Digital subtraction angiography (DSA) and selective embolization of the culprit vessel represent the preferred approach for unstable patients, with a high degree of success and low rebleeding risk [10, 11]. Surgery is indicated in cases when embolization is not available, the patient evolves to an ACS or the hematoma is infected, allowing for the evacuation of the hematoma, lowering the intraabdominal pressure and performing the ligation of the culprit vessel [5]. For patients in whom embolization or surgery was performed, postoperative follow- up with serial US examinations may allow practitioners to detect early rebleeding signs within the rectus sheath as well as to identify possibly infected contents, for which US-guidance diagnostic aspiration may be useful. An algorithm for the diagnosis and management of the patient with RSH is provided in Fig. 4.

Conclusions

RSH, although uncommon, should be considered in any patient presenting with abdominal pain. Abdominal POCUS, as the first-line imaging modality for the patient in the ICU or the emergency department, may allow practitioners to reach this diagnosis in most of the patients, avoiding the performance of unnecessary tests and the administration of wrong treatments, and allowing to selectively use more costly, sophisticated or potentially harmful methods, including the use of iodinated contrast media, in certain cases requiring so. POCUS should also be considered as a suitable method for the follow-up period.

Additional file

Additional file 1: Video 1. Abdominal ultrasound from the left coronal view showing a large complex cystic mass with multiple internal septations, corresponding to a large rectus sheath hematoma.

Abbreviations

RSH: rectus sheath hematoma; ICU: intensive care unit; POCUS: point-of-care ultrasound; CT: computed tomography; DSA: digital subtraction angiography; ACS: abdominal compartment syndrome.

Acknowledgements

This work has not been presented at any conferences.

Authors' contributions

GB observed the case, performed the ultrasound examinations, collected the data and drafted the manuscript. PB contributed significantly to the drafting and editing of the manuscript, performed the literature review and created the figures and edited the video. All authors read and approved the final manuscript.

Author details
[1] Intensive Care Unit, Hospital Central de las Fuerzas Armadas (DNSFFAA), 3060, 8 de Octubre Ave., 11600 Montevideo, Uruguay. [2] Intensive Care Unit, Clínica Cruz Azul, 2651, 60 St., Necochea 7630, Argentina.

References

1. Klingler PJ, Wetscher G, Glaser K, Tschmelitsch J, Schmid T, Hinder RA (1999) The use of ultrasound to differentiate rectus sheath hematoma from other acute abdominal disorders. Surg Endosc 13(11):1129–1134
2. Hatjipetrou A, Anyfantakis D, Kastanakis M (2015) Rectus sheath hematoma: a review of the literature. Int J Surg 13:267–271
3. Salemis NS, Gourgiotis S, Karalis G (2010) Diagnostic evaluation and management of patients with rectus sheath hematoma. A retrospective study. Int J Surg 8(4):290–293
4. Cherry WB, Mueller PS (2006) Rectus sheath hematoma: review of 126 cases at a single institution. Medicine (Baltimore) 85(2):105–110
5. Isik A, Peker K, Soyturk M, Firat D, Yoruker U, Yilmaz A (2015) Diagnostic evaluation and treatment of patients with rectus abdominis hematoma. Cir Esp 93(9):580–588
6. Gradauskas A, Venclauskas L, Pažusis M, Karpavičius A, Maleckas A (2018) Comparison of the different treatment strategies for patients with rectus sheath haematoma. Medicina (Kaunas) 54(3):38
7. Karapolat B, Tasdelen HA, Korkmaz HAA (2019) Conservative treatment of spontaneous rectus sheath hematomas: single center experience and literature review. Emerg Med Int 2019:2406873
8. Berná JD, Garcia-Medina V, Guirao J, Garcia-Medina J (1996) Rectus sheath hematoma: diagnostic classification by CT. Abdom Imaging 21(1):62–64
9. Pierro A, Cilla S, Modugno P, Centritto EM, De Filippo CM, Sallustio G (2018) Spontaneous rectus sheath hematoma: the utility of CT angiography. Radiol Case Rep 13(2):328–332
10. Rimola J, Perendreu J, Falcó J, Fortuño JR, Massuet A, Branera J (2007) Percutaneous arterial embolization in the management of rectus sheath hematoma. AJR Am J Roentgenol 188(6):W497–W502
11. Smithson A, Ruiz J, Perello R, Valverde M, Ramos J, Garzo L (2013) Diagnostic and management of spontaneous rectus sheath hematoma. Eur J Intern Med 24(6):579–582

Changes in speckle-tracking-derived mechanical dispersion index are associated with 30-day readmissions in acute heart failure

Mark Favot[1*], Robert Ehrman[1], Laura Gowland[1], Ashley Sullivan[1], Brian Reed[1], Aiden Abidov[2] and Phillip Levy[1,3]

Abstract

Background: The objective of the present study was to evaluate the relationship between speckle-tracking-derived parameters left ventricular (LV) mechanical dispersion index (MDI), defined as the standard deviation of the time-to-peak longitudinal strain of all segments analyzed of the LV, and global longitudinal strain (GLS) and 30-day post-discharge outcomes (death and readmission to the hospital) in patients with acute heart failure (AHF).

Methods: We performed a prospective observational study of selected emergency department patients with a primary diagnosis of AHF. Point-of-care echocardiograms were performed at baseline (prior to, or concurrent with the initiation of treatment) and 23 h post-enrollment. Offline speckle-tracking analysis was utilized to calculate GLS and MDI. The primary outcome was 30-day readmissions.

Results: A total of 31 patients were included, 13 of whom were readmitted within 30 days. Patients who were not readmitted to the hospital experienced an average relative improvement in MDI of 24% from baseline to 23 h (84 ms to 64 ms), while patients who were readmitted experienced an average relative worsening in MDI of 6% (66 ms to 70 ms) from baseline to 23 h.

Conclusions: MDI has promise as a treatment response variable in admitted patients with AHF; however, further study is needed.

Keywords: Longitudinal strain, Speckle-tracking, Mechanical dispersion index, Readmissions, Echocardiography, Point-of-care echocardiography

Introduction

Once a diagnosis of acute heart failure (AHF) has been established, conventional 2D and Doppler echocardiography techniques provide limited relevant information to guide treatment decisions at the point-of-care (POC) [1]. Left ventricular ejection fraction (LVEF) is the most extensively investigated echocardiographic parameter, but it does not appreciably change during the acute treatment phase of AHF [2] and it provides limited actionable information when it comes to the selection of specific therapies that may be most suitable for a given patient with AHF [3, 4].

LV strain utilizing speckle-tracking technology is a relatively new quantitative method for evaluating LV systolic function, and while it has been well studied in chronic HF [5–9], to date, there has been only one published report prospectively investigating its use, pre-treatment, in AHF [10]. Although there are numerous ways to measure LV strain utilizing speckle-tracking, global longitudinal peak systolic strain (GLS) is the most well studied [11]. GLS represents a summative measure of the degree of longitudinal shortening of each of the segments of the LV (typically 16–18 depending on the vendor and software being utilized) that are analyzed. GLS has been found to be associated with AHF readmission, independent of

*Correspondence: mfavot@med.wayne.edu
[1] Department of Emergency Medicine, Wayne State University School of Medicine, 6071 W. Outer Dr., Lourdes 447-D, Detroit, MI 48235, USA
Full list of author information is available at the end of the article

and incremental to clinical and basic echocardiographic parameters [12].

LV mechanical dispersion index (MDI) is the standard deviation (SD) of the time-to-peak longitudinal strain in each of the segments of the LV that are analyzed [13] and provides unique insight into mechanical dyssynchrony. While LV MDI has previously been shown to be a predictor of ventricular arrhythmias post-myocardial infarction, a predictor of adverse events following cardiac resynchronization therapy (CRT), and a discriminator of hypertrophic cardiomyopathy versus athlete's heart [13–15], it has yet to be considered as a potential measure of treatment effectiveness in AHF. A recent investigation by Chan et al. [16] found LV MDI to be an independent predictor of outcome in AHF patients after adjustment for baseline variables. The objective of the present study was to evaluate the relationship between the speckle-tracking-derived parameters LV MDI and GLS obtained pre- and 23-h post-treatment, and 30-day post-discharge outcomes (death and readmission to the hospital) in patients with AHF.

Materials and methods

Setting

This prospective observational study was conducted in the emergency department (ED) at 2 large, urban, tertiary-care centers serving approximately 80,000 and 100,000 patients per year, a majority of whom (> 90%) are African American. The study received approval by the Institutional Review Board (IRB).

Selection of participants

From February, 2015 to July, 2017 a convenience sample of eligible ED patients with a primary diagnosis of AHF treated with intravenous (IV) therapy were recruited during hours, where a study team member was available to perform a POC echocardiogram. Whenever possible, we attempted to enroll patients prior to administration treatment. The inclusion criteria were: 18 years of age or greater, primary admitting diagnosis of AHF (determined by the attending emergency physician) being treated with IV therapy, and the ability to provide informed written consent. Exclusion criteria were: the lack of immediate availability of a study team member capable of performing the echocardiograms, the need for emergent, resuscitative intervention (e.g., cardiopulmonary resuscitation, endotracheal intubation, and cardioversion), rapid atrial fibrillation/flutter or any other tachyarrhythmia requiring rate or rhythm control, heart rate persistently greater than 120 beats/min, poor image quality precluding speckle-tracking analysis, plans for emergent percutaneous coronary intervention (PCI) from the ED, pregnancy, incarceration, and plans for to another institution.

Potentially eligible subjects were identified by trained research assistants after discussion with the treating physician to enquire about the primary diagnosis and treatment plan so that all efforts could be made to enroll the patient, obtain consent and perform the baseline POC echocardiogram prior to the initiation of therapy. We allowed for a 20-min window from the initiation of therapy until the baseline POC echocardiogram—if images were unable to be obtained within this window, the patient was not eligible for enrollment.

Study design

At the time of enrollment, study subjects underwent a baseline POC echocardiogram that was performed by a study team member consisting of 2 ultrasound fellowship-trained emergency physicians with expertise in POC echocardiography and speckle-tracking, as well as a certified cardiac sonographer who is an employee of our department's division of clinical research. Vital signs and therapeutic interventions were recorded at the time of the baseline echocardiogram. Baseline demographic data, comorbidities, and home medications were also recorded at this time. Following the 1st echocardiogram, patients underwent usual care for AHF; a 2nd POC echocardiogram was performed 23 h following enrollment. Vital signs, laboratory findings, and further therapies and interventions up to this point were also recorded. Following the 2nd POC echocardiogram, subjects were tracked in-hospital until discharge at which time arrangements were made for a 30-day follow-up telephone interview to ascertain post-discharge outcomes (Fig. 1).

Point-of-care echocardiograms

All POC echocardiograms were performed using the same protocol with a portable ultrasound system (*Vivid q* by *GE*, Milwaukee, WI). Study echocardiograms were limited and included only the apical imaging window utilizing the 4-chamber, 2-chamber, and long axis views. After the recording of these ultrasound clips, the POC echocardiogram was considered complete and stored both in the ultrasound system and transmitted to our EchoPAC (*GE* Milwaukee, WI, USA) workstation for subsequent offline analysis by an investigator who was blinded to treatment, all clinical and laboratory variables and outcome.

Strain analysis

Offline analysis was conducted according to the recommendation of the American Society of Echocardiography and the European Society of Cardiovascular Imaging using commercially available software (EchoPAC version 110.1.1 BT 11, *GE* Milwaukee, WI, USA). We calculated GLS from the baseline POC echocardiogram and again

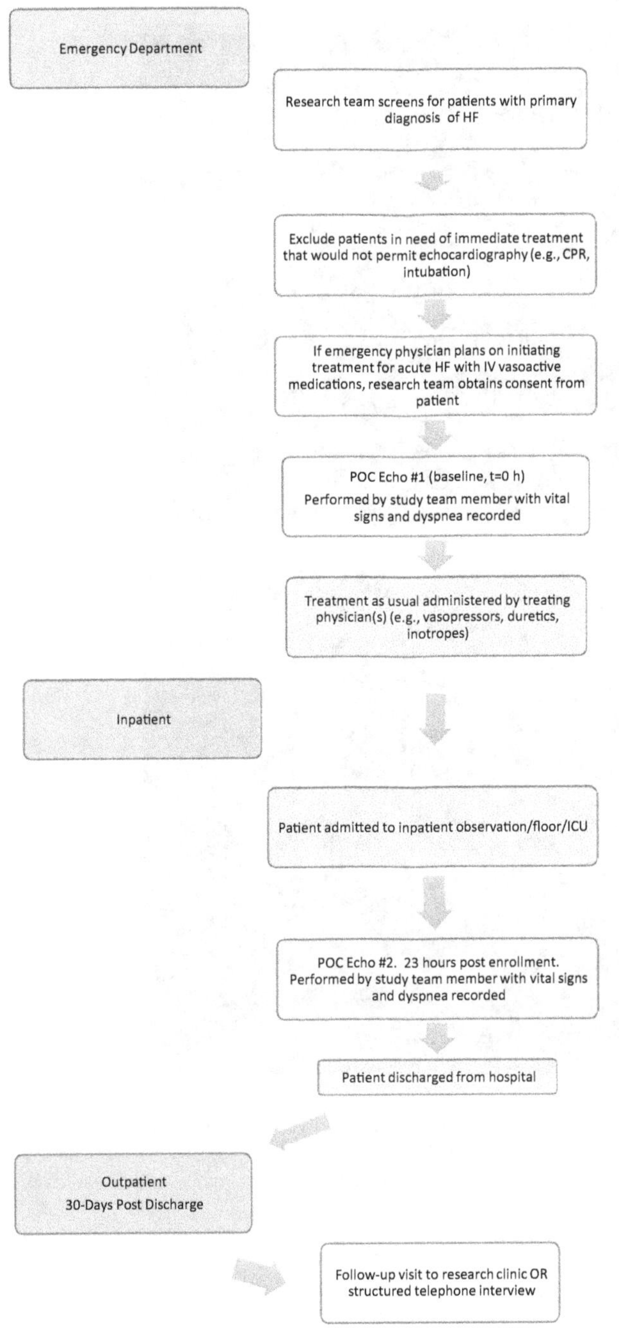

Fig. 1 Flow diagram for the study from enrollment in the emergency department to inpatient follow-up echocardiogram to outpatient follow-up at 30-day post-discharge

from the 2nd POC echocardiogram performed 23 h following enrollment using the embedded Automated Function Imaging (AFI) tool. Using the longitudinal strain tracings (Fig. 2), LV MDI was subsequently calculated for baseline and repeat POC echocardiograms by calculating standard deviation of the time-to-peak longitudinal (negative) strain for each of the segments analyzed. All of the strain analyses were performed by a single operator (MF) who was blinded to all of the clinical, radiological and laboratory data at the time of analysis. The automated tracings provided by the AFI software were utilized without any manual adjustments unless it was noted by the operator that the automatic tracings of the endocardial border were grossly inappropriate. Only echocardiograms with frame rates between 40 and 80 frames per second were included for analysis. Echocardiograms that had more than 1 non-trackable segment in a single imaging plane were excluded from analysis as GLS is unable to be calculated when any of the imaging planes are missing > 1 segmental strain. Our prior study demonstrated a very high inter-rater reliability between sonographers of with a concordance correlation coefficient of 0.993 [10].

Primary outcomes and data analysis

All statistical analyses were performed using SAS 9.4. Categorical variables were compared using Chi squared, or Fisher's exact test in cases were expected cell counts was insufficient, and continuous measures were compared using the paired *T* test and Wilcoxon Rank sum (both approaches were consistent in categorizing results at the 0.05 significance level). Logistic regression was performed to investigate the relationship between GLS, MDI, and our primary outcome which was readmission or death within 30 days of discharge. We assessed initial, final, and percent change to investigate whether absolute measure, or directional trends in MDI and GLS were useful predictors of patient outcome. Single and multiple logistic regressions were performed using measures of MDI and GLS individually, and in combination. The c-statistic [area under receiver–operator characteristic curve (AUC)] was reported as a measure of logistic regression performance, and Wald's Chi square was used to evaluate predictor significance in each model.

Results

Characteristics of study subjects

A total of 44 patients were enrolled, 13 were ultimately excluded from the final analysis because of technical issues that rendered one of their echocardiograms unsuitable for strain analysis (7 due to poor ECG tracing, 5 due to poor endocardial border definition, and 1 patient with a heart rate > 120 beats/min on the 23-h echocardiogram). This left a final cohort of 31 patients (all African–American), 16 of whom were male (51.6%) with a mean age of 56.6 years (SD = 11.5 years). All 31 patients had abnormally elevated NT-proBNP concentrations and chest radiograph findings compatible with AHF. Mean GLS at baseline for all patients was − 6.5% (SD = 3.3%) and the mean GLS at 23 h follow-up for all patients improved to − 7.6% (SD = 3.4%). Mean MDI at baseline for the entire cohort was 76 ms (SD = 29 ms),

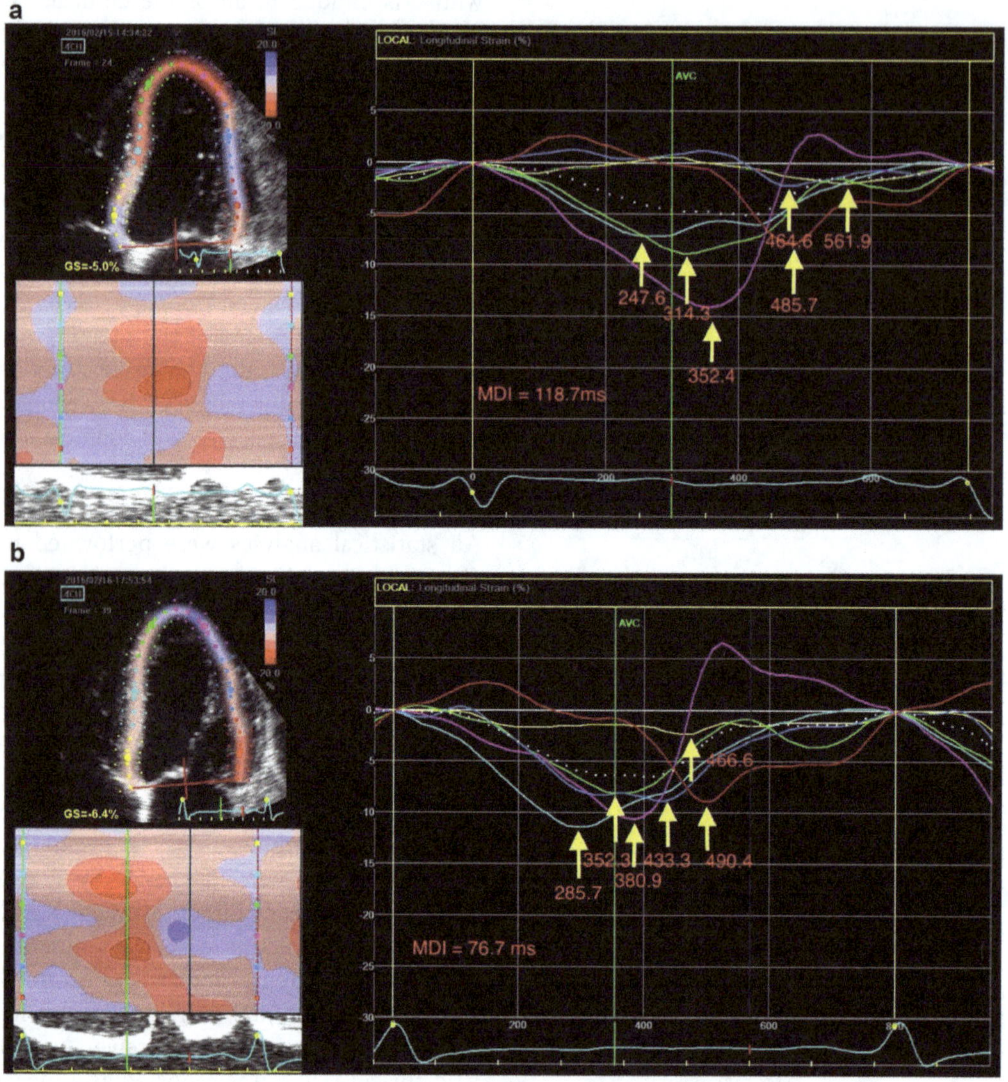

Fig. 2 Strain tracings from an apical 4 chamber view of a patient with acute heart failure at: **a** baseline and **b** 23-h follow-up. Each yellow arrowhead points to the peak longitudinal strain for one of the 6 segments of the left ventricular wall visualized in this view. The values adjacent to each arrowhead represent the time-to-peak longitudinal strain for the corresponding segment. Mechanical dispersion index (MDI) is calculated by calculating the standard deviation for the time-to-peak longitudinal strain values. After 23 h of treatment, the MDI has improved (decreased) by approximately 35% in this patient who had a favorable post-discharge outcome

while the mean MDI at 23 h follow-up for all patients had improved to 66 ms (SD = 16 ms). Thirteen (41.9%) patients were readmitted within 30 days and none died.

Data for the study cohort are presented in Table 1. To evaluate the representativeness of the cohort, we included data for a sample of 235 AHF patients from our institution who were enrolled in an on-going, ED-based AHF registry between March 2016 and August 2017. Overall the convenience sample that we enrolled for the present study was similar to this large registry with a high prevalence of elevated blood pressure, underlying hypertension and diabetes mellitus.

Main results

As shown in Table 1, with the exception of findings on strain imaging, there were no significant group differences between subjects that had a favorable post-discharge outcome and those who were readmitted. Regarding the strain findings, among patients who were not readmitted, the baseline GLS was − 5.7% (SD = 2.7%), while the 23 h follow-up GLS had improved to − 7.1% (SD = 2.9%) with an average absolute improvement in GLS over 23 h of 26%. For patients that were readmitted within 30 days, the mean baseline GLS was − 7.7% (SD = 3.8%), while the mean GLS at 23 h follow-up was −8.2% (SD = 4.0%) resulting in an average absolute

Table 1 Clinical and echocardiographic characteristics of study subjects

Parameter	30-day outcome		*p* value	Comparison EMROC cohort (n=235)
	Favorable (*n*=18)	Readmission (*n*=13)		
Age, mean in years	57.2	55.9	0.77	58.5
Gender, female *n* (%)	7 (38.9%)	8 (61.5%)	0.29	116 (49.4%)
African American, *n* (%)	18 (100%)	13 (100%)	1.0	218 (92.8%)
DM, *n* (%)	7 (38.9%)	4 (30.8%)	0.72	100 (42.6%)
CAD, *n* (%)	9 (50.0%)	10 (76.9%)	0.16	
HTN, *n* (%)	16 (88.9%)	11 (84.6%)	1.0	224 (95.3%)
CKD, *n* (%)	5 (27.8%)	2 (15.4%)	0.67	76 (32.3%)
COPD, *n* (%)	7 (38.9%)	5 (38.5%)	1.0	109 (46.6%)
Systolic BP at baseline, mean	165.3 mm Hg	172.9 mm Hg	0.51	160.0 mm Hg
NIPPV support	4 (22.2%)	2 (15.4%)	0.63	10 (4.3%)
NT-proBNP, median	6787 pg/mL (IQR 3353–9077)	6022 pg/mL (IQR 2179–10,434)	0.61	3345 pg/mL (IQR 1335–8413)
Any troponin in first 23 h > 99th percentile limit, *n* (%)	10 (55.6%)	8 (61.5%)	0.74	140 (59.6%)
Creatinine, mean	1.88 mg/dL	1.68 mg/dL	0.78	1.2 mg/dL
Vasodilator therapy, *n* (%)	5 (27.8%)	6 (46.2%)	0.45	77 (32.8%)
Inotropic therapy, *n* (%)	0 (0%)	0 (0%)	1.0	1 (0.4%)
Diuretic dosage in first 23 h, mean	63.3 mg	67.7 mg	0.75	42.6 mg
Echocardiographic data				
LVEF (%), mean (95% CI)	32 (26, 41)	33 (26, 41)	0.98	43%
Baseline GLS (%), mean (95% CI)	− 5.7 (− 7.0, − 4.3)	− 7.7 (− 10.0, − 5.4)	0.09	N/A
23-h GLS (%), mean (95% CI)	− 7.1 (− 8.6, − 5.7)	− 8.2 (− 10.6, − 5.7)	0.42	N/A
Absolute change GLS (%), mean (95% CI)	− 1.48 (− 2.5, − 0.43)	− 0.45 (− 1.49, 0.59)	0.09	N/A
Percentage change GLS (%), mean (95% CI)	− 61.9 (− 126, 2.3)	− 8.1 (− 27.3, 11.1)	0.08	N/A
Baseline MDI (ms), mean (95% CI)	84 (67, 101)	66 (55, 76)	0.07	N/A
23-h MDI (ms), mean (95% CI)	64 (57, 70)	70 (59, 81)	0.26	N/A
Absolute change MDI (ms), mean (95% CI)	− 20 (− 34.6, − 5.4)	4.3 (− 6.8, 15.3)	0.007	N/A
Percentage change MDI (%), mean (95% CI)	− 16.7 (− 28.8, − 4.7)	11.0 (− 6.8, 28.8)	0.008	N/A

EMROC Emergency Medicine Research and Outcomes Consortium, *DM* diabetes mellitus, *CAD* coronary artery disease, *HTN* hypertension, *CKD* chronic kidney disease, *COPD* chronic obstructive pulmonary disease, *BP* blood pressure, *NIPPV* non-invasive positive pressure ventilation, *LVEF* left ventricular ejection fraction, *GLS* global longitudinal strain, *MDI* mechanical dispersion index

improvement in GLS over 23 h of 6%. For the patients with a favorable post-discharge outcome, the mean MDI at baseline was 84 ms (SD = 34 ms), with improvement to 64 ms (SD = 13 ms) at 23 h follow-up. This resulted in an average relative improvement in MDI of 24%. In patients readmitted within 30 days, the mean MDI at baseline was 66 ms (SD = 18 ms) and the mean MDI at 23 h follow-up was 70 ms (SD = 19 ms). There was an average relative worsening in MDI for the readmitted patients over 23 h of 6%.

Given the small sample size, we present individual patient data in Fig. 3a, b, plotting the normalized absolute change in GLS versus the baseline GLS in Fig. 3a and the normalized absolute in MDI versus baseline MDI in Fig. 3b.

From a technical standpoint, of the 62 echocardiograms that made up the final study cohort, 26 of them had all 18 segments with adequate endocardial border tracings (as determined by the internal quality control system in the AFI software package), 18 echocardiograms had 17 segments that were suitable, 13 had 16 suitable segments, and 5 of the echocardiograms had 15 adequate segments. The segments that were most commonly found to be poorly tracked by the AFI software were: the apical anterior segment (16 times), the apical lateral segment (15 times), the apical posterolateral segment (9 times), and the apical anteroseptal segment (8 times). None of the other segments were found to be inadequately tracked more than 3 times. The average frames per second (FPS) for all of the 62 study

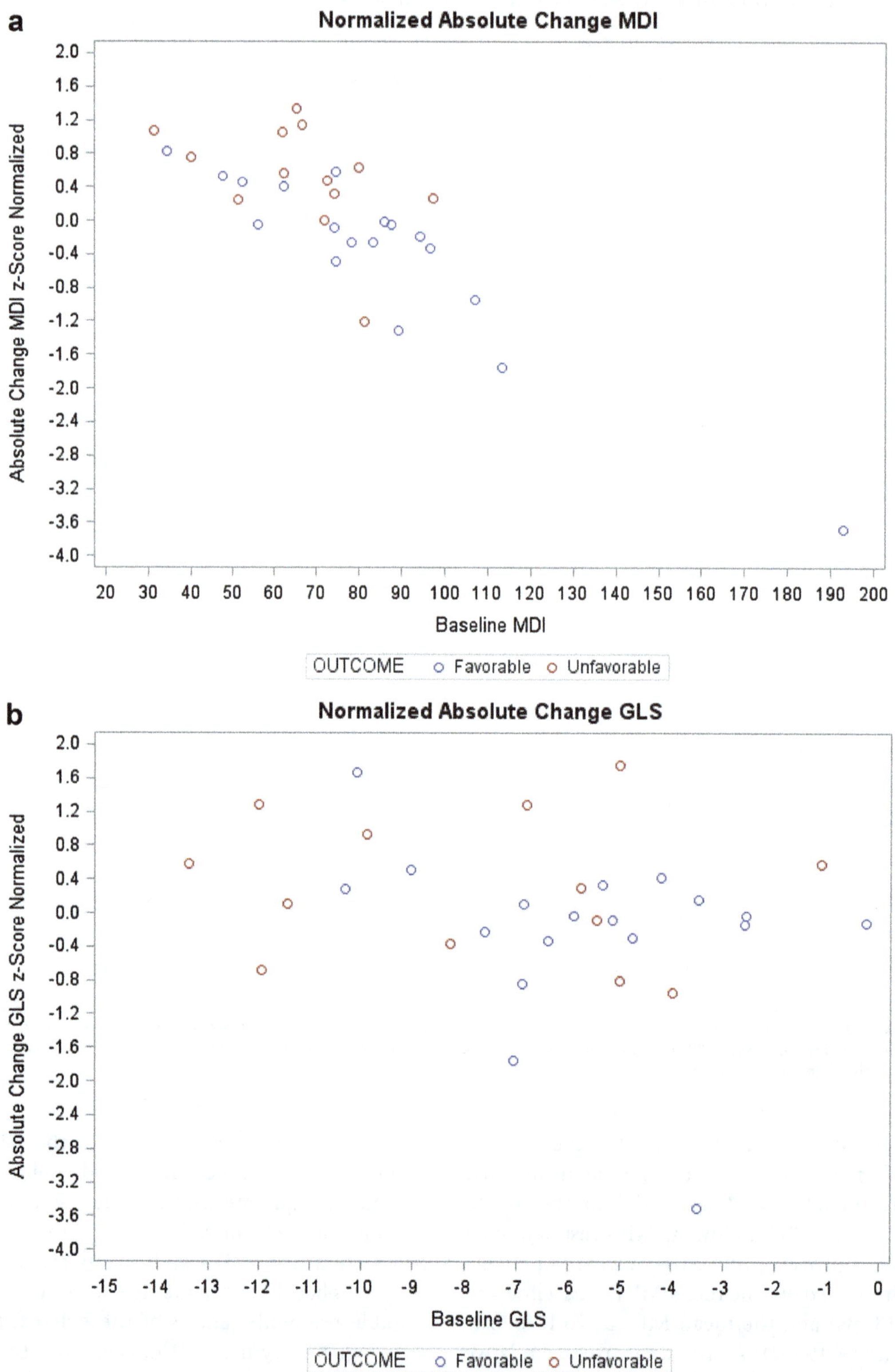

Fig. 3 **a** Scatter plot of baseline mechanical dispersion index (MDI) vs. z-score normalized change in MDI (Absolute). There is a fairly clear delineation between patients with favorable vs. unfavorable outcomes. The majority (10 out of 18) of those with favorable outcome tend to have baseline values of MDI larger than the mean (76.183 ms) and large normalized decreases over the 23 h period (13 out of 18), while the majority of patients with unfavorable outcomes (10 out of 13) had baseline MDI less than the mean and their MDI tended to increase (11 out of 13) over the 23 h period. **b** Scatter plot of baseline global longitudinal strain (GLS) vs. z-score normalized change in GLS (Absolute). Although the separation is not as pronounced as that of **a**, patients with favorable outcome (11 out of 18) tend to have a baseline GLS higher than the mean (−6.51%) and a decrease (11 out of 18) in GLS over the 23 h period. Patients with unfavorable outcomes had baseline GLS less than the mean (7 out of 13), and a majority (8 out of 13) had an increase in GLS over the 23 h period

echocardiograms was 68.3 with a frame rate range of 52 to 86 FPS.

Discussion

We present preliminary but highly promising data regarding the potential role of strain-based echocardiographic parameters in determining response to treatment and association with 30-day readmissions for patients hospitalized with AHF. To our knowledge, this is the first study of its kind prospectively evaluating MDI as a treatment response variable in AHF.

Our results are unique and informative, as they provide the first report of speckle-tracking-derived MDI data obtained from pre-treatment POC echocardiograms in patients with AHF. The change in MDI from the baseline echocardiogram to 23-h follow-up has never been reported in the published literature on AHF. Mechanical dispersion is an index of inter-segmental discoordination of contraction which evaluates the differences in time-to-peak shortening for each of the LV segments that are analyzed. A key strength of MDI is that it can be assessed using the same recording(s) as GLS and thus adds very little time to the interpretation.

Previous research has shown impaired GLS to be associated with poor outcomes in patients with HF, MDI, however, is far less studied in HF than GLS. In fact, until recently, nearly, all of the literature on MDI focused on its association with ventricular arrhythmias and its role in CRT [13, 17, 18]. A recent study by Chan et al. investigated both MDI and GLS as predictors of outcomes in hospitalized patients with HF with reduced ejection fraction (HFrEF), reporting that both GLS and MDI were independent predictors of long-term outcome after adjustment for baseline variables [16]. GLS > −7.8% and MDI > 72 ms were predictive of all-cause mortality or need for heart transplantation. Limitations of this study include the inclusion only of HFrEF subjects as well as the timing of echocardiograms with a median interval between admission and echocardiography of 10 days, rendering this measure less meaningful to the physician at the POC. This study does, however, lend support to the notion that MDI is a predictor of post-discharge outcomes in hospitalized HF patients, results that are consistent with our findings.

A potential mechanistic explanation for the observed change in MDI during treatment is that in patients with AHF, LV filling pressure is invariably increased. This elevated intra-cavitary pressure has the greatest impact on the subendocardial fibers as a result of their location immediately adjacent to the LV cavity. These fibers are oriented in a longitudinal fashion, thereby leading to the longitudinal strain parameters (including GLS and MDI) being the most sensitive of all the various strain measures [19]. Time-to-peak systolic strain for a given segment of the LV (the standard deviation of which is MDI) may be impaired by either: (1) decreased blood flow through the compromised small circulatory beds in the subendocardium which is the terminus of epicardial-to-endocardial coronary blood flow (the classical subendocardial ischemia model) or (2) pressure-induced decline in conduction velocity in areas with a high density of conducting fibers (i.e., the interventricular septum) [20, 21]. We suspect that during AHF episodes, a combination of these factors causes derangement in LV function. Thus, treatments geared towards reducing LV pressure (i.e., afterload reduction through vasodilation and non-invasive positive pressure ventilation) may be the key to maximizing improvements in GLS and MDI during the first 23 h of AHF therapy. In the present study, 23-h change in MDI proved to be a superior predictor than 23-h change in GLS; one reason for this may lie in the contractile potential of cardiomyocytes in AHF patients. There are likely limitations to the degree to which deformation (GLS) can improve with optimal treatment and thus many patients in our study exhibited substantially improved coordination of contraction timing (MDI) but only experienced small improvements in GLS after 23 h.

Our study has several important limitations, including small sample size and non-consecutive sampling of patients based on study team availability. Despite the relatively long time frame for the project, a study team member was available to enroll eligible subjects on average 2 days a month thereby placing significant limitations on our ability to capture patients. As previously mentioned, 13 patients had to be excluded from the final data analysis because of technical issues related to image quality or ECG-tracing quality. The majority of the ECG exclusions occurred early on during the study as our team was gaining familiarity with the precise timing necessary to capture clips that had three consecutive sinus beats with a good ECG waveform. The small number of subjects included for the final analysis thus raises the possibility of selection biases. To evaluate for this bias, we present data in Table 1 comparing the data from our study population with that of an AHF registry study also being conducted at our institution. The similarity between these 2 cohorts suggests that we captured a cohort of patients that was similar to the general population of AHF patients admitted at our institution.

We enrolled a fairly homogenous group of AHF patients, primarily a hypertensive, exclusively African-American cohort, and did not specifically evaluate or differentiate between patients with HFpEF versus HFrEF. It is possible that inclusion of a more diverse group of patients would alter our results; future studies are needed to address these questions. There were also differences in rates of CAD between the favorable outcome and readmitted cohorts (50% vs. 76.9%). Although this difference did not achieve statistical significance, it is certainly quite likely that CAD may have been the primary factor differentiating the primary outcome and this study was not powered to detect this difference. Future investigations would be wise to explore the role of CAD in LV longitudinal strain and how it influences short-term outcomes. Owing to the observational nature of this study, there is potential confounding from differences in treatments between patients. Another result of the observational and non-interventional design of the study is that invasive hemodynamic data (such as central venous pressure, pulmonary capillary wedge pressure, and central venous oxygen saturation) was not available for any of the patients in the study cohort. Comparison between the non-invasively derived indices of contractility using speckle-tracking and these established invasive parameters would have allowed for further hypothesis generation about the nature of the changes in speckle-tracking parameters that the study patients underwent. Future studies should ideally include these comparative data as well as echocardiography data on diastolic parameters obtained at the same time as the speckle-tracking data. Finally, there is some element of selection bias owing to the inherent limitations of speckle-tracking techniques—patients with atrial dysrhythmias or heart rate greater than 120 cannot be included; these limitations should not, however, preclude its use when feasible.

Conclusions

Based on the results of this study, the speckle-tracking-derived LV strain parameters MDI and GLS appear to undergo significant change during the treatment of AHF, and the magnitude of this change demonstrated an association with 30-day readmission rates. While our study is limited by a small sample size in a distinct patient population, data are promising, hypothesis generating only, and supportive of the need for further investigation of MDI and GLS as variables to help guide treatment and predict short-term outcome in AHF.

Authors' contributions

Study conception and design: MF, LG, and PL. Acquisition of data: MF, RE, LG, and AS. Analysis and interpretation of data: MF, RE, AS, BR, and PL. Drafting of manuscript: MF, RE, AS, and PL. Critical revision: RE, AS, AA, and PL. All authors read and approved the final manuscript.

Author details

[1] Department of Emergency Medicine, Wayne State University School of Medicine, 6071 W. Outer Dr., Lourdes 447-D, Detroit, MI 48235, USA. [2] Department of Internal Medicine, Division of Cardiology, Wayne State University School of Medicine, Detroit, MI, USA. [3] Cardiovascular Research Institute, Wayne State University School of Medicine, Detroit, MI, USA.

References

1. Long B, Koyfman A, Gottlieb M et al (2018) Management of heart failure in the emergency department: an evidence-based review of the literature. J Emerg Med. https://doi.org/10.1016/j.jemermed.2018.08.002
2. Gandhi SK, Powers JC, Abdel-Morsent N et al (2001) The pathogenesis of acute pulmonary edema associated with hypertension. N Engl J Med 344:17–22
3. Uriel N, Torre-Amione G, Milo O, Kaluski E, Perchenet L, Blatt A et al (2005) Echocardiographic ejection fraction in patients with acute heart failure: correlations with hemodynamic, clinical, and neurohormonal measures and short-term outcome. Eur J Heart Fail 7(5):815–819
4. Ponikowski P, Voors AA, Anker SD, Bueno H, Cleland JGF, Coats AJS et al (2016) 2016 ESC Guidelines for the diagnosis and treatment of acute and chronic heart failure. Eur Heart J 37(7):2129–2200
5. Cho GY, Marwick TH, Kim HS, Kim MK, Hong KS, Oh DJ (2009) Global 2-dimensional strain as a new prognosticator in patients with heart failure. J Am Coll Cardiol 54(7):618–624
6. Mignot A, Donal E, Zaroui A, Reant P, Salem A, Hamon C et al (2010) Global longitudinal strain as a major predictor of cardiac events in patients with depressed left ventricular function: a multicenter study. J Am Soc Echocardiogr 23(10):1019–1024
7. Ersboll M, Valeur N, Mogensen UM, Andersen MJ, Moller JE, Velazquez EJ et al (2013) Prediction of all-cause mortality and heart failure admissions from global left ventricular longitudinal strain in patients with acute myocardial infarction and preserved left ventricular ejection fraction. J Am Coll Cardiol 61(23):2365–2373
8. Stanton T, Leano R, Marwick TH (2009) Prediction of all-cause mortality from global longitudinal speckle strain: comparison with ejection fraction and wall motion scoring. Circ Cardiov Imaging. 2:356–364
9. Motoki H, Borowski AG, Shrestha K, Troughton RW, Tang W, Thomas JD, Klein AL (2012) Incremental prognostic value of assessing left ventricular myocardial mechanics in patients with chronic systolic heart failure. J Am Coll Cardiol 60:2074–2081
10. Favot M, Gowland L, Ehrman R, Gallien J, Khait L, Levy P (2016) Point-of-care strain echocardiography in acute heart failure. Am J Emerg Med 34(11):2234–2236
11. Gorcsan J 3rd, Tanaka H (2011) Echocardiographic assessment of myocardial strain. J Am Coll Cardiol 58(14):1401–1413
12. Saito M, Negishi K, Eskandari M, Huynh Q, Hawson J, Moore A et al (2015) Association of left ventricular strain with 30-day mortality and readmissions in patients with heart failure. J Am Soc Echocardiogr 28(6):652–656
13. Haugaa KH, Smedsrud MK, Steen T, Kongsgaard E, Loennechen JP, Skjaerpe T et al (2010) Mechanical Dispersion Assessed by myocardial strain in patients after myocardial infarction for risk prediction of ventricular arrhythmia. J Am Coll Cardiol Imaging 3:247–256
14. Aly MF, Kleijn SA, de Boer K, Abd El-Hady YA, Sorour KA, Kandil HI et al (2013) Comparison of three-dimensional echocardiographic software packages for assessment of left ventricular mechanical dyssynchrony and prediction of response to cardiac resynchronization therapy. Eur Heart J Cardiovasc Imaging 14(7):700–710
15. Schnell F, Matelot D, Daudin M, Kervio G, Mabo P, Carre F et al (2017) Mechanical dispersion by strain echocardiography: a novel tool to diagnose hypertrophic cardiomyopathy in athletes. J Am Soc Echocardiogr 30(3):251–261
16. Chan Y, Kuo C, Wu L, Wang C, Yey Y, Hsu L et al (2016) Combined global longitudinal strain and intraventricular mechanical dyssynchrony predicts long-term outcomes in patients with systolic heart failure. Circ J 80:177–185
17. Banasik G, Seglet O, Elwart M, Szulik M, Lenarczyk R, Kalarus Z, Kukulski T (2016) LV mechanical dispersion as a predictor of ventricular arrhythmia in patients with advanced systolic heart failure: a pilot study. Herz. 41:599–604
18. Bax JJ, Bleeker GB, Marwick TH, Molhoek SG, Boersma E, Steendijk P et al (2004) Left ventricular dyssynchrony predicts response and prognosis after cardiac resynchronization therapy. J Am Coll Cardiol 44:1834–1840
19. Feigenbaum H, Mastouri R, Sawada S (2012) A practical approach to using strain echocardiography to evaluate the left ventricle. Circ J 76:1550–1555

30

Fat embolism in right internal jugular vein: incidental ultrasound finding during internal jugular vein cannulation

Osman Adi[1*], Chan Pei Fong[1], Azlizawati Azil[1] and Shaik Farid Abdul Wahab[2]

Abstract

Background: We report a case study of fat embolism seen on ultrasound at right internal jugular vein during central venous cannulation in a patient diagnosed with fat embolism syndrome. This case demonstrates the importance of ultrasound for evaluation of trauma cases with suspicion of fat embolism.

Case presentation: A 23-year-old trauma patient with closed fracture of left femoral shaft and left humerus presented to our emergency department (ED). 11 h after admission to ED, patient became confused, hypoxic and hypotensive. He was then intubated for respiratory failure and mechanically ventilated. Transesophageal ultrasound revealed hyperdynamic heart, dilated right ventricle with no regional wall abnormalities and no major aorta injuries. Whole-body computed tomography was normal. During central venous cannulation of right internal jugular vein (IJV), we found free floating mobile hyperechoic spots, located at the anterior part of the vein. A diagnosis of fat embolism syndrome later was made based on the clinical presentation of long bone fractures and fat globulin in the blood. Despite aggressive fluid resuscitation, patient was a non-responder and needed vasopressor infusion for persistent shock. Blood aspirated during cannulation from the IJV revealed a fat globule. Patient underwent uneventful orthopedic procedures and was discharged well on day 5 of admission.

Conclusions: Point-of-care ultrasound findings of fat embolism in central vein can facilitate and increase the suspicion of fat embolism syndrome.

Keywords: Fat embolism syndrome, Fracture shaft of femur, Point-of-care ultrasound

Background

Fat embolism is a relatively under-recognized condition in patients with long bone fractures. When symptomatic, it can lead to serious effects on vital organs and even death. Diagnosis of fat embolism remains a challenge to clinicians today, as multiple diagnostic criteria exist. We report a case where the use of point-of-care ultrasound was able to visualize fat deposited at right internal jugular vein and increase the index of suspicion in diagnosis fat embolism syndrome. This case illustration demonstrates the importance of ultrasound as a tool to evaluate trauma cases with suspicion of fat embolism.

*Correspondence: osman.adi@gmail.com
[1] Department of Trauma and Emergency Medicine, Raja Permaisuri Bainun Hospital, 30450 Ipoh, Perak, Malaysia
Full list of author information is available at the end of the article

Case presentation

A 23 years old with no known medical illness presented to our emergency department after a head-on collision. He sustained closed fracture of the left femur (Fig. 1a), closed fracture of the left humerus, and multiple open fractures of the left foot. Patient was pink, not tachypneic and hemodynamically stable upon presentation. Patient was started on infusion tramadol for pain management and was planned for surgery.

11 h after ED admission, he was noted to be tachypneic and hypotensive with severe tachycardia. ABG showed hypoxemia and metabolic acidosis, despite O_2 given via non-rebreathing mask. He was intubated and mechanically ventilated. Extended Focused Sonography for Trauma was normal. Bedside transesophageal ultrasound revealed hyperdynamic heart, dilated right ventricle with

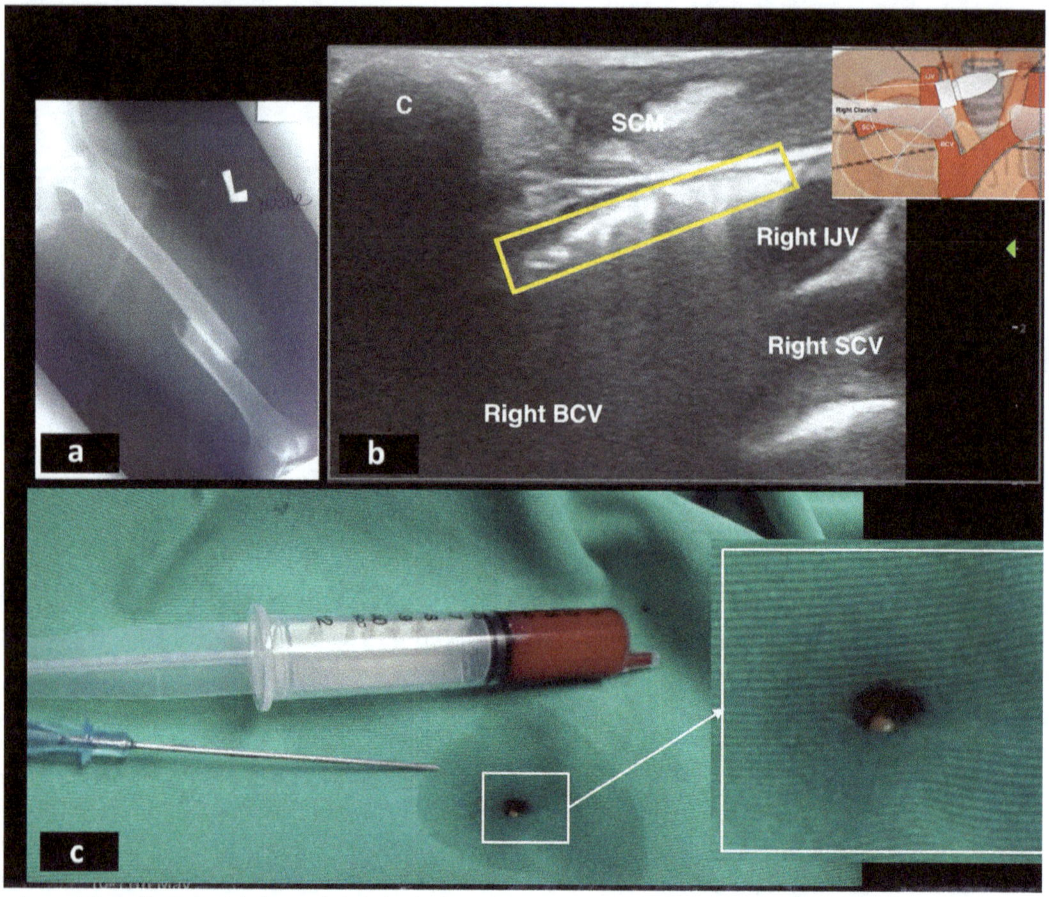

Fig. 1 **a** X-ray showed closed fracture right femoral shaft. **b** Ultrasound images revealed free floating mobile hyperechoic spots, located in the anterior part of the vein and cleared from the vein (yellow box). Small picture showing probe location in relation to clavicle, internal jugular vein, subclavian vein and brachiocephalic vein. **c** Fat globule was aspirated during cannulation of the IJV as shown in the white box. *C* Clavicle, *IJV* internal jugular vein, *SCV* subclavian vein, *BCV* brachiocephalic vein

no regional wall abnormalities and no major aorta injuries. Computed tomography of the whole body was also normal.

During central venous cannulation of the right internal jugular vein (IJV), we found multiple mobile and floating hyperechoic shadows deposited at the anterior part of the right IJV (Fig. 1b, Additional file 1: Video S1) Blood aspirated during cannulation from the right IJV revealed a fat globule (Fig. 1c). A diagnosis of fat embolism was suspected based on these incidental ultrasound findings in relation to the clinical presentation and background of multiple long bone fractures. Despite aggressive fluid resuscitation, patient was a non-responder. He needed intravenous noradrenaline infusion for persistent hypotension and tachycardia.

In the intensive care unit (ICU), patient's hemodynamic and respiratory status improved after continuous fluid and vasopressor therapy. Patient underwent multiple uneventful orthopedic procedures and was discharged well on day 5 of admission.

Discussion

Fat embolism is defined as evidence of fat globules found in the lung parenchyma and blood circulation usually occurring in trauma patients with long bone fractures [1]. A small number of these patients may develop fat embolism syndrome (FES), a potentially life-threatening condition characterized by the classic triad of hypoxemia, neurologic abnormalities, and petechial rash [2]. The onset of symptoms generally occurs within 12–72 h of the trauma [3]. Currently, to our knowledge, there is no literature discussing the difference between thrombus and fat embolism. Thrombus tends to be larger, mobile, be somewhat less echo-dense, and more commonly associated with spontaneous echo contrast. In contrast, fat embolism ultrasound images revealed free floating small, hypermobile and hyperechoic spots. Earlier literature classified fat embolism into 3 grades with grade III being the more serious clinical FES that leads to respiratory failure compared to grades I and II which are harmless [4].

In a retrospective study from 1979 to 2005 at the United States, Stein et al. reported incidence of fat embolism syndrome (FES) to be 0.12% to 0.7% in patients with fractures. Multiple fractures are found to increase the risk of FES compared to isolated fractures with femur being the most common cause [5]. An earlier 10-year review in New York also showed that 0.9% of patients with long bone fractures had clinically apparent FES. However, the true numbers of FES are probably underestimated because of the difficulty in making a definite diagnosis and the lack of specific testing [1].

Diagnosis of fat embolism syndrome remains a challenge to clinicians today, as multiple diagnostic criteria exist. The most commonly used Gurd and Wilson's criteria since 1974 proposed that 2 major criteria or 1 major and 4 minor criteria suggest a diagnosis of FES [6]. Major clinical features are (i) petechial rash (ii) respiratory symptoms plus bilateral signs on chest examination with positive radiographic changes, and (iii) cerebral signs unrelated to head injury or other condition. Respiratory findings were described as hypoxemia ($PaO_2 < 60$ mmHg) on FiO2 of 0.4. Minor features are fever >38.5, tachycardia HR>110 beats/min, retinal changes (fat or petechiae), renal changes (anuria, oliguria, fat globules), sudden drop in hemoglobin, sudden thrombocytopenia, high erythrocyte sedimentation rate, jaundice and fat globules in the sputum.

The limitations of the existing diagnostic criteria are the lack of laboratory markers or imaging tests to confirm the diagnosis of FES. Thus, the diagnosis of fat embolism is still based on clinical discretion of the treating physician after excluding other causes [7, 8]. This case may open up new possibility of point-of-care ultrasound as a triage tool in the emergency department to raise the suspicion of patients with suspected FES. The ultrasound identification of fat embolism with or without fat aspiration will definitely inflate the possibility of FES. Ultrasound can be amalgamated with the existing clinical criteria to confirm the diagnosis of FES.

The improvement of the quality of transthoracic echocardiography nowadays makes it a useful tool to assess for fat emboli in the circulation and heart of patients with long bone fractures as demonstrated in multiple case reports [9–11]. Fat emboli had been described as mobile, echogenic intraluminal mass in vessels [9] and "snowstorm"-like appearance in the chambers of the heart [10]. Fat emboli are usually spherical in shape, non-obstructive and show phasic flow with breathing [11]. This can be distinguished from a thrombus which adheres to the vein wall leading to a non-compressible vein and non-phasic flow with breathing.

It should be borne in mind that similar hyperechogenic spheres may also appear on ultrasound with infusion of blood products or agitated saline [12]. Another possibility for the echogenic materials is rouleaux formation due to stagnant red blood cells which is usually visualized at the junction of the valves and can be cleared away with compression of the vessel [13]. The right internal jugular vein in this patient was far from the valve area, compressible and the hyperechoic structures did not disappear immediately even with repeated scanning. Intraluminal air or air bubbles are another differential diagnosis for fat emboli. However, studies revealed that intraluminal air are short-lived (appear only within 3–5 of cardiac cycles) and diffuse in the lung when traversing the pulmonary circulation [14].

Based on our experience in this case, we propose searching for fat globules at deep veins near fracture sites such as the femoral vein in lower limb fractures and the IJV in upper limb fractures. There is currently no algorithm for point-of-care ultrasound in trauma patients to look for fat emboli. We will like to suggest scanning any vein proximal to the fracture site, followed by inferior vena cava and both sides of IJV. To confirm the diagnosis of fat emboli, ultrasound can serve as a useful tool to aspirate the fat globules under direct visualization. Larger systematic studies are needed to test out this hypothesis and determine whether diagnosis of fat embolism can be established earlier. This new idea may lead to prevention of FES complication and decrease in mortality.

To date, there is no proven treatment of FES, once it manifests in a patient. Prevention and high index of suspicion in high-risk patients are, therefore, needed to detect the condition early. Several measures had been identified as prophylaxis to prevent FES, but the quality of evidence is not strong. Hydration had been postulated to decrease the risk of FES due to the dilutional effect on the fat emboli and stress-related mediators [15]. Another recommendation is the use of corticosteroid for its anti-inflammatory effect to prevent FES [16] but its use remains controversial.

Although early operative fixation had been found to reduce the incidence of FES, the increased intramedullary pressure during fixation of fractures ironically increased the risk of FES [17]. Embolic materials were observed to pass through the heart by transesophageal echocardiography during orthopedic fixation of femur fractures with larger-size emboli (more than 10 mm) being more associated with increased mortality [18]. The mortality rate for fat embolism syndrome is around 7–20% in the literature [1, 19].

Conclusions

Point-of-care ultrasound findings of fat embolism in central vein can facilitate and increase the suspicion of fat embolism syndrome. Early diagnosis can help with prompt supportive treatment and improve outcome of this potentially fatal condition.

Additional file

Additional file 1. Multiple mobile and floating hyperechoic shadows deposited at the anterior part of the right IJV.

Authors' contributions
OA, CPF, SFAW and AA were in charge of the patient and collected the data. OA, SFAW and CPF wrote the manuscript. All the authors read and approved the final manuscript.

Author details
[1] Department of Trauma and Emergency Medicine, Raja Permaisuri Bainun Hospital, 30450 Ipoh, Perak, Malaysia. [2] Departments of Emergency Medicine, School of Medical Sciences, University Science of Malaysia (USM), Kubang Kerian, Kelantan, Malaysia.

Acknowledgements
The authors would like to thank the Society of Critical Care and Emergency Sonography (SUCCES) Malaysia, Ipoh Emergency Medicine Society (IEMS) and WINFOCUS, for their support and assistance.

References
1. Bulger EM, Smith DG, Maier RV, Jurkovich GJ (1997) Fat embolism syndrome: a 10-year review. Arch Surg. https://doi.org/10.1001/archsurg.1997.01430280109019
2. Johnson MJ, Lucas GL (1996) Fat embolism syndrome. Orthopedics 19:41–49
3. Gupta A, Reilly CS (2007) Fat embolism. Contin Educ Anaesth Crit Care Pain 7:148–151
4. Riska EB, Myllynen P (1982) Fat embolism in patients with multiple injuries. J Trauma Acute Care Surg 22(11):891–894
5. Stein PD, Yaekoub AY, Matta F, Kleerekoper M (2008) Fat Embolism Syndrome. Am J Med Sci 336(6):472–477
6. Gurd A, Wilson R (1972) Fat-embolism syndrome. Lancet 300:231–232
7. Kwiatt ME, Seamon MJ (2013) Fat embolism syndrome. Int J Crit Illn Inj Sci 3(1):64–68
8. Gurd A (1970) Fat embolism: an aid to diagnosis. J Bone Jt Surg Br Vol 52:732–737
9. Harris AC, Torreggiani WC, Lyburn ID, Zwirewich CV, Ho SGF, Munk PL (2000) CT and sonography of traumatic fat embolism in the common femoral vein. Am J Roentgenol 175(6):1741–1742
10. Huber-Lang M, Brinkmann A, Straeter J, Beck A, Gauss A, Gebhard F (2005) An unusual case of early fulminant post-traumatic fat embolism syndrome. Anaesthesia 60:1141–1143
11. Naddaf A, Andre J, Bly SJ, Hood D, Hodgson KJ, Desai SS (2016) Duplex ultrasound evidence of fat embolism syndrome. J Vasc Surg Cases Innov Tech 2(4):155–157
12. Summerfield DT, Cawcutt K, Van Demark R, Ritter MJ (2013) Fat embolism syndrome: improved diagnosis through the use of bedside echocardiography. Southwest J Pulm Crit Care 7:255–264
13. Blanco P, Volpicelli G (2016) Common pitfalls in point-of-care ultrasound: a practical guide for emergency and critical care physicians. Crit Ultrasound J 8(1):15
14. Attaran RR, Ata I, Kudithipudi V, Foster L, Sorrell VL (2006) Protocol for optimal detection and exclusion of a patent foramen ovale using transthoracic echocardiography with agitated saline microbubbles. Echocardiography 23(7):616–622
15. McDermott ID, Culpan P, Clancy M, Dooley JF (2002) The role of rehydration in the prevention of fat embolism syndrome. Injury 33(9):757–759
16. Schonfeld SA et al (1983) Fat embolism prophylaxis with corticosteroids. A prospective study in high-risk patients. Ann Intern Med 99(4):438–443
17. Giannoudis PV, Tzioupis C, Pape HC (2006) Fat embolism: the reaming controversy. Injury 37(4 SUPPL.):50–58
18. Pell AC, Christie J, Keating JF, Sutherland GR (1993) The detection of fat embolism by transoesophageal echocardiography during reamed intramedullary nailing. A study of 24 patients with femoral and tibial fractures. J Bone Jt, Surg Br
19. Robert J (1993) Fat Embolism Syndrome. Orthop. Rev. 22(5):567–571

Permissions

All chapters in this book were first published by Springer; hereby published with permission under the Creative Commons Attribution License or equivalent. Every chapter published in this book has been scrutinized by our experts. Their significance has been extensively debated. The topics covered herein carry significant findings which will fuel the growth of the discipline. They may even be implemented as practical applications or may be referred to as a beginning point for another development.

The contributors of this book come from diverse backgrounds, making this book a truly international effort. This book will bring forth new frontiers with its revolutionizing research information and detailed analysis of the nascent developments around the world.

We would like to thank all the contributing authors for lending their expertise to make the book truly unique. They have played a crucial role in the development of this book. Without their invaluable contributions this book wouldn't have been possible. They have made vital efforts to compile up to date information on the varied aspects of this subject to make this book a valuable addition to the collection of many professionals and students.

This book was conceptualized with the vision of imparting up-to-date information and advanced data in this field. To ensure the same, a matchless editorial board was set up. Every individual on the board went through rigorous rounds of assessment to prove their worth. After which they invested a large part of their time researching and compiling the most relevant data for our readers.

The editorial board has been involved in producing this book since its inception. They have spent rigorous hours researching and exploring the diverse topics which have resulted in the successful publishing of this book. They have passed on their knowledge of decades through this book. To expedite this challenging task, the publisher supported the team at every step. A small team of assistant editors was also appointed to further simplify the editing procedure and attain best results for the readers.

Apart from the editorial board, the designing team has also invested a significant amount of their time in understanding the subject and creating the most relevant covers. They scrutinized every image to scout for the most suitable representation of the subject and create an appropriate cover for the book.

The publishing team has been an ardent support to the editorial, designing and production team. Their endless efforts to recruit the best for this project, has resulted in the accomplishment of this book. They are a veteran in the field of academics and their pool of knowledge is as vast as their experience in printing. Their expertise and guidance has proved useful at every step. Their uncompromising quality standards have made this book an exceptional effort. Their encouragement from time to time has been an inspiration for everyone.

The publisher and the editorial board hope that this book will prove to be a valuable piece of knowledge for researchers, students, practitioners and scholars across the globe.

List of Contributors

Lorenzo De Marchi
Department of Anesthesia, Georgetown University, MedStar Georgetown University Hospital, 3800 Reservoir Road NW, CCC Building, Lower Level, Washington, DC, USA

Massimiliano Meineri
Department of Anesthesia and Pain Management, Toronto General Hospital, University Health Network, University of Toronto, 200 Elizabeth Street EN 3-400, Toronto, ON M5G 2C4, Canada

Jean-Eudes Bourcier, Emeric Gallard, Jean-Philippe Redonnet, Magali Majourau, Dominique Deshaie and Didier Garnier
Emergency, Anesthesiology and Critical Care Department, Lourdes Hospital

Jean-Marie Bourgeois
Avenue Alexandre Marqui, 65100 Lourdes, France. 2 CFFE (Centre Francophone de Formation en Echographie), Nîmes, France

Thomas Geeraerts
Anesthesiology and Critical Care Department, Toulouse University Hospital, University Toulouse III Paul Sabatier, Toulouse, France

Shihab Al Sheikh, Mariam Al Ali, Dhanya Sochel Kiran and Mohsen Al Tabatabai
Emergency Department, Rashid Hospital Trauma Center, Dubai, United Arab Emirates

Brian P. Lucas and Clay Block
Medicine Service, White River Junction VA Medical Center, White River Junction, VT, USA
Geisel School of Medicine at Dartmouth College, Hanover, NH, USA

Antonietta D'Addio
Geisel School of Medicine at Dartmouth College, Hanover, NH, USA

Harold L. Manning, Brian Remillard and James C. Leiter
Geisel School of Medicine at Dartmouth College, Hanover, NH, USA
Department of Medicine, Dartmouth-Hitchcock Medical Center, Lebanon, NH, USA

Babar Fiza, Michael Tang and Michael Maile
Department of Anesthesiology, University of Michigan Hospitals, 1500 East Medical Center Drive, Ann Arbor, MI 48109-5861, USA

Luís Magalhães
Hospital da Luz–Arrábida, Praceta de Henrique Moreira 150, 4400-346 Vila Nova de Gaia, Portugal

Sara Raquel Pereira Martins
Centro Hospitalar Universitário do Porto, Largo do Prof. Abel Salazar, 4099-001 Porto, Portugal

Ramon Nogué
Universitat de Lleida, Plaça de Víctor Siurana, 1, 25003 Lleida, Spain

William Beaubien-Souligny
Department of Anesthesiology and Intensive Care, Montreal Heart Institute, Université de Montréal, Montreal, QC, Canada
Division of Nephrology, Centre Hospitalier de l'Université de Montreal, 1000, Rue St-Denis, Montreal, QC H2X 0C1, Canada

Philippe Rola
Division of Intensive Care, Santa Cabrini Hospital, Montreal, QC, Canada

Korbin Haycock
Department of Emergency Medicine, Loma Linda University School of Medicine, Loma Linda, CA 92354, USA

Josée Bouchard
Division of Nephrology, Hôpital Sacré-Coeur de Montréal, Montreal, QC, Canada

Yoan Lamarche
Department of Surgery and Critical Care, Montreal Heart Institute, Université de Montréal, Montréal, QC, Canada

Rory Spiegel
Departments of Critical Care and Emergency Medicine, Washington Hospital Center, Georgetown University, Washington, DC, USA

André Y. Denault
Department of Anesthesiology and Intensive Care, Montreal Heart Institute, Université de Montréal, Montreal, QC, Canada
Division of Intensive Care, Centre Hospitalier de L'Université de Montreal, Montreal, QC, Canada

Paul Olszynski and Brent Thoma
Department of Emergency Medicine, University of Saskatchewan, Saskatoon, Canada

Daniel J. Kim
Department of Emergency Medicine, University of British Columbia, Vancouver, Canada

Michelle Clunie
Department of Anesthesia and Perioperative Medicine, University of Saskatchewan, Saskatoon, Canada

Peggy Lambos
Department of Pediatrics, University of Saskatchewan, Prince Albert, Canada

Tom Guzowski
Department of Internal Medicine, University of Saskatchewan, Saskatoon, Canada

Matthew Butz
Department of Family Medicine, University of Saskatchewan, Regina, Canada

Jonathan Wong
Department of Medicine, University of Alberta, Edmonton, AB, Canada

Steven Montague
Department of Medicine, Queen's University, Kingston, ON, Canada

Paul Wallace
Department of Medicine, University of Pennsylvania, Philadelphia, PA, USA

Kay Negishi
Department of Medicine, Massachusetts General Hospital, Boston, MA, USA

Andrew Liteplo
Department of Emergency Medicine, Massachusetts General Hospital, Boston, MA, USA

Jennifer Ringrose, Janeve Desy and Irene W. Y. Ma
Department of Medicine, Division of General Internal Medicine, Cumming School of Medicine, University of Calgary, 3330 Hospital Dr NW, Calgary, AB T2N 4N1, Canada

Renee Dversdal
Department of Medicine, Oregon Health & Science University, Portland, OR, USA

Brian Buchanan
Department of Critical Care, University of Alberta, Edmonton, AB, Canada

Ana Luisa Silveira Vieira
Department of Nephrology, Santa Casa de Misericórdia de Barbacena and University of Medicine of Barbacena Department of Point of Care Ultrasound, Minas Gerais, Brazil

José Muniz Pazeli Júnior
Department of Nephrology and Intensive Care Medicine, Santa Casa de Misericórdia de Barbacena and University of Medicine of Barbacena Department of Point of Care Ultrasound, Minas Gerais, Brazil

Marcus Gomes Bastos
Federal University of Juiz de Fora, Minas Gerais, Brazil
Faculty at School of Medicine, UNIFAGOC and SUPREMA, Minas Gerais, Brazil

Daralee Hughes, Irene Mynatt, Michael Prats, Creagh Boulger and David P. Bahner
Department of Emergency Medicine, The Ohio State University College of Medicine, 750 Prior Hall, 376 W 10th Ave, Columbus, OH 43210, USA

Michelle M. Corrado
Children's Hospital Colorado, The University of Colorado, Denver, CO, USA

Nelson A. Royall
Department of Surgery, The University of Oklahoma College of Medicine, Tulsa, OK, USA

Pablo Blanco
Intensive Care Unit, Clínica Cruz Azul, 2651, 60 St, Necochea 7630, Argentina
Department of Teaching and Research, Hospital "Dr. Emilio Ferreyra", 4801, 59 St, Necochea 7630, Argentina

María Fernanda Menéndez
Intensive Care Unit, Hospital "Dr. Emilio Ferreyra", 4801, 59 Ave, Necochea 7630, Argentina

Vigil James and Gene Yong-Kwang Ong
Children's Emergency, C/O KK Women's and Children's Hospital PTE. LTD, 100 Bukit Timah Road, Singapore 229899, Singapore

John Samuel
Department of Radiodiagnosis, Christian Fellowship Hospital, Oddanchatram, Tamil Nadu 624619, India

Chor Yek Kee
Paediatric Intensive Care Unit, Department of Pediatrics, Sarawak General Hospital, Kuching, Malaysia

Antoine Fasseaux
Department of Emergency Medicine, CHR Jolimont, 7100 La Louvière, Belgium

Philippe Pès
Department of Emergency Medicine, CHU Nantes, Nantes University Hospital, 44000 Nantes, France

Françoise Steenebruggen and Florence Dupriez
Department of Emergency Medicine, Cliniques Universitaires Saint Luc, 1200 Brussels, Belgium

Lisandro Montorfano and Matthew Wolfers
Department of General Surgery, Cleveland Clinic Florida, Weston, FL, USA

Marianna Sarkissyan, Federico Rodríguez, Fernando Pla and Miguel Montorfano
Department of Ultrasound and Vascular Doppler, Hospital de Emergencias "Dr. Clemente Alvarez", Av. Pellegrini 3205, Rosario, Santa Fe, Argentina

M. J Blans and E Bousie
Department of Intensive Care, Rijnstate Hospital, 6800 TA Arnhem, The Netherlands

J. G van der Hoeven
Department of Intensive Care, Radboud University Medical Center, 6500 HB Nijmegen, The Netherlands

F. H Bosch
Department of Internal Medicine, Rijnstate Hospital, 6800 TA Arnhem, The Netherlands

Diana Avila-Reyes
Department of Critical Care Medicine, Universidad Tecnologica de Pereira, Grupo de Investigacion Medicina Critica Y Cuidados Intensivos (GIMCCI), Pereira, Colombia

Andres O. Acevedo-Cardona
Department of Critical Care Medicine, Universidad Tecnologica de Pereira,, Pereira, Colombia
Master en Ecocardiografia en Cuidados Intensivos, Sociedad Espanola de Imagen Cardiaca/Universidad Francisco de Vitoria, Espana, Pereira, Spain

Jose F. Gomez-Gonzalez
Department of Critical Care Medicine, Universidad Tecnologica de Pereira, Pereira, Colombia
Grupo Investigacion de Medicina Critica Y Cuidados Intensivos (GIMCCI), Pereira, Colombia

David R. Echeverry-Piedrahita
Department of Critical Care Medicine, Universidad Tecnologica de Pereira, Pereira, Colombia

Mateo Aguirre-Florez and Adrian Giraldo-Diaconeasa
Department of Medicine, Universidad Tecnologica de Pereira, Pereira, Colombia

Matthew A. Taylor and Christopher H. Merritt
University of South Carolina School of Medicine, Columbia, SC 29209, USA

Philip J. Riddle Jr
Department of Internal Medicine, Prisma Health Midlands, University of South Carolina School of Medicine, Columbia, SC 29209, USA

Carter J. DeGennaro
Department of Emergency Medicine, Prisma Health Midlands, University of South Carolina School of Medicine, Columbia, SC 29209, USA

Keith R. Barron
Department of Internal Medicine, Prisma Health Midlands, University of South Carolina School of Medicine, Columbia, SC 29209, USA
Ultrasound Institute, University of South Carolina School of Medicine, Columbia, SC 29209, USA
Palmetto Health-USC Medical Group, 5 Medical Park Road, Columbia, SC 29203, USA

Conor McKaigney
Department of Emergency Medicine & Cumming School of Medicine, Emergency Physician, Calgary Zone, Alberta Health Services, University of Calgary, 7007 14th St. SW, Calgary, AB T2V1P9, Canada

Colin Bell
Department of Emergency Medicine & Cumming School of Medicine, Emergency Physician, Calgary Zone, Alberta Health Services, University of Calgary, 7007 14th St. SW, Calgary, AB T2V1P9, Canada
Department of Emergency Medicine, Queen's University, 76 Stuart St Kingston, Kingston, ON K7L2V7, Canada

Joseph Newbigging and Louise Rang
Department of Emergency Medicine, Queen's University, 76 Stuart St Kingston, Kingston, ON K7L2V7, Canada

Natalie Wagner
Department of Biomedical & Molecular Sciences, Queen's University, 74 Union St Kingston, Kingston, ON K7L3N6, Canada

Andrew Hall
Department of Emergency Medicine, Queen's University, 76 Stuart St Kingston, Kingston, ON K7L2V7, Canada
Office of Professional Development & Educational Scholarship, Queen's University, 68 Barrie St Kingston, Kingston, ON K7L3N6, Canada
Royal College of Physicians and Surgeons Canada, 774 Echo Drive, Ottawa, ON K1S5N8, Canada
Department of Emergency Medicine, The Ottawa Hospital and University of Ottawa, 1053 Carling Ave, E-Main, Room EM-206, Ottawa, ON K1Y4E9, Canada

Angelo G. Delmonaco, Irene Raffaldi, Emanuela Garrone and Antonio F. Urbino
Department of Pediatric Emergency, Regina Margherita Children's Hospital, A.O.U. Città Della Salute E Della Scienza Di Torino, Turin, Italy

Andrea Carpino, Francesco Del Monte and Lorenzo Riboldi
Postgraduate School of Pediatrics, University of Turin, Piazza Polonia 94, 10126 Turin, Italy

Giulia Pruccoli, Francesco Licciardi and Emilia Parodi
Department of Pediatric and Public Health Sciences, Regina Margherita Children's Hospital, A.O.U. Città Della Salute E Della Scienza Di Torino, University of Turin, Turin, Italy

Daniel S. Brenner, Rodney Omron and Tiffany C. Fong
Department of Emergency Medicine, Johns Hopkins School of Medicine, 1830 East Monument St Suite 6-100, Baltimore, MD 21287, USA

Gigi Y. Liu
Hospitalist Program, Division of General Internal Medicine, Department of Medicine, Johns Hopkins School of Medicine, Baltimore, MD, USA

Olive Tang
Medical Scientist Training Program, Johns Hopkins School of Medicine, Baltimore, MD, USA

Brian T. Garibaldi
Department of Pulmonary and Critical Care Medicine, Johns Hopkins Hospital, Baltimore, MD, USA

Maryam Al Ali and Salma Alrajaby
Arab Board in Emergency Medicine, Rashid Hospital Trauma Center, Dubai Health Authority, oud metha, Dubai, United Arab Emirates

Sarah Jabbour
Emergency Medicine Resident, Rashid Hospital Trauma Center, Dubai Health Authority, oud metha, Dubai, United Arab Emirates

Naima Kilhamn
Department of Perioperative Medicine and Intensive Care, Karolinska University Hospital, Solna, 171 76 Stockholm, Sweden

Mårten Renberg, Claire Rimes-Stigare, Max Bell and Daniel Hertzberg
Department of Perioperative Medicine and Intensive Care, Karolinska University Hospital, Solna, 171 76 Stockholm, Sweden
Department of Physiology and Pharmacology, Karolinska Institutet, Stockholm, Sweden

Olof Jonmarker
Department of Radiology, Karolinska University Hospital, Huddinge, Stockholm, Sweden

Osman Adi and Azma Haryaty Ahmad
Department of Emergency and Trauma, Raja Permaisuri Bainun Hospital, Jalan Raja Ashman (Jalan Hospital), Jalan Raja Ashman, 30400 Ipoh, Perak, Malaysia

Kok Meng Sum
Department of Anesthesiology & Intensive Care, Beacon Hospital, No. 1, Jalan 215, Off Jalan Templer, Section 51, 46050 Petaling Jaya, Selangor, Malaysia

Mahathar Abd. Wahab
Department of Emergency and Trauma, Kuala Lumpur Hospital, Jalan Pahang, 50586 Kuala Lumpur, Wilayah Persekutuan Kuala Lumpur, Malaysia

Luca Neri
A.O Niguarda Ca' Granda' Hospital, Piazza dell'Ospedale Maggiore, 3, 20162 Milan, MI, Italy

Nova Panebianco
Division of Emergency Ultrasound, Department of Emergency Medicine, Hospital of the University of Pennsylvania, 3400 Spruce St, Philadelphia, PA 19104, USA

Michaëla A. M. Huson
Department of Microbiology and Infectious Diseases, Erasmus Medical Centre, Rotterdam, The Netherlands

Dan Kaminstein
Department of Emergency Medicine, Medical College of Georgia, Augusta University, Augusta, GA, USA

Daniel Kahn
Department of Internal Medicine, University of California, Los Angeles, CA, USA

Sabine Belard
Department of Paediatric Pulmonology, Immunology and Intensive Care Medicine, Charité-Universitätsmedizin Berlin, Berlin, Germany
Berlin Institute of Health, Berlin, Germany

Tom Heller
Lighthouse Clinic, Kamuzu Central Hospital, Lilongwe, Malawi

Prakash Ganesh
Lighthouse Clinic, Kamuzu Central Hospital, Lilongwe, Malawi
International Training and Education Centre for Health, University of Washington, Seattle, WA, USA

Vanessa Kandoole-Kabwere
Department of Internal Medicine, College of Medicine, University of Malawi, Blantyre, Malawi

Claudia Wallrauch
Division of Infectious Diseases and Tropical Medicine, University Hospital, LMU, Munich, Germany

Sam Phiri
Lighthouse Clinic, Kamuzu Central Hospital, Lilongwe, Malawi
Department of Global Health, University of Washington, Seattle, USA
Department of Medicine, University of North Carolina School of Medicine, Chapel Hill, NC, USA
Department of Public Health, College of Medicine, School of Public Health and Family Medicine, University of Malawi, Lilongwe, Malawi

Benno Kreuels
Department of Internal Medicine, College of Medicine, University of Malawi, Blantyre, Malawi
Department of Tropical Medicine, Bernhard Nocht Institute for Tropical Medicine, I. Department of Medicine, University Medical Center Hamburg-Eppendorf, Hamburg, Germany

Matthew Jefkins and Barry Chan
Division of General Internal Medicine, Department of Medicine, Queen's University, Kingston, Ontario K7L 3N6, Canada

Veronica Sepulveda-Ortiz, Fred Warkentine, Rebecca Starr-Seal and Anna Rominger
Division of Pediatric Emergency Medicine, Department of Pediatrics, University of Louisville, 571 S. Floyd Street, Suite 412, Louisville, KY 40202, USA

Gabriela Bello
Intensive Care Unit, Hospital Central de las Fuerzas Armadas (DNSFFAA), 3060, 8 de Octubre Ave, 11600 Montevideo, Uruguay

Mark Favot, Robert Ehrman, Laura Gowland, Ashley Sullivan and Brian Reed
Department of Emergency Medicine, Wayne State University School of Medicine, 6071 W. Outer Dr, Lourdes 447-D, Detroit, MI 48235, USA

Aiden Abidov
Department of Internal Medicine, Division of Cardiology, Wayne State University School of Medicine, Detroit, MI, USA

Phillip Levy
Department of Emergency Medicine, Wayne State University School of Medicine, 6071 W. Outer Dr, Lourdes 447-D, Detroit, MI 48235, USA
Cardiovascular Research Institute, Wayne State University School of Medicine, Detroit, MI, USA

Chan Pei Fong and Azlizawati Azil
Department of Emergency and Trauma, Raja Permaisuri Bainun Hospital, Jalan Raja Ashman (Jalan Hospital), Jalan Raja Ashman, 30400 Ipoh, Perak, Malaysia

Shaik Farid Abdul Wahab
Departments of Emergency Medicine, School of Medical Sciences, University Science of Malaysia (USM), Kubang Kerian, Kelantan, Malaysia

Index

www.ingramcontent.com/pod-product-compliance
Lightning Source LLC
LaVergne TN
LVHW082159200926
848484LV00008B/2186